MEDICAL MAN

Helen Webster

◆ FriesenPress

Suite 300 - 990 Fort St
Victoria, BC, Canada, V8V 3K2
www.friesenpress.com

ISBN
978-1-4602-7877-2 (Hardcover)
978-1-4602-7878-9 (Paperback)
978-1-4602-7879-6 (eBook)

1. Fiction, Historical

Distributed to the trade by The Ingram Book Company

This story is fascinating. The medical facts are correct for the times, too. The chapter about the appendicitis death is particularly interesting because Dr. Ross describes the correct management of an appendiceal abscess before the era of IV antibiotics. Also, he describes well the ethical dilemmas that can occur when doctors disagree about treatment. Such situations today would take place in a hospital, which would have department chiefs to bring a resolution that would be in the best interests of the patient. The case of the insane farmer shows Robert's quick thinking and inventive mind. Paranoid psychoses still occur at the same rate today. However, the medical profession no longer has to face the same distance and communication limitations. Police response times have also improved. We still use morphine - it is the same as it was then - but not for psychiatric use and Dr. Ross uses it as a sedative, which it can be. He also describes its other common side effect - nausea. Hyoscine has much more limited use now.

A lot has changed in fewer than one hundred years. This volume is an opportunity to reflect on earlier times... I always learn from history and this is good history.

- Dr. Gerrard A. Vaughan

"The Province of Alberta was only four years old when a young doctor arrived with his wife and two sons to begin a remarkable life of service in the new pioneer community. The story of Dr. T. Robert Ross is a compelling account of a man driven by an unselfish instinct to help and to heal.... *Medical Man* is set against a background of momentous events: the Great War, the Spanish influenza pandemic, crippling prairie droughts, and the Great Depression, all challenged the fortitude and skill of Dr. Ross. His courage, dedication and daring are all a part of this surprisingly dramatic story of frontier medicine, and his life is truly defined by the title of this excellent book."

- Colin M. Ross Legacy of The Caliph

Laughter, tears and just the plain inability to put the book down...all markings of a good book that describe my experience reading *Medical Man*. I'm so glad to have had the opportunity to read this manuscript and get a glimpse into the world of medicine, and the travels, hardships and joys of Dr. Robert Ross's life and family. Some of the medical stories were truly amazing and I can't imagine living through some of those experiences. This story is full of discovery, perseverance, bravery and appreciation for life. Helen Webster has done a great job with the writing and organization. and a marvellous job of character development, transitions and keeping the reader engaged. *Medical Man* is rich with experiences from Dr. Ross's life as a doctor in the early to mid 1900's. The characters have depth and come to life on every page. The research and time put into this manuscript are evident and well done. Truly a pleasure to read.

- Editor, Friesen Press

TABLE OF CONTENTS

CALGARY 1950-1962

ACKNOWLEDGEMENTS

APPENDICES

To

My mother, Elizabeth,

Who in her wisdom kept Robert's original writing,
which provided the genesis for this book

and

My daughter, Lisa,

Her constant support and patient editing ensured
that the whole story would be written.

PREFACE

This is a true story about a real man and his family who lived in remarkable times in Canadian, world, and medical history. It is based on the stories, both written and oral, of Thomas Robert Ross: his own written records of his medical stories; fragments of his actual case notes; his correspondence, and that of his wife, Jennie; letters written to and about them by friends and family, including their descendants; and stories told by their acquaintances, their children, and their grandchildren.

While all patients' names and sometimes the location of their cases have been changed to protect confidentiality, the medical stories are otherwise factual.

The events of Robert's and his family's lives really happened, as did all the historical events included. With the exception of the names of his patients as noted above, these are real people.

Finally, the author asks the reader's indulgence in accepting that in some instances, factual accuracy must be balanced against serving the interests of the story. And, of course, the necessary fictional liberties have been taken with conversations or when describing the thoughts that express Robert's and Jennie's hopes and dreams.

Thomas Robert Ross was born in 1871, four years after Confederation and the formation of the Dominion of Canada. He grew up as the son of a Hudson's Bay Company (HBC) trading post manager and became an HBC trader himself, living and travelling in the wilderness of Quebec and Northern Ontario until the age of twenty-eight.

At that time, Robert decided to marry and to also fulfill his lifelong dream of becoming a doctor. Accordingly, he travelled to Sudbury where, in 1900, he married Jennie Louise Ryan, the young cousin of a family friend. Four years later, he was accepted at Queen's University in Kingston, where he graduated in 1908 with his Doctor of Medicine and Master of Surgery (MDCM).

Upon completion of his internship in Montreal, Robert returned with his wife and two young sons to northern Ontario to take up his duties with the HBC until he secured a medical position. But he did not wish to live in a large city, such as Toronto or Montreal; he was unwilling to look for a shared practice as a doctor in rural Ontario or Quebec; and he was far too restless to settle again for continued employment with the HBC.

Robert knew that medical men, especially surgeons, were needed in the new western provinces of Alberta and Saskatchewan. In 1909, determined to establish a medical practice of his own and eager to assume the role and responsibilities of a doctor, T. Robert Ross, MDCM, packed up his young family and, along with thousands of other immigrants looking for new lives on the prairies, boarded the Canadian Pacific Railway (CPR) to travel to the West.

PROLOGUE
1954

"...the death of someone you love is always a shock..."

Robert lifted his hands from the typewriter keys and rubbed his temples and the bridge of his nose, where his new glasses pinched. It was kind of people to write and offer their sympathy on the death of his wife, but sometimes it was difficult to put his own feelings about her death into words. She had been ill for a very long time.

Robert paused to consider his next words to his old friend, Reverend Moss, and looked out the window of his study at the snow covered yard of his Calgary home. It was a bright February day with a high thin overcast and quick clouds scudding ahead of a winter storm. The clouds parted briefly, and a quick flash of gold at the edge of his desk caught his eye. Jennie's letter seal lay there, a tiny, pretty thing that she had worn on a chain around her neck. The face was incised with a thistle and the words "Dinna Forget."

"Dinna forget, dinna forget...." How could he forget? There was so much to remember, so many journeys, so many stories.

What did the flash of gold remind him of? Robert smiled and leaned back in his chair, letting his mind drift back over half a century to a grand home in Sudbury, Ontario....

PART ONE
Ontario and Quebec
1900-1909

THE FIRST DECADE

Chapter 1
Marriage and Medicine

The firelight winked on the gold wedding bands of the two remarkable women as they sat over their afternoon tea in the newly decorated parlour of Dr. Helen Ryan's large comfortable home. Maggie McLeod Ross McKenzie, who had moved from Sudbury to Montreal upon her marriage to her second husband, Peter McKenzie, a chief factor of the Hudson's Bay Company, had travelled by rail to visit her old friend.

After Maggie had admired Helen's new baby boy and commented favourably on the deep burgundy of the new wallpaper and the glow of the beautifully finished mahogany wainscoting, the women caught up on news of family and friends. They discussed the growing prosperity of the town, the political career of Helen's husband, TJ Ryan, who was the mayor, and the changes that were happening in northern Ontario following completion of the Canadian Pacific Railway.

Maggie knew that Helen, called "Nell" by her family, still missed her younger brother who had been killed in a railroad accident five years earlier, so was relieved to see her friend could speak more easily of the tragedy.

They also touched on the changing role of women in the country and the world with hopes that the new century would see more women in non-traditional roles. Nell, who had a large and very busy practice in Sudbury and the surrounding area, was one of the first woman doctors in Canada. She was also the first woman doctor to become a member of the Canadian Medical Association (CMA).

Nell had known Maggie for many years, and their friendship had deepened when Maggie and her family of ten children had lived in the HBC Post at Whitefish Lake with her trader husband, TB Ross. The post was about two miles into the wilderness north of the town, so visits had been frequent. When Maggie had left her first husband, she had stayed with Nell until her second marriage.

"And what of your news from Montreal, Maggie?" Nell smiled. "Are you enjoying your new life as a Montreal society matron?"

Maggie laughed. Her home was located on a tree-lined street in an affluent suburb of Montreal. "Dearest Nell, I cannot tell you how different it is from my former life, but, yes, I am enjoying it."

"It is hard to imagine the changes in your life."

"Born in the wilds of Northern Quebec, married at seventeen, then after living for over thirty years in trading posts in the North woods to living in great comfort in Montreal? Yes, darling Nell, it has been a most interesting but very welcome change. And I am particularly pleased for Sybil's sake. I know my daughter will make a good marriage in the city."

They both chuckled at the irony of that statement. Making a good marriage was still very important for a woman, even if the times were becoming somewhat more enlightened.

Nell brought the conversation back to the original intent of Maggie's visit. "And since we are speaking of marriage, old friend, is that not one of the purposes of this visit?"

"Of course, Nell. I think, don't you, that we should continue our earlier discussion of the possibility of a marriage between your young cousin Jennie and my son Robert?"

Jennie Louise Ryan was a pretty, well-educated school teacher, who had lived with Nell in Sudbury for several years. She was a spirited young woman nearing twenty-five, and, to date, she showed little interest in the young men her cousin had arranged for her to meet. Much as Nell loved Jennie's presence in the household, she was becoming concerned that her cousin might be on the way to spinsterhood.

Thomas Robert Ross, Maggie's third son of her first marriage, was a handsome man of twenty-eight years. He was well established in his position as a trader for the Hudson's Bay Company with good prospects for advancement. To his mother's great pleasure, he had recently told her that he was ready to consider marriage.

Both Nell and Maggie were aware that over the past while, Robert's trips from his HBC post in Biscotasing to visit Sudbury and especially to call on his mother's friend, Dr. Ryan, had become more frequent. Strong-willed Jennie Louise, who had firmly refused the attentions of other suitors, was definitely pleased when Robert came to call.

Nell put down her teacup and turned to Maggie. "Jennie is a little older than most young women looking for a husband. But that means she is past the silly stage. She comes from a solid respectable farming family in Mt. Forest and knows how to manage a household. She is excellent with the children. She adores baby Horace and wants a large family of her own. I would, of course, certainly see that she received an appropriate marriage portion. She is very bright, well educated, and quite pretty. Although others have found her cleverness and bookishness off-putting, I appreciate intelligence in a woman, as I'm sure do you."

Maggie smiled, "Well, Nell, you yourself are a clever strong woman, so it is natural that you are a fierce supporter of a woman who thinks for herself. I, too, believe Jennie's quick mind and education will be an asset."

"An asset to Robert? Do you mean as a trader's wife?"

"Of course, how do you suppose my own children were educated? And who ran the posts while my first husband was away? But, I have some other news, just between us at the moment."

Nell waited. Her friend often surprised her.

"Robert is going to pursue his dream of becoming a doctor, so he may not spend too many more years in the northern bush. I will certainly encourage him to attend the medical school at McGill in Montreal. The university is near my home."

Nell was delighted with this news. "Well, I didn't know he had those plans," she said. "Jennie would make an excellent doctor's wife. I, of course, would be most willing to assist Robert with his studies." She paused, "Maggie, you know that I received my medical degree from Queen's College Medical School. The faculty there is very fine. Kingston would also be a good choice for Robert, as would Toronto."

The maid came in to remove the tea tray, and Nell smiled her thanks before returning to the conversation about marriage. "Maggie, are you at all worried by Jennie's fragile physique and sometimes questionable health? She suffers badly with rheumatism in the winter's cold. Will that not be a problem in the North woods? They will surely have to live at Robert's place of work at an HBC post until he is accepted at McGill or another university?"

Maggie and Nell were both physically robust, strong women who seemed never to be ill.

Maggie wasn't worried. "As long as she can bear children, Jennie's health won't be a concern. They can afford a nursemaid for the babies on his HBC salary, and she will always have help with the housekeeping, probably an Ojibwe or Metis girl. Bear in mind that life as a post manager's wife is much more comfortable now than it was when I raised ten children in the wilderness."

The women smiled at one another, the decision made. Provided they were both willing, Robert and Jennie would be married.

For Robert, there was never any question that Jennie was the perfect choice. The young couple went for long, carefully chaperoned walks through the small city and along the railways tracks. Jennie spoke of her pleasure in teaching young children and her love of books and poetry. Robert told her how much he wanted to be married and have a large family and also something of his life growing up in the northern wilderness of Quebec and Ontario.

Jennie shared something of her own childhood. She, like Robert, was one of ten children. Her own mother had died when Jennie was barely a year old, and her father had remarried a year later. Her step-mother had then borne five more children whose care had fallen to Jennie and her older sister Bertha. Jennie Louise's older cousin Nell had helped with the children until she had left Mt. Forest to go to college. Jennie worshiped her cousin who had been the constant in her life, and she was happy to be living with Nell in Sudbury.

Robert confided his plans to go to Queen's University in Kingston to become a doctor, rather than McGill as his mother hoped, telling Jennie that Queen's had been his dream since he was fifteen. At that time, a tutor hired by his mother had come from Kingston to their home at Whitefish Lake to teach the children the sciences, and this inspired the young man with his own dreams of a medical career.

Jennie spoke of her own academic achievements, her career as a school teacher, and how she had always been supported in those endeavours by Nell.

Robert was utterly enthralled by this scholarly young woman and said, "I think you are the prettiest school teacher I have ever seen, and I would be honoured if you would become my wife."

Jennie readily consented. She knew that she had to marry, she was already very fond of Robert, and this handsome, confident young man promised to be the ideal match. It was impossible for Jennie to under-stand what this marriage meant for her future. Robert was an ambi-tious young man who had lived for many years as a solitary traveller in the wilderness and who would remain a restless, untamed searcher for the rest of his life. But for now, thoughts of life as a doctor's wife settled in Kingston filled Jennie's dreams.

"I am very pleased to think that you plan to become a doctor, Robert. If you wish me to do so, I will be able to help you with your studies."

Jennie had visions of establishing a home in Kingston, a university town that would be ideal for her own academic pursuits. She also knew that her own educational background, which included Latin and mathematics, and her quick mind would allow her to help him succeed in his medical studies. She would be involved in learning alongside her new husband.

Robert smiled, well content with this agreement. "We will do very well together, Miss Ryan."

And Jennie happily agreed.

***

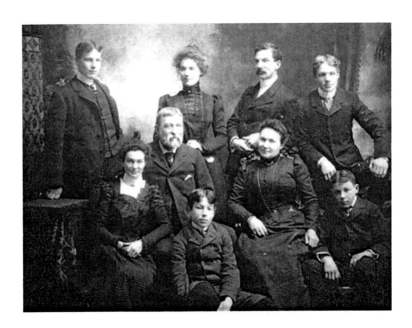

Robert and Jennie's Wedding Photo, Montreal, Quebec, 1900
Back Row l to r
Alexander, Sybil, Robert, Colin
Middle Row
Jennie, Peter McKenzie, Maggie
Front Row
Arthur, Donald

Following their marriage in 1900, the couple set up a home in the village of Dinorwic in northern Ontario. Robert continued to work for the HBC while waiting for news of his admission to Queen's. They had written his application letter together. Meanwhile, Jennie began to understand more of the life her new husband had lived for the past thirty years.

Their residence was a two-story house not far from the village where Robert managed the Hudson's Bay Company store. Jennie would walk with him into the village each day, and while she sometimes found the nearness of the dark woods intimidating, she enjoyed as many comforts as village life allowed. She had hired a young Ojibwe girl to help with the house, and to her great joy, Robert had arranged for her piano to be moved to Dinorwic, where she soon found a woman to give her piano lessons. Nell's family visited from Sudbury, as did Robert's younger brothers, Arthur and Donald. Jennie made muslin curtains for her new home, unpacked her dishes into the china closet, and soon made friends with the local merchants' wives.

Jennie and Robert supported the small church in Dinorwic; Jennie became a member of the church women's group and settled into the role of a trader's wife. She quietly began to assist Robert with financial matters at the post as well as doing her own household accounts. It gave her pleasure to do this for him, and although he always had a clerk, her help was welcome.

They went camping with groups of friends on nearby lakes. Jennie loved travelling by canoe in summer and, in winter, enjoyed slipping through the hushed white woods by dog sled. When the Ojibwe set up their winter camp near the post, a small group of their children joined Jennie's classes to have their lessons along with the village youngsters.

All the time, Jennie and Robert waited for news that his application to study medicine at Queen's would be accepted, and Jennie dreamed of a home in Kingston.

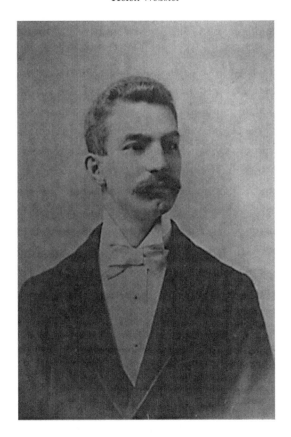

Robert at Queen's University, Kingston, Ontario, 1904

In 1904, Jennie gave birth to their first child, a son, whom they named Gordon McLeod. It had been a very difficult pregnancy for her, and there was concern that she might not survive the birth. But Gordon was a healthy infant, and Jennie gradually regained her health. They adored their baby boy, and to make life even happier, Robert was accepted at Queen's in that year and the family moved to Kingston, a beautiful university town. They set up a small home, and though she was lonely at first and missed her friends and family, Jennie soon made new friends and was content to live there. She loved looking after Gordon, a quiet, happy little boy, and spending her time studying medical texts and assisting Robert with his papers and exams. Her husband had always been an outdoorsman. He chafed at bookwork and the enforced sitting in classrooms. However, Robert enjoyed the laboratory work and the surgical classes and especially learning from real people with real illnesses. He became a superb diagnostician and surgeon in the process but always found it difficult to sit and study.

Jennie's patient tutoring and revision were invaluable. In later years, Robert was to say she could easily have passed any exams set; he had the bedside manner and technical skills, but Jennie had the knowledge.

Then, in Robert's final year at Queen's, Jennie found herself again with child. They were pleased, although once more she endured a difficult pregnancy. She longed for a baby girl and struggled to cope with her constant nausea and pain while still helping Robert with his crucial final year papers.

In the spring of 1908, Robert graduated with his Doctor of Medicine and Master of Surgery, and in September, their second son, Douglas Robert, was born. Again, Jennie was near death. Her physician told Robert that she must never have another child. Robert, already mourning the children who would never be, nodded his understanding and consent.

Jennie, unutterably saddened, moved into her mother-in-law's home in Montreal with the children and their nurse while Robert completed his internship at a hospital in that city.

The family received the best of care. Maggie was delighted to have her son and his family staying with her, but Jennie was ill, lonely, and bitter that she had another son rather than the daughter she had wished for. Knowing now that she would never have more children, and frail after the birth, Jennie fell into a profound depression, which was to linger for many years. Maggie was sympathetic towards her daughter-in-law's illness and depression, commenting in a letter to Jennie's cousin Nell that *"Jennie does her best but has more heart than strength."* However, Robert had not told his mother that Jennie would never be able to have more children, and Maggie, ignorant of this devastating news, finally lost patience with Jennie for her continuing sadness.

"My dear woman, you have two beautiful boys, and you will have more children. It is your duty to your husband, and you know he wishes to have a large family."

The young couple was plunged into deeper despair when it was suspected that Gordon had a heart condition. Jennie's depression worsened, and Robert began to fear for her sanity, especially when she tried to treat her baby son as if he was a girl.

Her husband, who believed in the healing power of the wilderness and who was now worried about a typhoid epidemic in Montreal, determined to get his wife and children out of the city and back to the woods.

Their departure was hastened as another tragedy struck. Maggie's husband, Peter, was showing early signs of dementia, and as the disease progressed rapidly, the household was plunged into sadness with the realization that he would have to be institutionalized.

As soon as Robert completed his internship, he and Jennie and the children moved back to northern Ontario where he resumed his work as a Hudson's Bay Company employee while looking elsewhere for a position as a doctor.

Jennie, relieved to be back in Dinorwic where she had been very happy, slowly began to improve. She spent some time each day in prayer, calling on her faith to sustain her, telling her husband, who was also grieving, that this was God's will and would only make them stronger. But it would be months until she regained her strength.

She desperately missed her cousin Nell, who had been like a mother to her. Dr. Ryan had moved to the West Coast in 1907, and the letters Jennie wrote to her spoke eloquently of the younger woman's sadness.

While Robert was thrilled with his new son and loved both his boys deeply, his wife did not seem able to show the same love for her second son as she continued to lavish on Gordon. Douglas was a colicky baby, screaming in pain all night long and constantly testing his mother's limited strength. Even with help through the day, Jennie's exhaustion and frustration with the new baby worried Robert, but there was little more he could do, and he wanted to begin his new medical career.

Remembering that his wife had at one time expressed a desire to go to the Western Territories, he quietly decided to look to the new provinces of Alberta and Saskatchewan for the family's future. He had heard at Queen's that doctors were needed in the new settlements to the west and hoped a complete change of scenery would help Jennie put this sad episode behind her and regain her verve for life.

Robert also recognized that he was too restless to settle permanently again with the HBC. So, quite sure that they would all be much happier in the West than in Ontario or Quebec, he began to plan, determined to learn all he could about Alberta.

Chapter 2
Alberta Bound

The eastern newspapers of the early 1900s, especially the *Toronto Globe,* were full of news of the great immigration to the rich and fertile lands of the southern prairies. Astonishingly inexpensive parcels of land were being offered to anyone interested in settling and farming in the new provinces of Saskatchewan and Alberta.

The Canadian Pacific Railway, which benefited from unprecedented government largesse, supported the idea of the fertility of the desert; all those agencies involved, including the governments of the two provinces, conveniently forgot the devastating droughts of the previous decades and pointed only to the rainy years of 1897 to 1900. Pamphleteers, newspapers, and government agencies all published information that sent young and old westward to the promise of a new life in the prairie provinces. There were "dryland specialists" and just plain land speculators who stated that hard times would never afflict southern Alberta, and others who claimed that the more the land was ploughed, the more moisture would be available.

Robert read all this with great interest. He had never been and never would be interested in becoming a farmer, but he longed for new adventures. He was dissatisfied with the sameness of his life with the HBC and realized that he had absolutely no interest in a medical position in an eastern city. Each week, the papers and those travellers who passed through Dinorwic brought more news of thousands heading west; one had only to watch the trains moving through to see the railcars jammed with hopeful settlers. His restlessness and the need to travel grew more insistent.

Robert knew that the claims of moisture coming up through the ground were nonsense, and his reading had informed him of the heat and drought that were common in southwestern Alberta, but, like many others, his need for change and adventure was fuelled by the dreams of Canadian Expansion. He was sure that his services as a doctor, and especially as a surgeon, would be in demand. He kept in touch with his contacts at Queen's University and the University of Toronto and soon discovered two items of information that pushed him towards a decision.

The first was news of a medical man in a small town called Lethbridge, in Alberta, who was making a name for himself as a daring surgeon in the Wild West. The second was news of a place not far from Lethbridge called Bow Island. This village was considered to have great promise for growth, both as the centre of a farming community and a future centre for the distribution of natural gas. The papers were full of news that natural gas had been discovered in plenty in southern Alberta.

In 1909, Bow Island #1 was the largest gas well in Canada. In one year, the community had grown from a tiny flag station on the Canadian Pacific Railway line to a village with three hotels, four general stores, and other small businesses, and the population was close to the numbers needed to be incorporated as a town. A bank was being constructed, and lots were for sale for one hundred pounds apiece. The flood of immigration continued seemingly unabated to southern Alberta, and Bow Island seemed to be very well situated for the future.

Robert firmed up his plans. He would need to determine exactly what his savings from the Hudson's Bay Company years amounted to and also ensure that his HBC pension would follow him wherever the family travelled. Jennie had again taken over the post accounts, and

Robert was confident that his wife could, at any time, provide an accurate accounting of their personal financial circumstances.

Robert would need nurses for a private practice, which he had decided was his goal. Since he was unsure whether any nurses would be available in the unknown place called Bow Island, he sent an advertisement to Queen's and the University of Toronto asking for two young and adventurous women trained as nurses to accompany the family to Alberta. The advertisement promised rail fare, housing, and employment for two graduate nurses who were looking for new lives in the West. Part of their duties would involve caring for Jennie, still recovering from Douglas's birth, and acting as nursemaids to Gordon and the baby on the train trip.

Finally, Robert negotiated a contract with the Canadian Pacific Railway as a CPR doctor, which meant he would travel at much lower fares and also guaranteed work for him anywhere the CPR had employees, which by this time, was all across Canada.

Satisfied that he had all his plans in place, Robert sat one evening with his wife and informed her that he had decided to look to the new province of Alberta for the family's future.

"Alberta? Alberta?" Jennie's response was close to a cry of alarm, but she quickly composed herself and marshalled what few arguments she had to dissuade Robert. "Douglas is barely five months old, I am not well enough yet to travel, and Gordon...what about Gordon? What about school? And a church? And our families and friends?"

"Gordon won't be going to school for at least a year; we'll be settled somewhere by then," was the blithe reply. "And I have arranged for two nurses to accompany us on our journey to look after you and the boys."

Jennie was ever practical. "Money, Robert. What do you plan to do until you are working again?" She had not been best pleased with their return to HBC postings, but at least it was a secure income.

"You know very well that our finances are just fine. We have some savings, and I will receive a small pension from the Company when I leave. I have also negotiated a contract with the CPR, which will give us much lower fares and hotel rates and ensure that I have some income to add to what I will earn when I set up a practice in Alberta. Now let me tell you about Bow Island and our trip to the West."

His wife barely heard him as he spoke at length about the new place, just catching fragments of information as she struggled with the whole idea. "About the same size, maybe a bit larger than Dinorwic; stores and houses and a bank, a blacksmith shop, several congregations, plans to build a new Presbyterian church — I can help with that Jennie..." his voice went on enthusiastically.

Jennie knew the matter was settled and that she could not bear to be parted from Robert, so began once again to think of everything that would need to be done to prepare for another move.

Within a few months, household goods had been packed for shipment, with good silver and china sent to Montreal to be stored, goodbyes had been said to friends and families, and the two nurses from Kingston had arrived in Sudbury. Then the four adults and two children, along with thousands of other immigrants looking for a new life, boarded the train at Sudbury and headed west.

PART TWO
Alberta
1909-1962

BOW ISLAND 1909

Chapter 3
By CPR to Bow Island

The natural world Jennie knew was either tall dark trees on the edge of villages or towns, such as Dinorwic or Sudbury, or the lovely parks of Kingston or Montreal. In Mt. Forest where she had grown up, her travel by horse-drawn carriage or train from town to town had been through green areas interrupted by neatly fenced farms and orchards. While living in Dinorwic and visiting HBC posts, she journeyed through the wilderness by canoe in summer and dog sled in winter, usually on day trips. With the exception of their honeymoon trip to Montreal, train travel had been limited to short excursions, with any journey of more than one day being broken by an overnight stay with friends or at a pleasant traveller's inn along the way.

Now she and Robert and their two little boys, along with the two nurses, Misses Emma and Mercilla Veale, had embarked on a journey west to Alberta that would take them over two weeks, leaving everything familiar behind.

They boarded the Canadian Pacific Railway train with its great steam engine puffing billows of smoke into the clear morning light. It was early on a fine summer morning in 1909 when the train, hauling freight cars, passenger cars, and a Pullman car with a small observation car at the rear, pulled out of the Sudbury station. With several stop-overs planned along the way, the Ross family and the two nurses hoped to arrive in Bow Island in late July.

They settled into their assigned places in the rear of the Pullman car. Their seats faced one another beside the windows with a small table that could be set up in between for their meals. Berths would be made up each night, and the boys would each sleep with a nurse, one with Emma and one with Mercilla.

At nine months, Douglas spent most of his time on one of the nurses' laps or playing on a thick blanket on the floor, but for five-year-old Gordon, the excitement was overwhelming, and he had great difficulty sitting still. Very soon he got his "sea legs" and was able to march up and down the aisle between the seats or sit with his mother while she told him stories.

Just along the aisle from where they sat, there was a water closet and a storage area for their baggage with the clothes they had chosen to wear on the train and the medical bags belonging to the doctor and the nurses. As Robert was now under contract to the CPR, he could be called on if any illness or accidents occurred during their trip, but fortunately, he was to remain untroubled on this journey. Embracing his new role as a doctor, Robert had left behind his trader's garb and was now more appropriately attired in vested suits, shirts, and ties.

The women all wore similar travelling costumes of long dark skirts and belted jackets. Jennie had at first attempted to wear her usual high-necked white blouses, but soon found the dust and fine soot from the coal-fired engines made wearing white impossible and changed to more sensible dark grey.

The train had moved smoothly away from Sudbury, heading across the expanse of the Canadian Shield north of Lake Superior on its journey west. It slowed down to pick up mail from hanging stanchions at small railway flag stops beside the tracks and through-out the journey. There were also frequent stops at small way stations to load travellers into the other passenger cars. The majority of those who caught the train were immigrants heading west to the unclaimed lands of the three new prairie provinces, and their hopes and fears were written on their faces. A few of the passengers were businessmen travelling to Winnipeg or Regina or even on to Calgary, and the Ross party was happy to hear what they had to say about any previous trips to the West.

By the close of the first day of the trip, the huge metal wheels were still clickety clacking around the top of the vast, grey, rocky expanses of the Canadian Shield, and they were just passing through their old home in Dinorwic. The endless, uninhabited landscape was heavy with scrub trees, huge rock outcroppings, and dark, impenetrable ranks of firs. For Robert, the journey west meant returning to the familiar wilderness of his youth, and he was content to see the miles roll by and the terrain grow wilder.

When they awoke on the second day of their journey west from Sudbury, the harshness of the Shield had given way to rolling brown and green hills that went on seemingly forever under a cold blue sky.

The family and the nurses gazed out the window, entranced by the miles of huge country rolling past and talked about their adventure into the unknown. Jennie was quite enjoying train travel, the novelty taking her mind off her recent sadness. She and her husband had many hours to talk together, the service was excellent, and the food was good. It was possible to either have their meals brought to them or go along to the dining car. This was a new innovation in rail travel, and on a number of occasions Robert and Jennie enjoyed this opportunity to dine in a more formal setting.

Transfixed by the view, Jennie's geography lessons seemed to be coming to life before her eyes. However, those lessons had come nowhere close to preparing her for the experience of their journey across the immensity of this land that was Canada.

"My goodness, it is vast and empty. Where are the people, Robert? Where are the farms? Is this all there is, miles and miles of hills and trees and rocks? I find it all somewhat overwhelming." Jennie was determined to be calm and brave and had rather liked sleeping in a comfortable berth in their carriage, but the sight of the great unpeopled distances was much more than she had expected.

Robert chuckled, "Remember, we're still in Ontario. Later today, we will cross the border into the province of Manitoba, and then you will all see the Great Plains, the prairies. There will be small settlements as we approach the capital city of Manitoba, called Winnipeg. I have spoken to you about the head office of the HBC, and I've been there before on Hudson's Bay Company business. It is a small but cosmopolitan city on the Red River. You will all enjoy the time there."

Robert continued to prepare them for what they would experience. "Tomorrow we will arrive in Winnipeg, and we'll spend a few days there before we carry on to Alberta. This prairie city has much to offer, including a new opera house. Now look, there is a little village on the edge of the rail line. We will stop there for coal and for water for the train and supplies of food. If you wish, you and Miss Emma and Miss Mercilla and the boys may accompany me onto the platform to walk and get some fresh air. I would advise this, ladies. Wear your bonnets and shawls, of course."

So with Robert enjoying every minute of the trip and Jennie and the nurses somewhat apprehensive but willing, they continued on to their first destination. By now, they were all awed by the sheer scale of the prairies that spread out on all sides. The landscape was not flat, but the space was so large that it was hard to see the dips and valleys in the harsh light of day.

As evening of the second day approached, a dusty haze blurred the horizon, and the evening light of a glorious prairie sunset played over the curves and contours of the lands to the west placing the low hills and shallow valleys in sharp contrast. Then the shadows gradually spread and utter darkness covered the land.

This was always when Jennie felt most vulnerable. There were no lights to show her where homes might be and people might reside, only blackness as the train moved through the night. Emma came to her to say that her berth was ready and to help prepare her for bed. Despite her sadness and anxiety, and her loneliness when she thought of leaving her family and all that was familiar behind, Jennie was eating better and sleeping well, and Robert was well pleased with her improving health.

Jennie was enjoying the company of the two nurses, both strong-minded women who were also leaving all that was familiar behind and travelling to a new life in an unknown part of the country. Jennie's admiration for their courage was boundless, especially for Mercilla who was nearly ten years her senior. The three women were becoming friends. Their conversations ranged from discussion about the failing health of King Edward VII and events across the country, to training for nurses and medical matters. The nurses were eager to hear Dr. Ross's opinion on the first successful human-to-human blood transfusion. Robert's cautious reply was that much more needed to be learned about this advance.

Robert was more than willing to regale them with stories of his years with the HBC, and they enjoyed hearing about the man who had suffered a really sad day when he had tried to wed a young woman in Dinorwic. Her brothers had run him out of town when they discovered his previous wives had all died under mysterious circumstances. For hours on end, though, the Rosses and their companions were content to simply sit and gaze in wonder at the changing countryside outside the windows.

On the third morning of their trip, Robert talked to them about the time they would spend in Winnipeg.

"You will find Winnipeg to be a very welcoming city. I have booked two rooms for us; the Misses Veale and the boys will have one bedroom, and we will have the other. It is a new CPR hotel called the Royal Alexandra, and I stayed there on my most recent trip to Winnipeg. We will be very comfortable. The staff is excellent, and you will be well looked after."

He spoke to Emma and Mercilla. "Mrs. Ross and I will be dining with several officers of the Company and the CPR and their wives. I have people to meet with at HBC Headquarters, and I wish to visit the new Faculty of Medicine at the University of Manitoba. We will also attend Sunday worship at St Stephens Presbyterian Church. You three ladies may hire a carriage to explore the city in the mornings, and then, Jennie, you must rest in the afternoons before dinner. I think you will all find it an enjoyable few days before we continue our journey to Alberta."

The Ross party was indeed well looked after, and the women were pleasantly surprised by the city on the Red River. They enjoyed the carriage rides through the leafy streets in the cool of the mornings, admiring the neighbourhoods shaded with bright summer leaves and the parks where they stopped to stroll while Gordon ran and played on the grass. And Jennie enjoyed having the children looked after, which allowed her to spend time alone with her husband, something that she had missed since the children were born. She was also regaining her strength, though she was still subject to periods of dark depression and worry.

In the afternoons, when Robert went about the business of finalizing his departure from the HBC and arranging for his monies to be paid into accounts in Calgary, Jennie slept in the shadowed quiet of her hotel room.

They dined out each evening, and the usually reserved Mrs. Ross discovered that she was the centre of attention. She found, however, that it was easy to converse with the HBC wives. They cared little about the new provinces of Saskatchewan and Alberta, speaking instead of the recent opening of the new Winnipeg Grand Opera House and other events in their city of which they were very proud. They were also interested in the fashions and social life of the eastern provinces, and Jennie was happy to chat with them about that, and everyone was much impressed by Robert's acquiring a medical degree in Kingston.

Many of these women had also spent time in the wilderness of HBC posts and were pleased to now be living in the civilization of Winnipeg. They had nothing to say about Bow Island, and were not too impressed by the Ross's trip to Alberta beyond expressing admiration at the courage it would take to start a new life in the "Wild West."

As they were preparing to leave the hotel on their last morning, and the chambermaid was packing under Jennie's supervision, Robert sat in a chair and they talked about their time in Winnipeg and their upcoming stay in Regina.

"Jennie, my dear, your colour is much better. I think the travel and the fresh prairie air are having a good effect on your health. Are you not feeling better as I predicted?"

"Yes, I am. You were wise to insist that we seek a new life in the West. I'm sorry, though, to leave Winnipeg. It's a charming place, not at all the frontier city I expected. Will Bow Island be somewhat similar, do you think?"

"No, not nearly so large, my dear, not really even a town yet. A much younger and smaller settlement, but there will be good people there, as everywhere. And remember, we will not stay there long, only until I can secure a position in Lethbridge. I will tell you what I know about Bow Island as we travel."

When they left Winnipeg, Jennie looked back longingly as the train pulled out of the station with much blowing of whistles and gusts of steam from the engine. It seemed to her that they had already come so far, and now they had several more days and nights before they reached their final destination in Alberta. The nurses, on the other hand, were glad to be embarking on the last legs of the journey and were excited at the idea that Bow Island was so close.

They did have another overnight stay in Regina, the capital of the new province of Saskatchewan. Again, a lovely town, this time built on the banks of the swiftly flowing South Saskatchewan River. To Jennie, the green trees and blue water, and particularly the rows of neat brick homes she watched from her window as the train passed through the city, were a welcome relief from what was beginning to look like an absolutely deserted landscape. To Robert, the rolling golden open spaces of the prairies were a promise of room to grow, of endless miles to explore, and above all, of the freedom to set his own path.

Unlike the two nurses, who were visibly excited about this new land, Jennie grew quieter and quieter as the miles of prairie slipped by the window, the loneliness broken only by the occasional tiny settlement clinging close by the railway. Despite her best resolve, she began to feel somewhat anxious as they travelled through endless grasslands. As she had when they traversed the Canadian Shield in Northern Ontario, she was distressed about the absence of towns and visible farms.

"Robert, there is no one here. Where will we live?"

It was quite true that her physical health had improved, but the rapid pulse beating in her temples betrayed her growing fear. Concerned, her doctor husband, who knew what lay ahead on their journey, spoke to one of the nurses. "Miss Veale, Mrs. Ross needs to lie down. I will give you some of her medication to help her sleep for a time." He leaned towards Jennie and murmured, "My dear, of course you are worried and overwhelmed. It is huge, this Canada of ours, but we will have our own home on the prairies, and it will be a fine place to live and raise our sons."

***

When the train stopped in Medicine Hat, the Ross party enjoyed a brief walk on the platform while passengers and goods, including a large quantity of mining equipment, were unloaded. The station was a place of constant activity, and the travellers caught snatches of conversation in many languages as men loaded carts with workers and machinery for the mines. Gordon clung closely to his father's hand as the shouts and noise swirled around them. Then it was time to board the train again for the last stage of their journey.

The rails stretched out across the empty plains ahead and behind. There was a thin high cloud overhead and the wind blew dust devils across the land on either side, rippling and flattening the yellow buffalo grass. The passengers peered hopefully through the grimy windows, hoping it would not be long until they reached Bow Island.

They arrived shortly before noon. The train slowed to a stop at the station, which was no more than a boxcar without wheels set by the track. They disembarked, leaving the now familiar comforts of the train to begin their new lives in this tiny prairie hamlet.

For a few moments as they neared Bow Island, Robert had seriously considered carrying on to Lethbridge. That city was where he hoped eventually to practise with a surgeon he had heard of and admired, named Dr. F. H. Mewburn. However, he knew a doctor was needed in Bow Island right now. He was also eager to get his family settled into their lodgings. He had sent a telegram ahead to secure places for them all at a boarding house that took in CPR crew members as well as other travellers.

Robert had every intention of renting furnished rooms in Bow Island where they would live until he could secure the position he desired in Lethbridge, but the boarding house seemed the best option until they found a place. Robert could see that Jennie, who had always had her own possessions, was not happy with the idea of staying in a boarding house, but he assured her that they would send for their household goods when they were more settled.

Meanwhile, Robert needed to establish his own practice here and begin earning some money. They had been able to travel quite inexpensively with Robert's CPR privileges, but the fares for the two nurses and the money needed to set up his own medical clinic here would use up all their savings.

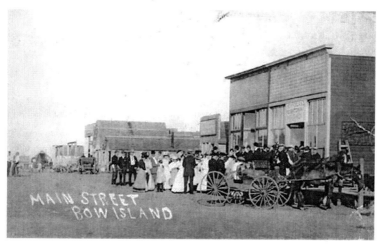

Main Street, Bow Island, Alberta 1909

The three women looked around in stunned silence at the townsite with its rutted, dusty street and a few widely spaced wooden buildings. Having lived in Dinorwic, Jennie was prepared for a small village, but she had not envisioned this flat treeless place.

Their baggage was loaded into a cart, and wordlessly, the doctor, the three women, and the children walked the short distance from the station to their destination on Railway Street. A hot dry wind was blowing and the prairie dust was soon part of their clothes and clinging to every bit of exposed skin. Even with scarves over their faces, dust collected in their nostrils and mouths and throats.

They kept their heads down; Emma carried the baby with his face pressed firmly into her shoulder, and Mercilla had a firm grip on Gordon's hand as the group trudged along the dirt road to their new home. Everything looked raw and new to the family from the East.

Robert, carrying his medical bag, his face alight with curiosity and excitement, strode along beside them, taking in the little prairie settlement with its well-spaced buildings and new construction. He was exhilarated by the trip and the great open spaces. Heat and dust and flies meant nothing to him, and the windswept land was infinitely preferable to the claustrophobia of cities. He drank in the vastness of the land, and although it was far removed from the icy coasts of Labrador or the forested wilderness of Northern Ontario where he had lived for over thirty years, he surveyed the Great Plains around him and felt that he had come home.

Bow Island had been settled in 1900 when natural gas wells were drilled in the area. It was a typical prairie community with a general store, a feed store, a farrier, and a farm equipment supplier. Plans for the new Presbyterian church, St Andrews, were underway, and Robert, thinking of construction of a medical clinic, took note of the Pioneer Lumber Yard. As soon as the women and little boys had been settled into the boarding house, he left them to their unpacking and set out to explore this new village.

The most notable characteristics of the townsite were that it was flat and dusty and exposed to the elements on every side. Although there were coulees with green trees in the surrounding countryside, and the Saskatchewan and Bow Rivers were not far away, the boxcar railway station and buildings themselves were situated on a level stretch of ground. The streets were wide, the buildings set far apart, and the wind seemed to blow constantly from all directions.

The village had its beginnings with the gradual settlement of the grasslands between Lethbridge and Medicine Hat by cattle ranchers in the late 1800s. In 1903, the CPR placed a section house, a boxcar minus wheels, on site, thus dividing the long stretch between two other flag stops, Winnifred and Burdett. One of the ranchers, a Mr. James Olquist, filed for land just north of the railway line, and part of his land became the townsite. More settlers, most from the United States, which was less than one hundred miles to the South, arrived in Bow Island, and homesteaders began to locate around the townsite.

Coal was plentiful in the coulees nearby, and over the next few years, natural gas was discovered near Medicine Hat. Shortly thereafter, drilling for gas began in the Bow Island area. Drillers joined farmers and coal miners as citizens of this new community.

In February of 1909, a strong flow of gas was struck, and the little settlement was on its way to becoming a very prosperous town. Soon there was a livery stable, a lumber yard, a general store, a boarding house, several hotels, a binding company, a blacksmith, a hardware and trading company, and a meat market, all to be followed by a jewelry store and photography business.

For the Ross family and the Veale sisters, Bow Island was familiar in that it was about the same size and composition of many eastern towns, but it was vastly different in geography and climate. The change from the tree-lined streets and the rolling hills of Ontario towns to the vast grasslands of Alberta was enormous. Robert loved it, but even the years spent alone in the Northern Ontario HBC posts could not have prepared anyone for this unending sweep of land and the unbroken arch of sky above.

The rhythms of small town life were also familiar to the family, but they quickly noted one important difference, and that was the strength and warmth of the welcome they received. Everyone else here was also a newcomer. The settled traditions and reserved behaviours of their previous homes had been left behind; most were young and eager to make new lives for themselves, and old ways were set aside in an atmosphere of openness and friendliness. Everyone helped everyone else, all the time.

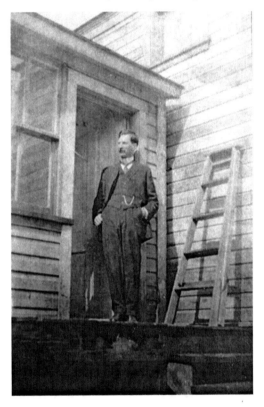

Robert on front porch of medical clinic, Bow Island, Alberta, 1909

During his exploratory walk, where he was greeted warmly by everyone he met, Robert discovered an empty grocery store in the two-story Clyde Bell Building. This business had closed just prior to the family's arrival in Bow Island, and Robert recognized that this empty building would be ideal for his purposes. He hired some village men, who were always looking for extra work, to construct a two-room hospital on the ground floor where he would have his office.

He also rented the existing simple living quarters on the second floor for the family and the nurses. It was far too small for a family of four and two adults, so the young women quickly found accommodation of their own nearby.

The townsfolk were delighted that they would now have a doctor and nurses living in the centre of the village, and who would all be available on a minute's notice. One of the two nurses, Emma, was also qualified to care for mental patients, so with the hospital and the doctor's office downstairs, and his living quarters upstairs, Bow Island was well served.

Robert immediately became involved with the building committee for the new St Andrews Presbyterian Church and served as the treasurer for the church's board of managers, offering his clinic for their meetings.

His wife, once she got over her shock at how different Bow Island was from her expectations, tried to establish a home above the hospital. They were not able to afford to hire a girl to assist with laundry and with caring for the children. Jennie was still very weak, and Douglas was frequently ill with stomach trouble and earache, often keeping her up through the night. Gordon, now five years old, was a tall, quiet boy. He missed going to kindergarten, but the school was a mile away, and Jennie simply couldn't manage to walk him there while carrying a squirming baby.

Their rooms above the clinic were cold and draughty, and their furniture had been damaged so badly during shipping that it was unusable. Upon opening the packing crates and discovering the shattered remains, Jennie had remarked unhappily that what was left was only good for kindling. With no money to purchase new furniture, they made do with what discards the previous owners had left behind.

Water had to be purchased by the barrel and was kept at the side of the building, so when Robert came upstairs for his noon meal, he always carried a few pails of water for household use. In winter, when everything was frozen, their only water supply came from snow that they melted in a metal pail on the stove top.

During these lunch breaks, Robert was able to mind the children, so Jennie could shop for their food. A young fellow from the grocery store was happy to carry her purchases home and up the stairs to their rooms.

Since of necessity she was out every day, Jennie quickly began to know the people of her new town. Often Gordon would accompany his mother, she in a wide hat, shirtwaist dress, and trim black boots, and he in his boots, short pants, and long sleeved shirt. As had been her practice in Dinorwic, she also managed the accounts for the new medical practice and quickly became a member of the church women's group, taking her children with her, as was the custom.

Jennie's friendship with the nurses, begun on the train, grew deeper, and with their company and her own activities, she started to build a life in Alberta. She also continued a lifelong habit of letter writing, describing her new life to her old friends and family back East, and to her cousin Nell on Vancouver Island.

Robert's boundless energy was evident from the first day of their arrival as he began building the new hospital and tending to his new patients. An aspect of his practice that he enjoyed greatly was the obstetrical work; inevitably, he was busy in a new town full of young people. In the next few months, assisted by a midwife, Mrs. Whitfield, he was called to the surrounding homesteads, where he delivered many babies, including the son of Mr. and Mrs. George Thomas. But, although there was plenty of work, there was little cash, so barter doctoring was employed, with chickens and produce exchanged for his services on many occasions.

Unfortunately, as Jennie tartly observed, this didn't pay the rent or buy coal, and it was growing increasingly colder as winter neared. She found it harder and harder to stretch his earnings and small HBC pension to pay rent, purchase food, and buy fuel, which, at five dollars per ton, was very expensive and seemed to be gobbled up by their stove without producing much heat in their living quarters.

The town was growing in every sense of the word. The usual illnesses were always present, although often exacerbated by the hard work and difficult conditions everyone endured.

Even before the two-room hospital was completed, Robert was called upon to see patients in their homes, often rough shacks or sod huts, called soddies, which were set bravely on their homesteads.

A sad beginning to his career in Bow Island was the death of a young woman. She was just twenty-one and had been very ill for some time when Robert began to care for her. All he could do was make her as comfortable as possible at her home about a half mile west of town. He rode by horseback out along the dirt track to see her every day, and it grieved him to watch such a young woman die.

"This is a hard life for both men and women, Jennie," Robert said as he shared his sorrow over the young woman's death. "She was only twenty-one, and her grieving young husband is working two jobs, trying to make a go of farming as well as working for the gas company. It has been a heartbreaking end to their dream of a new life here in Alberta."

Jennie said nothing, but simply sat with the sick baby on her lap and gazed around their shabby, cold rooms, thinking of her own dreams.

By far, the largest part of Robert's practice was taken up with mining and farming injuries. Many times men who were brought to him after serious accidents should have remained in the little hospital for a few days, but with farms to manage or jobs at the gas wells to return to, they often insisted on leaving too soon.

Robert soon realized that his practice would involve many trips to homesteads to do follow-up visits for these men and for their wives and children. He had always loved being out-of-doors, so his horseback rides or trips by sleigh were a pleasure to him, even in the wind and cold as the winter came. However, before the snow arrived that year, he would experience a very disturbing case.

Chapter 4
Paranoid Psychosis

This strange case, which occurred shortly after the hospital building was opened, promised to be the most unusual event Robert would experience during his time in Bow Island. It would challenge the expertise he had gained as a Bay Man, as well as test his medical training.

It happened to be a day when Robert was alone in his office, as both Emma and Mercilla were out on calls to nearby farms. Since the nurses travelled in horse-drawn buggies, they would often have to stay overnight with the family who had called for them. The nurses were not expected to return until the following morning, nor did Jennie expect Robert to return at a specific time. His medical work often involved tending to patients who lived some distance from the village.

Just after Robert opened the clinic for business that morning, a large and loud-voiced man dressed in typical farmer's garb of overalls and heavy shirt came into the office. He announced his name as Smith and showed the doctor a deep wound across the fleshy part of his thumb. Robert indicated that the man was to sit down in the surgery and then examined the gaping, dirty wound.

"I'll wash this out with antiseptic solution, Mr. Smith, and then I'll probably have to use an anaesthetic while I stitch it."

"No anaesthetic. I don't feel pain. Just do it, Doc."

"Don't you want me to use an anaesthetic before I put in the stitches?"

"Nah, just go ahead and sew it up. I told you. I can stand any amount of pain."

Robert was skeptical, but he insisted on cleaning the wound with antiseptic and began to close it with stitches. The man did not flinch at either the cleansing solution or the needle piercing his flesh, but began muttering words that Robert could not understand. As the doctor worked on his hand, Smith continued to mumble incoherently, giving the impression that he was recovering from a bout of drunkenness.

Robert said nothing but thought, "This fellow is a drunkard and must still be drunk as this cut is very deep and the stitching must hurt fiercely."

Oddly, there was no odour of liquor on the farmer's breath, and he sat stolidly throughout the entire procedure.

Robert covered the thumb with a neat dressing and wrapped a firm bandage around the farmer's hand. "Come back tomorrow, as I am concerned about infection, even blood poisoning since the wound was so dirty. If there is any problem, I will have to clean the wound again, and you may have to spend some time in the hospital so that I can keep an eye on it."

"All right, Doc. I'll see you tomorrow. Here's your pay." The farmer placed a twenty-five cent piece on Robert's desk and left.

"Well," Robert said to himself. "That was interesting. I have done a lot of surgery free of charge, but that is the smallest fee I have ever received."

Robert soon put the matter of the farmer's thumb to the back of his mind as more patients needing his attention arrived at his office. Working on the farm and on the gas wells meant accidents and injuries were common, and the townsfolk were glad of the new doctor's skills. He spent a busy afternoon and gave no more thought to his stoic morning patient.

But that evening, just as Robert was about to close the office and head upstairs for his supper, the same farmer walked in and declared, "Look at my thumb, doctor. The stitches are out."

To Robert's surprise, the dressings were off the hand, and the wound gaped as badly as before it had been stitched. "What happened?"

"Oh, I took the stitches out to show my friend what a good job you had done. Now I need you to do it again."

The doctor was furious. "You are either drunk or crazy. You will have a serious infection in that hand if you do not look after it as I told you, and you have already made it worse by tearing it open again."

The man roared at Robert, towering over him with his bloody fist in the air. "I am not a drunk. I never touch alcohol. I am a Mormon, and my church forbids drinking. And don't call me crazy. My wife and son have already told me I am crazy, and I am going to get them for that when I return home."

Robert thought quickly as he now believed that he was dealing with a case of insanity. He realized that the first thing he needed to do was calm the man down and then find out what he meant by "getting" his wife and son.

"I am sorry for what I said just now. Of course you are not crazy. That was my mistake. Please sit down and I will sew up your thumb again."

This he proceeded to do, again without anaesthetic and once more to the accompaniment of incoherent rambling. By now, Robert was thoroughly worried for his own safety, as well as for the man's wife and children.

When the hand was once again bandaged, the farmer stood up to leave, and as he did so, he asked the doctor, "Are you a Mormon?"

Robert replied that he was not, and the farmer said, very calmly, "I wish you were a Mormon because then I could tell you a secret."

Hoping that he would learn something that would safeguard the wife and son, Robert said," I would certainly like to become a Mormon and listen to your secret."

Smiling happily at this, Smith said, "Get down on your knees and pray, and I will make you a Mormon and tell you my secret."

Not wanting to kneel in the presence of such madness, and equally reluctant to disturb Smith any further, Robert spoke carefully. "But I am a Presbyterian, and Presbyterians always stand when they pray. I cannot kneel until you make me a Mormon."

To his relief, Smith accepted this with little objection. "Oh, well, that is all right then. I will kneel and pray for both of us. You must not move, though."

The man then knelt and prayed quite coherently and very beautifully.

Robert, who was mentally searching for ways out of this dilemma, recalled something from his medical training. He had learned that the subconscious mind is often in control of the speaker. This was apparently true, for Smith's memory of his religious studies was evident as he calmly recited his prayers.

When the farmer finished praying, he rose from his knees and stated that Robert was now a brother Mormon. "So I can tell you my secret."

They both sat down, and Smith told Robert that he had left his farm early that morning and walked to town, a distance of about four miles. He had needed to have someone look at his hand, and he had heard that there was a new doctor in town. "I just finished digging a well close to my house. It has sixteen feet of water in it, and I am going to drown my family."

To Robert's horror, the farmer continued the story in the same calm voice. "I will return to the farm about midnight tonight. They will all be fast asleep, and when they wake up in the morning, they will all be floating in the well."

Robert listened anxiously, running through possibilities in his head. He had not seen a policeman in the time he had been in town and he knew of no telephone in the whole place, certainly not one in his office. It was now late in the evening, and the street by his building was deserted. He wished fervently that he had brought his revolver down to the office with him this morning.

Meanwhile, the madman went on in a cold voice, showing no emotion as his dreadful plan unfolded. "There are five children and the wife. I will start with the youngest child, the baby. Then the older ones 'til I get to the oldest boy. He is a husky lad of fifteen and may give me quite a tussle, but I am larger than he is. The wife will be last. She will put up a fight, but I am much stronger than she is, and I will get her into the well with the kids all right."

The time by now was within an hour of midnight, and Robert had no way of notifying anyone in authority, but he knew he had to do something. "You know, that will be a big job for one man alone. As your brother Mormon, I think I should go with you and help you."

"All right, as a brother Mormon, you can come along with me."

"First, though," Robert suggested, "we should go to the restaurant and get something to eat. It will give us the strength we need to do this job."

Pleased that Robert was not opposed to his plan, Smith replied, "Yes, you're right. I'm very hungry."

"Come with me and we will go to Chuck Chen's place. I know he is open very late and I see there is still light in the windows."

The rest of the village was in darkness, but the restaurant was still open, although there were no other customers inside when the doctor and the farmer went in and sat down. When Chuck Chen appeared from the kitchen, Robert ordered two large steaks, some dessert, and coffee.

Rising from their table, Robert told Smith "I need to show the cook how to fix our steaks."

As calmly as he could, he walked toward the kitchen, where he hoped to speak to Chuck Chen alone. However, the big farmer was right behind him, so Robert was unable to ask the proprietor to notify the authorities.

In a few minutes the steaks were done and brought to the table, and Smith started to eat ravenously. It was obvious that he had not eaten in some time, and his attention was occupied by the food, so again Robert made an effort to speak to the restaurant owner on his own. "I want to get my steak cooked a little more. I will be right back; you just keep eating."

This time, the farmer remained at the table, which gave Robert the opportunity he needed to talk privately to Chuck Chen. He spoke quietly but urgently, watching the table where Smith sat. "Are there any police in the area? The man I am with is a madman and a possible killer. He has told me that he intends to drown his wife and five children."

"There are no police in town, but there is a policeman who lives on a farm about three miles distant," Chuck Chen answered just as quietly, looking nervously into the restaurant and glancing at his knives on the counter.

"Could you get someone to go and get the policeman?" Robert asked. "I will look after the shop till you return, and I'll keep the madman here with me."

"I know very few persons in town as I have only been here myself for a short time, and I don't know anyone here who knows where the policeman lives. Who would believe this strange story in the middle of the night?" Chuck Chen thought hard for a few moments, then, "I'll have to go myself. I know where the policeman lives. It would not take more than two hours there and back, but the country is not fenced and the trail is very hard to find."

Robert agreed that this was the only option and said he would think of a way to keep the farmer occupied while Chuck was gone.

They both looked at Smith, still placidly eating his steak. Chuck Chen made his decision. "Go and sit down. I'll serve your coffee and dessert. Then I'll go and tell the policeman your story, as long as you are willing to stay here and be sure nothing happens to my business while I'm gone."

Chuck Chen served the two men their dessert and coffee, and left, after saying loudly that he had a short errand to run, but if the men stayed behind to look after the restaurant, he would be right back to bring them more coffee and another dessert.

Robert promised they would.

Smith ate his pie and drank his coffee but soon began to fret about leaving. "We must get on our way to the farm at once as I want to finish my plan while the family is sleeping soundly."

"But we promised to look after the cafe until Mr. Chen returns. He fed us well, and we need to keep our promise as good Mormons." Robert tried without success to persuade Mr. Smith to stay.

The farmer announced, "You can wait and look after the shop if you like, but I must go now. I'll do the job on my own."

Robert had been thinking hard about what to do in this eventuality and had a plan that he had first considered in the office but had seen no way to implement at that time.

"If you are determined to go alone, that is all right with me. I'll stay here as I promised Mr. Chen. I think we should have another cup of coffee before you go so that you can be sure to stay awake and do a good job."

"All right, but just one cup, and then I must go before they waken."

"I'll make the coffee. Please sit down again; it will only take a few minutes." In his medical case, which he had brought with him, Robert had a number of tablets of apomorphine. He always had the case with him, and carrying it had aroused no suspicion from the farmer. The doctor took two tablets out of the case while he was in the kitchen and, when the coffee was ready, carried it to the table. As he poured the coffee into the farmer's cup, he surreptitiously added the two tablets along with sugar and stirred it thoroughly. "Here you go. Drink this, and you will be all set to go out to the farm."

In about ten minutes, the farmer shook his head and complained. "Say, I'm getting sick." He became pale and began to perspire profusely.

"Let's go outside and get some fresh air. That should help."

As soon as the two men reached the sidewalk, the farmer began to vomit and was very weak. Robert, pretending great concern, said, "One of the first symptoms of blood poisoning is nausea and vomiting. I'm afraid that you're going to have a severe attack of blood poisoning unless I can stop it at once. I have an injection in my doctor's bag that

I can give you and you will feel better very soon afterwards. You can then go about the urgent business you have on hand."

"Please give it to me, Doc. I have to drown them tonight."

The two men came back into the shop, and Smith staggered to his chair, where he slumped, weak and exhausted by the vomiting and beginning to feel the effects of the apomorphine. Robert dissolved a tablet of hyoscine in a teaspoon of water and injected it into the man's arm.

"This will make you relax and feel sleepy for a bit, but you will then feel much better." From his experience in the hospitals in Montreal, Robert knew that hyoscine was a potent sedative and had seen it used to good effect with maniacal cases during his internships.

"I must keep this man quiet until the policeman arrives," were the doctor's worried thoughts as he watched the farmer relax and then slide further into a state of semi-stupor. "Now, please let Chuck Chen and the police arrive soon. This sedative will last for a few hours, but what I'll do if they don't come in time, I'm not altogether sure."

Just before two hours had passed, the man began to stir, but Chuck and two burly men, both dressed in civilian clothes, arrived at the shop.

"I am very glad to see you. My name is Doctor Robert Ross, and I hope you're here to take this man into custody."

"Yes. I'm with the police. Here is my badge," said the more senior of the two men, raising the lapel of his jacket to show Robert. "Come outside and tell me what this is all about, Doctor."

Smith remained quiet and tractable, so, leaving him in the care of the younger man and Chuck Chen, Robert went outside with the policeman.

"The man is insane and has stated his intention of killing his wife and five children by dropping them into the well on their property while they're sleeping." Robert went on to recount the full story, beginning with the arrival of the farmer at his medical office early that morning.

"My God, man, you could have been killed," the policeman exclaimed, shocked at all Robert had told him. "It's a good thing you figured out what to do, and that Chuck Chen knew where I lived. I'll go right now and send a wire to Lethbridge asking them to send a couple of mounted police on the soonest train."

Robert, who by now was well past exhaustion himself, volunteered to keep watch over Smith with Chuck Chen and the younger man until the senior policeman returned from sending the telegram.

The officer was not gone for long, and he arrived back on the scene with news that the Mounties were on their way. He told Robert that he would take charge of Smith. Relieved at this news, Robert told the officer that Smith would need to walk off the drugs while they waited for the train.

Turning to Chuck Chen, he said, "Here is the money for our meal, Mr. Chen. Thank you for all of your assistance. I will see you again." Chuck Chen smiled and nodded but said nothing more as the men left, and Robert gratefully set off for his bed, hoping to get a few hours of sleep before the train arrived.

Twice during the night, Robert heard the farmer and his guards passing on the wooden sidewalk below his window. The farmer was shouting, "Let me go! Let me go! I have done nothing."

"Be quiet, man, you threatened to drown your entire family. We will let you go when the train comes in and not before."

A few hours later, Robert arose and made his way through the early morning quiet to the boxcar station to wait for the train. The policemen and a now calm Smith were already there. When the train arrived, and the farmer saw the mounted police step off, he bolted away from his guards and dashed across the open prairie. Fortunately for the police and for the man's family, it was already light enough that they could see him as he ran across the unfenced fields. One of the Mounties soon caught up with the fleeing farmer and brought him down with a rugby tackle. The madman was handcuffed and put on the train, which was heading for Ponoka and the insane asylum.

The next weeks passed uneventfully. Robert's practice grew rapidly, and he and his wife became busy and well-respected citizens of Bow Island. The people of the community and surrounding area were good friends and good neighbours to the family; the incident with Smith was forgotten, though Robert would be forever grateful to the brave proprietor of the cafe.

Chuck Chen's unselfish act not only rescued the doctor from a terrible situation, but it also saved the lives of a young mother and her five children. Robert greatly appreciated the man's quick and intelligent comprehension of the mortal danger that had threatened the family at the hands of a murderous maniac, and the courage Mr. Chen had shown by volunteering to go out on such a hazardous mission. It had been the middle of the night in a little known and sparsely populated prairie countryside, and the man had done his utmost to secure help.

Robert had been besieged by the good wishes of the small population of Bow Island in the days following the incident, but, although he told the townspeople of Mr. Chen's bravery, the man never received the public recognition he deserved for his quiet heroism. "I wish I had gone back to see him, to say thank you again," Robert mused as he went about his daily rounds, "he probably did not expect it, but, still, I wish I had."

Chapter 5
A Prairie Winter

Winter in Ontario had been the Rosses' favourite time of year. Bundled in furs, the family would travel by dog sled to visit friends and neighbours, moving easily over the snow-covered paths and frozen lakes and rivers. The heat and black flies of summer were absent, and everyone was more relaxed now that the hard work of autumn was over.

In Bow Island, winter was also a time of relative leisure, and the people of the village enjoyed the social activities offered to all. Many of the settlers brought small musical instruments with them when they moved to Alberta, so groups quickly came together, and winter was the time to practise and perform. An evening of playing and singing in someone's home was a common event, and guests, well wrapped in warm buffalo robes, arrived by wagons or sleds drawn by teams of horses or oxen to enjoy music or a homegrown drama or recitation. Card parties held in church basements were also well attended as were concerts in the schoolhouse.

When baby Douglas was well, which seemed to be very rarely, Robert and Jennie and the children enjoyed several of these gatherings, and they all welcomed the company and the warmth.

They usually went to these events in the company of the two nurses and their new friends, and on one or two occasions, they were able to hire a local girl to look after the children. This gave Jennie a much-needed break, and besides enjoying the evening out, she believed it was important for Robert's practice to go to these social events. She knew that, in addition to valuing his skills as a physician and surgeon, the townsfolk appreciated Robert's help in building the new church as well as taking on the position of treasurer.

The highlight of the Rosses' first winter in Bow Island was the Masquerade Ball held on January 1, 1910. Jennie had never learned how to dance, but she and Robert attended and enjoyed the music and admired the costumes. Jennie always dressed modestly, but her dark green woollen dress this evening had the elegant touch of fine pin tucks over the bodice. It flared out from her tiny waist to a full skirt that just brushed the insteps of her shiny black boots. The understated dress was enhanced by a high-necked lace inset. She put on her serviceable, long black woollen coat, as she had left her fur coat, a gift from her husband, in storage back East.

"Even if you don't have your fur coat here, Jennie, you should carry your mink hand warmer. It is very warm and sensible," Robert suggested, and she agreed. Not in the least worried about being too showy himself, Robert elected to wear his beautifully embroidered and fringed deerskin coat over his suit and vest. Along with Jennie's fur coat and hand warmer, Robert had acquired the deerskin coat during his HBC days.

The two nurses, who had chosen to wear costumes, smiled happily at the couple, and the foursome set out under a cold black sky filled with stars to travel to the Lundquist Hall. A girl had been hired to look after the boys for the evening, and she would remain until the Rosses' return and then would join her own family at the dance.

Their arrival at the masquerade was greeted with warm calls of welcome, handshakes, and invitations to enjoy the food set out on long tables to one side of the room. The hall was packed with clowns and hoboes, witches and ghosts, flower girls, and characters from fairy land. Children and parents alike moved around the hall in colourful costumes. The adults soon settled onto benches while the youngsters sat on the floor to enjoy the evening's entertainment.

The presentation included a minstrel show, choral singing, and a wonderful band concert. By ten o'clock, the stirring band music ended, and the thirsty musicians took a brief break before switching to the gentler strains of waltzes and polkas.

As couples began to whirl to the music, Robert and Jennie retrieved their coats and, smiling to friends, made their way to the exit. Robert would have loved to stay for the dancing but, knowing Jennie could not participate, chose to leave with his wife. They agreed that it had been a most successful evening. Despite the hardships they all suffered, the people of Bow Island were among the kindest Jennie had ever met, and she could not help but think that with a better house, she could have made a life in Bow Island. But, she knew that this was not to be.

***

One afternoon in early December, Robert rode across the frozen prairie towards home. He had attended a birth at a homestead about four miles from the village.

Now, as his reliable horse trotted along the narrow path through the wheat stubble, Robert kept a wary eye on the steel grey sky and lowering dark clouds to the northwest. He knew a blizzard was coming, and the buffalo trail he was following could be quickly obliterated when the rising wind and snow reached his path.

When they moved to Alberta, Robert had brought with him in addition to his beaver coat, a heavy fleece-lined, waxed canvas coat, called a duster, which he wore over his woollen suit. The duster had a slit up the middle in the back that extended from hem to saddle height. This deep vent allowed his legs to be covered when riding. The coat, plus his heavy woollen mittens and muffler and felted-wool Stetson hat, ensured that he was warm.

Nevertheless, Robert well knew how easily anyone, even someone with his excellent sense of direction, could get lost in the fury of a blizzard. The cold and wind were a constant presence in their lives, to be considered and respected at all times.

There had been no wind when he left for his hour's ride home, but the sky was now a milky grey, and the flurries of hard dry snow were increasing. Robert urged his willing mount to a little more speed, patting the horse's heavy coat and murmuring words of encouragement.

He had another reason for wishing to be home early this evening. He needed to have a talk with Jennie about his plans. Last week, he had sent off more telegrams to the universities back east looking for information about possible surgical positions in Alberta. In particular, he hoped for an opportunity to work with the surgeon in Lethbridge whom he so admired.

Robert enjoyed life in Bow Island. He was a busy and happy member of the community and the Presbyterian Church, where he served as treasurer. He could already see that despite the hardships, Jennie was putting down roots in the small community, and he knew how much she valued her friendships with the Veale sisters and the other families who had welcomed them so warmly to the place. But he had never pretended that Bow Island would be a permanent residence, so when Jennie began to talk seriously about finding a more permanent home for them there, he decided to remind her of his plans.

Robert chatted for a few minutes with the young fellow at the livery stable where he kept his horse, then walked home along the snowy streets. He loved to be outdoors and enjoyed his rides across the plains, and he wasn't usually bothered by any weather, but this evening he was glad to be home before the blizzard's full fury struck.

Robert stamped the dry snow off his boots as he climbed the outside stairs to their quarters above the little hospital. Jennie, dressed in a warm, floor-length woollen dress with long sleeves and a high neck, was sitting close by the stove with the weekly mending in her lap, and the children's laundry hung to dry on lines above its heat. Gordon played with his blocks on the carpet at her feet, ignoring the cold drafts that reached icy fingers in through every crack in the walls. Douglas, who even when ill was a very active one-year-old, was finally sleeping peacefully in his makeshift cot in the corner of the room, well wrapped in blankets to ward off the chill.

Robert looked at his wife and thought that even though he knew she was exhausted, she looked very pretty in the deep blue dress. The colour suited her fair skin and black hair. The dress, a favourite of his, had been made for her by a dressmaker during their last winter in Kingston. This cold afternoon she also had a warm shawl around her shoulders and fingerless gloves on her hands. As usual, she wore her gold wedding watch on a heavy grosgrain ribbon at her waist and glanced at it as her husband came in the door.

"Good evening, Robert, you are home earlier than usual. Your dinner is on the back of the stove; shall I get it for you?"

"In a few minutes, thank you." Robert placed his rifle on the rack over the door and hung up his coat and hat and set his boots behind the stove to dry.

"I'll have my tea sitting by the warmth with you," he said, and moved to his chair across from his wife. For this important conversation, Robert had chosen an evening when he knew there were no overnight patients in the hospital and the two nurses would have gone to the homes where they boarded.

As soon as his father sat down, Gordon, delighted that Robert was home early, promptly climbed up into his lap and requested a story.

"In a few minutes, Son. Your mother and I have some things to discuss. Play with your blocks. That is a fine house you are building." The little boy slipped obediently to the carpet, and Jennie put aside her mending and somewhat apprehensively clasped her hands in her lap. "What is it, Robert?"

"I sent another telegram to the University of Toronto last week asking about Doctor Mewburn and the possibility of a surgical position in Lethbridge. It is only a matter of time now. I'm sure that I will receive news within days. Lethbridge is growing rapidly, and more doctors will be needed. Remember, working with Mewburn is one of the reasons I came to the West."

Jennie drew a long breath then released it in a deep sigh but said nothing. It had been twenty degrees below zero for seven weeks, she was desperately concerned for her children, and the thought of another move to another unknown place left her in despair, but she simply looked at her husband as he went on.

"You know that we will move as soon as I hear from Toronto. There is little point in looking for a house here. Even if I can't get on the staff at the Galt Hospital, we will still go to Lethbridge. This is not a surprise, Jennie."

"No, it is not a surprise, but I didn't think it would be so soon. Surely things will get better here. I was looking forward to Christmas with our new friends. I know we can't afford our own Christmas tree, but there are plans for a community tree for all to enjoy on Christmas night, Nell has sent presents for the children, and we are all looking forward to the New Year's Masquerade." Jennie responded wistfully.

"We won't be moving to Lethbridge until February at the earliest, so we will be able to attend that party, and our friends can visit us in Lethbridge. You will enjoy living in a larger city. Also, the men who come into my office tell me that winter has only just begun, and the Farmer's Almanac says it will be bitterly cold in Bow Island this year. Times will continue to be hard for everyone." He paused, but Jennie said nothing, so he went on. "Keep in mind that we are leaving to go to a position I have been waiting for since we left Dinorwic. Our financial affairs will improve as I will earn a good salary at the Galt Hospital, and I will be part of an established medical practice. So no looking for a house now. I know these rooms are cold, but they will have to do until such time as we move."

"What about Emma and Mercilla? Do they know about this plan?"

"I'll talk to them tomorrow. They may wish to find employment in Lethbridge as well. But that is their choice, of course."

"Oh, I think they will stay here. Both of them have made very good friends, and Bow Island is now their home."

Jennie, knowing there was no choice but to move if Robert secured the position, asked, "And will we find a house in Lethbridge, Robert? These rooms are small and cold, but at least they are clean. I don't think I could bear another flea-infested boarding house."

Robert shrugged, "Jennie, I simply don't know. I will have to go ahead and see if I can find something if I get the position. We'll see."

He looked around the cold little room with the castoff furniture left by the previous inhabitants, the only comfort a deep red, patterned rug covering the wooden floor. The carpet was the one large item of their own furniture that had survived being shipped to Bow Island.

He sighed and thought to himself, "I hope Lethbridge will see us in warmer housing, but we're moving, even if we have to rent furnished rooms again."

Gordon looked up expectantly at his parents, and Robert smiled at him and motioned for him to climb up into his lap for a story. The matter of moving to Lethbridge was settled.

Jennie, knowing further discussion was pointless, made them both a fresh cup of tea and took up her mending again. The only sounds in the room were the soft hissing of the gas lamps and the quiet crackle of the coals settling in the stove and Robert's voice as he read to Gordon. The five-year-old was enthralled by Barrie's Peter Pan, and the illustrated copy his father held was well worn with reading and re-reading. Outside, the wind of the blizzard buffeted the walls, and the building shuddered under its blows, and the room became even colder. When the story was finished, Jennie reluctantly left her place by the stove and took Gordon's hand, helping him down from her husband's lap.

"Come along now, Gordon. Time for bed. We'll tuck you in under the buffalo robe beside Douglas. Don't disturb him. It is a blessing that he is still asleep. Your father will kiss you goodnight when you are settled."

Robert sat in his chair, enjoying the peace of the evening, satisfied that his conversation with Jennie had gone well. He did not enjoy upsetting her, but she had always known about his desire to work with the famous surgeon. He would talk to the nurses tomorrow about his plans to move.

His thoughts turned to the day ahead. There was a Dr. Paterson from Western Hospital in Toronto who wanted to come out west. He could take over the practice here in Bow Island.

Robert knew that he would need to leave Bow Island as soon as he heard from Lethbridge. An assistant to Dr. Mewburn was a coveted position, and he would not miss this opportunity by delaying.

Within weeks of his conversation with Jennie, he received a response from his University of Toronto contact. Dr. Mewburn was not only looking for a surgical assistant, he also wanted a locum to take his place while he went on a leave of absence. Robert immediately sent a telegram to the Galt Hospital applying for the position. He also decided to go on his own to Lethbridge as soon as Dr. Paterson arrived in early February. The rest of the family would move when he had secured the position and found a new home for them.

LETHBRIDGE
1910

Chapter 6
The Galt Hospital

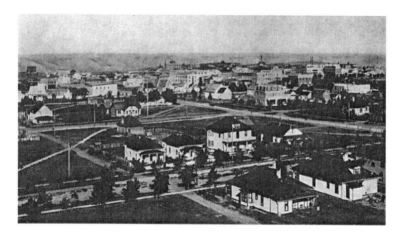

Lethbridge, Alberta, 1910

The red bricks of the Galt Hospital glowed in the last light of the late winter afternoon when Robert reined his horse to a stop. As was his habit in a new town where he planned to work, he was surveying the city of Lethbridge from the seat of a buggy he had hired that morning. He had arrived from Bow Island on the early train, and the day had been spent exploring Lethbridge, a bustling prosperous community of red brick buildings, neat white framed houses, and the usual miners' shacks on the outskirts of town.

In 1910, Lethbridge was a substantial small city, its wealth derived from the surrounding coal mines and from its location as a distribution centre for the Canadian Pacific Railway. The surrounding farmlands were undergoing rapid settlement by the flood of immigrants brought to the West by the railway to open up southern Alberta.

There was a plentiful water supply from the Oldman River, which cut through the centre of town. Seeing the river's location, Robert felt a worm of anxiety as he suspected the water was probably already contaminated by the runoff from farmlands, factories, and sewage from the town. He felt sure that there would be a typhoid epidemic in the near future. However, that kind of pollution was common enough in cities all across the land, so Robert, always a pragmatist, pushed that worry out of his mind for now.

The appeal of the town for him lay not in its size or wealth or people, but in the opportunity it offered him to work first as a locum, then as a surgical assistant and physician with Dr. Frank Hamilton Mewburn.

By 1910, Dr. Mewburn was well known throughout the western provinces as one of the first surgeons to operate in Alberta. His most famous early surgery took place in Fort Macleod in 1890, where he had attempted a bone graft using bone from a dog. Dr. Mewburn had established a medical practice in Lethbridge in 1886 and his fame had spread quickly. He maintained his ties with the Medical Schools of eastern Canada and, in the spring of 1910, let it be known that he was looking for another surgical assistant.

Shortly after Robert had sent his telegram to Dr. Mewburn, he had received a favourable reply and had set up an interview. He had quickly settled his affairs in Bow Island, leaving his nurses instructions for the few patients in the small hospital, and had informed Jennie that he would send for her as soon as he was settled. He was confident both that he would get the position offered and that, once she had seen Lethbridge, his wife would be happy with the move to a larger place. It was, after all, just a short train ride to Bow Island to visit her friends.

At the end of his day of exploring, Robert was well pleased with the prosperous city. He felt Jennie and the boys would do well here, and the move appealed to his restless, adventurous spirit. It also satisfied his desire to learn more surgical techniques as well as to advance his career. Bow Island had been a good beginning, but his interview with Dr. Mewburn was the chance he had been looking for to make his mark in Alberta.

He looked once again at the hospital. It had a pleasing aspect from the road, with a wide front door and many windows set into its red brick facade. He knew it was large enough to accommodate over fifty patients and that the annex to the left was a School of Nursing. To the rear of the building, the land dropped sharply down to the river, and on the opposite banks Robert could see through the winter bare trees to open land. Beyond that was farmland and low hills, now fading in the early evening light.

"Good," he murmured, "a teaching hospital and an excellent surgeon with whom to work. This will suit my needs very well." At no time did he doubt that he would obtain the position; his qualifications and experience were too good to be turned down.

Robert clucked to the sleepy horse and made his way back in the dusk through the quiet streets to his hotel. Tomorrow he would go to his interview, arrange for a boarding house for himself and his family, and, once settled, contact Jennie.

The interview went exactly as Robert had expected. When Dr. Mewburn rose from behind his large mahogany desk to shake Robert's hand, the young doctor saw that Mewburn was a small man, about five foot six inches, to Robert's near six feet, but the senior doctor exuded confidence and authority. He indicated that Robert should sit down in a chair in front of the desk and then questioned him thoroughly regarding his medical training and surgical experience. He followed this up with a few blunt and probing questions about Robert's age and his life before Queen's.

"You have excellent recommendations from Queen's and the other universities I contacted, and your initiative at Bow Island impresses me," he stated, "but your age is a puzzle. You are a good ten years older than most of the doctors who apply for work in Alberta. Why is that?"

Robert quickly reviewed his life with the Hudson's Bay Company and his unusually late application to Queen's University.

"Hmmmph! You have led an interesting life, young man. Your experience with the Hudson's Bay Company and your proven ability to manage men will serve you well."

Stating that he was satisfied with the answers Robert gave him, he showed no further interest in the younger doctor's personal life, beyond remarking that Robert would need to find a place to stay that was close to the hospital as he would be on call all hours of the day and night.

Mewburn rose again, shook Robert's hand, and dismissed him. "You'll begin tomorrow morning. Be here at six o'clock. We'll do surgical rounds together, and then I expect you to go to the medical practice office where you will meet my other assistant, who is also the anaesthesiologist for the hospital. You will find him a most amiable and worthy young man. Good day."

And with that, the interview was over. Robert left Mewburn's office and stood in the brightly lit white painted hall outside the senior doctor's office for a few moments while he considered the personality of the man he had just met.

"Hmmm," Robert thought. "Mewburn likes to be in charge and certainly has a very abrupt manner, but...he's supposed to be a wonderful and daring surgeon. He may be brusque, but I'm here to learn, so I can put up with his manner as long as he's as good as described. We'll see."

Before Robert left the hospital, he had a long look around and was excited by what he saw. This was a fine place, clean and bright and new, with excellent facilities. However, right now he needed to find temporary lodgings close to the hospital so that he and his family could settle into their new life in Lethbridge.

On his way back to his hotel, he stopped at the telegraph office to send a telegram to Jennie letting her know that his interview had been successful. It said simply, *"Interview successful. Come to Lethbridge. Will find house soon."*

Jennie's reply was equally succinct and its brevity surprised Robert. *"Congratulations. Will come when house found."*

Although she was driven almost to distraction by the fierce cold and winter winds and the dust of life in Bow Island, Jennie had no desire to uproot the children and move again so soon.

They had only been in Bow Island for six months, but in their short time there, the family had made good friends and had enjoyed the winter activities, and Jennie had become a member of her church women's groups. She was busy with Robert's bookkeeping and the friendship with Emma and Mercilla, which had begun on the long train trip and had been cemented in the hard work of establishing the hospital and Robert's practice. It was an important part of her life.

The thought of moving again to another boarding house in an unknown city where she knew no one had little appeal. Unlike her gregarious husband, Jennie was reserved, and meeting new people was always an ordeal. She also understood very well that she would hardly see Robert in Lethbridge as he would be working all hours of the day and night while he established himself in that new city.

When Robert's telegram arrived on the day of his successful interview, all these thoughts went through her head as she wrote her daring reply. Robert frowned when he read it, though it was not unexpected. He knew that Jennie was just now beginning to regain her strength after Douglas's birth, so she would be reluctant to move after only six months in one place, but he believed his wife and family should follow him wherever his employment took him.

He was also well aware that he would be extremely busy. Having little time and less desire to look for a suitable house right now, he simply arranged for money to be sent to Jennie to meet her household needs in Bow Island for the time being.

"I'll take the train and go back to Bow Island soon to sort this out," he thought and then immediately forgot his mild concern as he began to consider his first day at the hospital.

When he arrived the next morning, Robert discovered that the operating room on the second floor of Galt Hospital was small but very clean and bright. Dr. Mewburn was one of the first doctors in the West to insist upon the importance of aseptic surgery, which pleased Robert very much, as this had been emphasized in his medical training at Queen's and reinforced through the work of Joseph Lister. The surgery had whitewashed walls, exceptionally large windows that allowed for ample daylight, a simple table on which to operate, and several standing lamps to provide light at night. It also had the look of being scrubbed frequently with carbolic soap.

In pride of place in a small room next to the surgery stood an X-ray machine, which, though it had to be hand-cranked for power, would make the bone setting jobs much easier. As Robert had foreseen, there was also a supply of young, well-trained, and very hardworking nurses who put in their twelve-hour shifts and then went back to the residence next door to write reports and fall exhausted into bed.

As in all coal towns of the time, mining accidents were frequent, and broken limbs and terrible injuries were regular occurrences. These accidents made up the bulk of the surgical work, and, attended by these skillful nurses, Robert was in the operating room almost every day. Robert enjoyed the hard work and also the experience he was gaining. He looked forward to learning even more after Mewburn returned.

The days were long. Upon completion of the morning surgeries, the doctors spent time on the necessary paperwork and sometimes even managed a short break for luncheon. This was followed by afternoon office hours, where they tended to patients until late in the day. After a short break for supper at home, they returned for evening office hours.

Immersed in his work, Robert had little time to dwell on his absent family.

***

Most days, the work followed the prescribed routine and the days and weeks, full of interesting surgeries and new patients with ordinary ills, passed quickly. Robert liked the town, with its neat white framed houses, the bustle of downtown, the hardworking farm folk and miners, and the businessmen he met in the course of his daily rounds. There was little time for thoughts of Jennie and the boys until just before sleep when Robert longed for his family to be with him.

For a time, he had been content to remain in the boarding house where he lived and was well looked after by his landlady, who admired the handsome young doctor, but he was surprised by how much he missed his wife and children. Although he had lived in relative isolation as a Bay Man until he was nearly thirty, his life had changed, and he wanted the comforts of family. It was time for Jennie and the boys to come to Lethbridge.

Robert engaged the services of a merchant who found small but furnished rooms near the hospital so that the doctor's family could join him. They were situated on a pleasant street, and Robert knew that they would suit their needs until he was quite sure he wanted to remain in Lethbridge. He was determined to bring his wife and children to join him in Lethbridge within the fortnight and a telegram was sent to Bow Island saying all was in readiness.

Jennie, knowing the move was imminent, packed up their few household goods and said her regretful goodbyes with many promises to come back for a visit and invitations for her friends to visit them in Lethbridge. Robert travelled to Bow Island to accompany his family on their journey, and as the train carried them on the short trip to Lethbridge, he told Jennie about their cozy new rooms.

The family moved into their new accommodations near the Galt Hospital. The previous tenant had been a businessman who had moved with his family to the West Coast. His wife had been a gardener, and the place was surrounded by a pretty yard. Robert had seen that the rooms were clean and freshly painted. There were two bedrooms and a tiny kitchen.

As always, Jennie kept Robert's medical accounts as well as those of the household. She soon became involved in the local Methodist Church and slowly made new friends in the women's groups.

Robert, as she had correctly surmised would be the case, was extremely busy both at the hospital and in the medical office. He returned home late each evening, often too tired to do more than eat his dinner and go to bed.

On the rare days when he had a few hours away from the hospital or the office, he often chose to saddle a horse and ride out into the countryside. There were few signs of habitation along the roads and paths he chose, with farmhouses far distant from one another. The prairie landscape was completely unlike the huge dark forests of his youth, but the windswept grasses and gently sloping hills had their own beauty. Watching the clouds racing across the bright blue of the prairie skies, Robert smiled, enjoying the vast open spaces and contemplating his future in this new land. For now, the family was settled, Robert was earning a good salary at the Galt Hospital and in the medical practice office, and they were able to put some savings aside.

Chapter 7
Insanity at the Hotel and a Hanging

Evening office hours usually lasted until about ten o'clock. This accommodated those people, mostly men, who were unable to leave their farms or the mines throughout the day. The miners were never given leave to go to the doctor's during the day, and it was a rare man who would dare to take time off without permission from the boss, because it would mean loss of his employment.

One evening Dr. Mewburn, who had returned to the practice, asked Robert if he could take a call that had just come in for him as he himself was unable to leave the patient he was tending to at the time.

The man asking for a doctor was registered in a room at the Lethbridge Hotel, and when Robert arrived and tied his horse to the rail, the waiting desk clerk urgently sent him up the staircase to the room. Robert knocked on the closed door saying, "My name is Doctor Ross. I believe you have a patient here who requires medical care?"

He was answered by a trembling voice from within, "Is it the doctor? Come in, come in quickly."

The room Robert entered was very small, and the door opened inward. On his left was a single bed jammed up against the wall with a man lying on it, his face to the wall. On the opposite side of the narrow room there was a washstand on which stood a basin for water and a jug. The remaining space was a path leading to the window.

At the far end of the room, two men, dressed like farmhands, sat stiffly in small chairs that had been shoved against the wall below the window. It was one of these men who had asked Dr. Ross to come into the room, and once he was inside, both men frantically began telling him about their friend.

"He has been having head trouble for days, complaining of pain and strange noises. We thought we had better bring him into town to see Doctor Mewburn."

Robert apologized for Dr. Mewburn's absence, explaining that the senior doctor had not been able to come but had sent him instead. The two men were quite agitated but agreed that Dr. Ross would do as a substitute.

Moving into the small room until he was standing quite close to the seated men, Robert turned and calmly addressed the patient on the bed, who had not moved and was lying silently, facing the wall. "How long have you been ill?"

Without answering him, the man abruptly turned over and leapt up to stand between Robert and the door.

"Didn't I tell you?" he yelled at his two friends, "If you brought a doctor here, I would kill him. I am the Lord God Almighty, and you have disobeyed me."

As he shouted, his friends, expecting to see a killing, took refuge by diving under the bed. The infuriated man grabbed the water pitcher and raising it aloft, brought it down swiftly towards the startled doctor's head.

Robert, who had been a member of the boxing club at Queen's, was still quick on his feet. He ducked his head to one side, allowing the jug to crash in pieces against the wall. He slipped past the man and reached for the door knob, twisting it desperately, but nothing happened. The door was stuck. Hard as he pulled, Robert could not get it to open.

The crazed man still gripped the broken handle of the jug in his hand and struck again at Robert's head. As the doctor ducked sideways to avoid this second attempt on his life, he threw himself against the door to avoid the slashing handle. But he was unable to avoid the blow completely, and the sharp edge struck him between the shoulders, slicing a long gash in his coat. At the same moment, Robert kicked backwards, and his foot caught the wild man in the abdomen, sending him crashing into the chairs so recently abandoned by his friends.

Robert slammed his weight into the door once more, and to his relief, it finally came unstuck. He flung himself out of the room and into the safety of the hallway. Turning, he quickly pulled the door tightly shut behind him.

The maniacal man, yelling obscenities, bounced back from the end of the narrow space in the room and pounded on the door. His two friends cowered under the bed while a frightening tug of war ensued with Robert straining to hold the door shut on the hall side and the enraged patient yanking on it from within the room.

Another hotel guest, disturbed by the commotion, rushed down the hall shouting, "What's going on? What's all the noise about?"

"There is a crazy man in this room." Robert gasped at her, holding the door tightly shut. "I'm a doctor. Call the police. Hurry! I can't hold this door shut much longer."

Shocked to hear this, the frightened woman immediately ran down the stairs to the front desk, and in a matter of minutes, though it seemed much longer, two mounted police officers came bounding up the stairs.

Robert, still braced to hold the door shut, quickly told them the story.

"Thank you, Doctor Ross. We'll deal with this. You may let go of the door knob now, sir."

Robert did so, gladly, and the madman inside, who was still pulling on the doorknob, crashed backwards into the room. The mounted police were on him before he could get up, but such was his strength that it required the efforts of both officers to restrain and handcuff him. Seeing that all was now safe, his two friends emerged from under the bed and accompanied him as he was led away by the police.

Robert, still a bit shaken from this encounter, also took his leave and rode back through the quiet dark streets to the office where he showed Dr. Mewburn his coat and told him the story.

"I am thankful it was not me who went to see him," Dr. Mewburn commented when Robert finished his tale, "he could have killed me. I'm glad you are all right, Doctor Ross. We'd better close up now. No doubt you will have to talk to the police about this tomorrow. I wonder why the man's friends didn't call the police to begin with if he was so obviously mad."

Robert wondered the same thing, knowing that although he was unhurt, he would need his coat mended, and this day's adventures would leave him somewhat sore on the morrow.

***

Several busy weeks passed, and Robert was mulling over his newest case as his horse and buggy carried him to the medical office through the cool air of the early morning. He felt uneasy about the patient he had seen the night before and berated himself for not going to the police at the time, though he doubted that anything would have been done at two o'clock in the morning. Still, he had stopped at the police station on his way to work this morning and dropped off the bottle, telling them the story and his suspicions. The officer had asked him if the man was going to press charges and Robert had replied, "I certainly hope so. The fellow was too ill to talk last night, but I will encourage him to do so when I check on him later today."

Robert also knew that he was short of sleep and realized that was contributing to his unease, but he rarely second-guessed himself about his decisions. Suddenly, he flipped the reins and turned his horse back in the direction of the miner's shack, thinking, "If nothing else, it will ease my mind to see that the fellow is still alive. I really think his wife tried to poison him, but how the devil can I prove it?"

The previous night, Robert had been called out at about midnight to go to the home of a coal miner named Romanchuk. The miner, who worked at Number Three Mine, had returned from the eleven o'clock shift and had then become violently ill. His next-door neighbours, two young men, had offered to stay with him while his wife went to call the doctor from the telephone office.

Upon Robert's arrival at the miner's home on the north side of the Oldman River, he had been met by one of the friends. This man led Robert to the miner's bedside in the dark, one-room shack. It was instantly obvious from the stench that Romanchuk had been vomiting frequently. Robert called for more light, and when it was supplied by lanterns, he could see that the miner's face was pallid, even under the coal dust that was ground into his skin.

The fellow groaned, "I can't bear this pain in my gut, Doc, make it stop." And with that, he again vomited violently.

As he bent over to examine the patient, Robert snapped at the others, "Get some rags and water and clean this mess up. While you're at it, find a cleaner blanket to cover the poor fellow after I examine him. And bring me a pail of clean warm water as well."

He turned back to the miner. "What have you been drinking, man?"

"My wife said that I had been looking very tired and gave me a drink from my whiskey bottle." He weakly waved his hand towards the shelf, where Robert could see a grimy bottle. "I was sick as soon as I drank it. She said the whiskey would do me good, but oh, oh...." He retched once more with great painful heaves.

Robert immediately seized the whiskey bottle which smelled very strongly of sulphur and secured it in his medical bag, asking the miner, "Where is your wife?"

"Not back from the telephone office. She went to call you. Please, please, help."

"I'm sure you've been poisoned. I need to talk to your wife, but right now I will try to flush the poison out of your system." Robert inserted a tube down the miner's throat and down into the stomach and placed a funnel on the end in his hand. He then poured some warm water from the bucket into the funnel, and watched it disappear down into the man's gut. He knew this would flush out everything the miner had consumed. The water came back up in a few seconds and, stomach now empty, the convulsive vomiting finally stopped. Robert then gave the man a mild sedative.

"Thanks, Doc, I already feel much better," said the man. Then, exhausted by the violence of his illness, he dozed off.

By now, at least an hour had passed, and still the man's wife had not returned. Robert left the miner with his friends and gave instructions to come and get him if there was any change for the worse. He also took the whiskey bottle with him as he left, saying to the friends, "I will turn this over to the police who will no doubt want to make an investigation."

Robert was relieved the next morning when he arrived at the shack and found his patient not only still alive but resting fairly comfortably. His wife was there. Robert thought her a hard-faced, mean looking woman as she sat in the corner of the room, weeping copiously.

"Have you reported this to the police?" The miner was very anxious.

"Yes, I took them the bottle this morning. I believe you should also press charges against your wife. She tried to kill you, man."

"Please," the miner begged. "Please do not say that. The police will arrest my wife, and then what will my poor children do? She has promised me that it will not happen again. I'm not going to accuse her, and I beg you not to go on with this. I'm begging you, Doc."

Robert glanced at the woman, who immediately increased the volume of her wailing. He shook his head in disgust. Her flow of crocodile tears could soften neither her vicious expression nor his suspicious heart.

"I am sure this woman tried to poison you last night, and you have no guarantee that she will not try to do it again. I certainly don't trust her and believe that you should press charges both for your protection and the protection of your children."

The woman acted as though she could not speak English, but Robert suspected that she understood every word he spoke. Again, she increased her wailing, taking an occasional sideways glance at the doctor to observe the effect.

The miner pleaded with Robert, "Doc, I cannot manage without her. I cannot work and also look after my children. They will starve. It was a mistake, and it won't happen again. For my children's sake, if the police come, I will say it never happened."

Robert, who knew that it was very likely true that the children would starve without their mother, realized that he could not force the man to say anything against his wife, so he grudgingly agreed. "But know this," he spoke bluntly to the woman, "I will keep an eye on this whole situation."

Three weeks passed, and Robert continued to fret about the case. He learned that the police had visited the miner's home but had been sent away by the miner who denied anything had happened. Robert dropped in unannounced to see the man on several occasions and checked up on him through other miners whom he met, and all seemed to be well. Nevertheless, he was still worried, believing that somehow, the wife would try again.

Sure enough, about a month after the incident, he received a midnight phone call from the power house at Number Three Mine. Right away, Robert thought of the miner and the earlier poisoning attempt.

"Doctor Ross," the foreman begged, "you have to come as fast as you can. A miner has been shot. He was on his way home after the eleven o'clock shift. He crawled back here through the dark to the power house. He's in a bad way, Doc."

"I'll be there as fast as my horse can carry me." And with that, Robert hung up the phone, rushed out to the stable behind the house, readied his horse, and set off for the mine. He urged his mount to its best speed along the now familiar trails. As soon as he arrived, he knew his worst fears had been realized when he recognized the miner lying on some planks on the floor.

The injured miner, seeing that the doctor had arrived, groaned, "Oh, Doctor Ross, I should have listened to you when you told me to report my wife to the police. They got me this time."

"Hush man, you can tell me all about it in a minute. For now, I can give you something for the pain and have a look at your wounds."

As Robert prepared an ampoule of morphia, he quietly instructed the foreman who had originally called him to get an ambulance and get it quickly.

The miner, writhing in pain, gasped out his story. "When I was walking home through the darkest part of the coulee, I met another miner...his name's Dominic I think. He asked if I was Romanchuk. When I said I was, he got real close and shot me in the stomach. The shot knocked me down, but I was able to crawl back here." In agony by now, he moaned, "She got me, Doc, she got me!"

The morphia began to take effect, and the miner could no longer speak coherently but now lay more comfortably on the planks. It was obvious to Robert that there was little he could do for him there in the power house, and that the man was so badly wounded and had lost so much blood that he might not live long enough to get him to the hospital.

The horse-drawn ambulance arrived shortly thereafter, and as the miner was carefully loaded into the wagon, Robert telephoned the police and told them what had happened. "Romanchuk is on his way to the hospital, but he is probably not going to live long, so you had better get his statement quickly."

"Thank you, Doctor Ross, we're on our way to the hospital now to do just that. Then we will go to inform his wife and look for the man who shot him."

After obtaining Romanchuk's statement, the police began the hunt for Dominic. They found him comfortably ensconced in Romanchuk's bed with the latter's wife. They also found a revolver in Dominic's clothing, which the police were sure Dominique had used to shoot Romanchuk.

Meanwhile, Robert had ridden back to town, again urging his horse along the dark trail as fast as he could safely travel. He went directly to Dr. Mewburn's home and reported the matter to him. The senior surgeon immediately got up and headed to the hospital where they met for the surgery. By now, it was two o'clock in the morning, but Mewburn ordered the operating room prepared for the emergency surgery. Robert would assist, and Dr. Ireland, another assistant, would administer the anaesthetic. When all was ready, Dr. Mewburn walked into the room.

Romanchuk, who had regained consciousness by this time, recognized the surgeon and pleaded, "Oh, Doctor Mewburn, you have to save my life for the sake of my poor children."

Ether anaesthetic was used to put the miner to sleep for the duration of the surgery. However, practically nothing could be done for the patient. The bullet had torn ghastly holes through the intestines. That dreadful injury, combined with the accompanying blood loss meant that the prognosis was grim, even under the skilled hands of Dr. Mewburn. The anaesthesiologist was very concerned about the patient's thready heartbeat; however, there was no choice but to go ahead. It took considerable time to get the intestines sewn up and their contents cleaned from the abdominal cavity. Finally, Robert closed the incision, and the patient was sent back to the ward under the watchful eyes of the charge nurse. Despite receiving such excellent care, the miner died a few hours after the operation.

Robert left the hospital as dawn was breaking over the quiet city, angry that the situation had come to such a tragic conclusion.

How he wished that Romanchuk had come to his senses and pressed charges for the whiskey incident. That may have saved him from a painful death.

"And what now for those children?" Robert muttered to himself as his horse patiently clip-clopped him home through the silent streets.

The days passed, and news came that neighbours had taken in the children as Romanchuk's wife showed no interest in their welfare. She had found another man, abandoned her family, and moved on, leaving no clue as to her current whereabouts.

When it was time for Dominic to stand trial for murder, Dr. Mewburn and Robert were both called to give evidence. The deceased's dying statement to the police was read to the jury, and it seemed very evident that Dominic would be found guilty.

Robert then gave his evidence, which included his suspicions that Romanchuk's wife had attempted to poison her husband.

"And when did this alleged attempted poisoning take place, Doctor Ross?" the judge inquired.

"About three weeks before the shooting. I have the exact date in my notes if you require it, Your Honour. I handed over the tainted whiskey bottle to the police the following morning."

"And why did you decide not to pursue the matter further?"

"Romanchuk refused to press charges, saying he would deny it ever happened. He also denied it to the police when they went to his shack. He pleaded with me not to pursue the matter for the sake of his youngsters. Also, his friends assured me that they would keep a close eye on Romanchuk's wife."

"Thank you, Doctor Ross. That will be all."

Dr. Mewburn was then called to the stand.

The defence counsel asked Dr. Mewburn if Romanchuk had said anything to the doctor before the operation began.

"Yes," he replied. "As soon as I walked into the operating room, Romanchuk begged me to save his life for the sake of his children."

As soon as the doctor made this statement, the presiding judge stopped the trial, dismissed the jury, and adjourned the Court, explaining, "The jury has heard the deceased's dying statement as part of the Court's evidence against Dominic, and that evidence has been invalidated by what Dr. Mewburn has testified, under oath, that Romanchuk said to him. It shows that Romanchuk believed that he would not die and thought that Dr. Mewburn's operation would save his life; therefore, it was not a dying statement."

Disappointed with this unwelcome turn of events, the two doctors left the courtroom.

Dr. Mewburn had a motorcar, and the men, both furious about the mistrial, got into the car to drive back to the office.

Robert sardonically commented, "Well, Doctor, it looks as though your comment about Romanchuk's last words may have saved another man's life."

Dr. Mewburn, who was known for his shortness of temper and intolerance of even implied criticism, was very heated, and he used strong language in his reply to Robert.

"I didn't want to save that bastard's life, Doctor Ross, so don't suggest that I did!"

To no one's surprise, a new trial with a new jury was held roughly four weeks later. It had been determined that the miner's statement imploring Mewburn to save his life for the sake of his poor children, which had been attributed to Romanchuk at the first trial, was not relevant to the guilt or innocence of Dominic so it didn't matter whether or not it was a dying declaration. Thus, a new trial was ordered.

Dr. Mewburn and Robert were summoned again and gave their evidence. It was a very busy day at their medical office, so the two doctors left immediately after they had testified and thus did not hear the other witnesses.

"We've spent enough time on this, Doctor Ross. We have other important work to do. We can only hope they get it right this time." With that, Dr. Mewburn got in his car to drive back to the office.

Robert had several house calls to make so had arrived at the courthouse by horse and buggy. When he returned to the office later in the afternoon, he was relieved to hear that Dominic had been found guilty and sentenced to be hanged, so although delayed, justice would be done.

Dr. Mewburn's only comment was a resounding, "Excellent."

Robert, though pleased with the verdict and the sentence, was not entirely happy and remarked grimly, "What about the wife? Does she get off scot-free? She probably planned the whole thing."

Later that summer, Robert's thoughts were echoed. He learned that when the hangman's noose had been placed around Dominic's neck, and he had been asked if he had anything to say, the condemned man had replied, "Yes. If the woman who got me to shoot her husband was standing beside me with a noose around her neck, too, I would die satisfied."

Chapter 8
Not a Country Gentleman

Dr. Mewburn soon became very confident in the new doctor's abilities and decided to put Robert in charge of his maternity cases. The senior doctor had a large and growing surgical practice, and once he was convinced of Robert's capabilities, gradually switched his mothers-to-be over to Dr. Ross. This worked well for both of them; Mewburn could concentrate on surgery and was freed from night calls for maternity cases, and Robert, who didn't mind the night calls, was pleased with the rapid increase in his own practice.

Lethbridge was growing rapidly, new families meant new babies. Robert was to bring many babies into the world in the time he was in Lethbridge, and obstetrics was an aspect of his medical practice that he always enjoyed.

Maternity cases were not normally admitted to either of the two hospitals in Lethbridge. Instead, as was the custom of the day, all confinements took place in the patient's own home where the mother was attended by a midwife or a graduate nurse and a doctor.

One evening shortly after their decision to have Robert take on Mewburn's obstetrical cases, both doctors were busy working in the medical practice office. At about nine o'clock, the senior doctor asked Robert to go to the home of Mrs. Eliza Miller, one of the first maternity cases they had reviewed. The mother-to-be had called earlier to say that her labour pains had begun, so Mewburn suggested that

Robert go to the house to get acquainted with her and meet the nurse who was already there waiting for the birth. Robert went in his buggy rather than on horseback so that he would have a conveyance for the mother should it become necessary to take her to the hospital, though Mewburn assured him that he did not anticipate any complications.

The house was a well-kept dwelling on a treed lot. It was a two-story building with bedrooms above a living room and kitchen. Robert was greeted at the door by a nervous little housemaid and shown into the living room to his right where he was met by a well-dressed, elderly lady who had been sitting quietly knitting.

"My name is Doctor Ross, and I am here to see Mrs. Miller, who is expecting her baby. Could you tell me where she is?"

"Of course, Doctor Ross, just go up the stairs you saw as you entered the house, and you will find her in the first room on the right."

Robert followed her directions to find the young woman resting quite comfortably under the care of the nurse. The bedroom was cheerful and brightly lit, and all necessary arrangements for the birth had been made, so Robert introduced himself, examined the mother-to-be and chatted with her for a few moments.

"Doctor Mewburn told me that you would be coming," the young woman said. "I'm pleased to see you, though Nurse has been very good. My husband is out of town and not expected back for a few days, and this is my first baby." She smiled, but Robert could see that she was a little apprehensive.

"You are in excellent health, Mrs. Miller, and Doctor Mewburn assured me that all was well. And you have a very fine nurse here with you. Have you had any more labour pains?"

"None in the last hour, Doctor, but I hope the nurse will stay."

"Yes, of course she will, and as soon as the contractions begin again, she will call me, and I will return immediately."

"Thank you for coming to meet me. I think I will sleep a little now."

Robert went home and, feeling sure that he would be called soon, had a little sleep himself. About two o'clock in the morning, the nurse phoned to say that the pains had begun again, so Robert harnessed his horse to the carriage and returned to the Miller house. The pains were severe but came and went, until about four o'clock when it became necessary to use forceps to turn the baby. Within minutes, the child was born, a fine, healthy baby boy.

When all had been done for the comfort of mother and baby and they were both asleep, the elderly lady who had directed him upstairs earlier that evening invited the nurse and Dr. Ross to have coffee and cake with her as a little celebration. The invitation was gladly accepted, and they all sat in the living room and enjoyed their early breakfast.

"I am Eliza's aunt, Mrs. Enid Miller. I arrived just two days ago to be with her on this auspicious occasion. Just in time, too." She smiled at Robert. "When you came in this evening, I knew you were a doctor. You look like a doctor, but when I met Doctor Mewburn, I didn't think he was a doctor. He doesn't look like a doctor, he looks like a country gentleman."

They all laughed at this description, and Robert thanked the nurse before he left. "You are an excellent midwife," he chuckled. "And you look like a nurse."

At the office next day, Dr. Mewburn spoke to Robert. "I would like you to continue with the case. I phoned the Millers, and they were very happy with your service." Robert, pleased, agreed to make the usual follow-up calls.

That afternoon when he arrived at the house, Aunt Enid was sitting with her niece and the baby while the nurse rested. After checking that all was well with Eliza and her baby, conversation turned to where the senior Mrs. Miller lived.

"Ontario," she replied. "We have just been sitting here comparing Ontario to Alberta."

"Where in Ontario? What town?"

When she named the town, Robert laughed. "Do you know a doctor there named Beggs? He is a fellow graduate from Queen's University. I visited him in that very town just a few years ago."

"For goodness' sake, Doctor Beggs is our family doctor," Aunt Enid exclaimed.

Thinking of her earlier remark, Robert asked, "Would you say that Doctor Beggs dresses like a gentleman?"

"Oh, Doctor Ross, you misunderstood me last night. What I really meant was that Doctor Mewburn looked and dressed like an English gentleman...like a country squire."

They all chuckled, and when Robert returned to the office, he related the story to Dr. Mewburn, who was pleased and much amused to be compared to a country squire.

"It would be surprising with your wild Canadian background, Doctor Ross, if you looked like an English country squire, but you will do very well here in Alberta."

Jennie's pithy comment when Robert told her the story that evening was very much to the point. She laughed as she remarked, "Imagine what she would have said if she had seen you in your Hudson's Bay trader garb, Robert. A long, long, way from an English country squire."

***

On fine Sunday afternoons after church, the family often enjoyed a buggy ride through the streets and out into the countryside. Douglas, now a toddler, sat proudly beside his father on the driver's seat of the buggy, his little legs sticking straight out, his black curls shining in the sun. Gordon, very grown-up at six, shared the seat behind his father and brother, sitting beside his mother with her parasol providing shade. He knew he would sit in the front seat on the way home.

"I find it hard to believe how much this city has grown even in the short time we have lived here, Robert." Jennie spoke as she admired the houses and gardens. "Each week, it appears there are more houses and businesses springing up."

"Yes, one of the new doctors at the hospital said that the population has doubled and doubled again in the last five years. Lethbridge now has about eight thousand people and more are coming all the time. I have some concerns about how well the farms will do if we have a dry year. There just won't be enough water."

Jennie replied, "Everything I have read in the *Edmonton Bulletin* praises this land as ideal for settlers and says there will always be plenty of water for growing wheat. There is certainly enough water this year. Even in August, the streams are still flowing down to the river."

Robert, thinking about the wind and dust they had experienced in Bow Island, was not convinced, but it was too fine a day to discuss his growing concerns about drought.

Gordon spotted some children playing in a small park and slid to the side of the buggy, looking with longing at their game.

Jennie patted the seat beside her. "Sit quietly, Gordon, we'll soon be out in the country, and we'll find a place to have a picnic and a walk."

Gordon, knowing how sedate the walk would be, sighed but obeyed his mother as his father commented on the passing country-side. "Have you noticed, my dear, how much longer it takes us now to get out of the city and find some open space? I know you enjoy your walks along the shady streets, but I sometimes feel quite hemmed in by all this building."

Jennie looked intently at her husband for a long moment before answering. "Yes, I have noticed that as well, but surely growth cannot continue at this pace. And the city has set aside space for new parks, so there is always open green space nearby."

Robert put an arm around Douglas who had begun to fidget. The younger boy usually had a nap about this time, it was hot, and enforced sitting made him restless. "Lean against me, Douglas, and rest a little," his father instructed, but the toddler was too excited by the buggy ride to rest and continued to wriggle.

They travelled up a long sloping incline, and now were into open country overlooking the city. A fresh breeze blew away the mosquitoes, bringing some relief from the heat while a grove of trees by the road-side promised a shady spot for the boys to run off some of their energy.

"Here's a perfect spot for our picnic," Robert said, as he reined the horse to a halt and jumped out of the buggy. Gordon and Douglas promptly scrambled after him, and he helped Jennie out of the buggy and spread a blanket for her. "I'll look after the horse while you lay out our lunch," he said. Douglas began to scamper towards the nearby field, but Robert captured him with one arm and, laughing, said, "Boys, stay with your mother."

Their horse contentedly cropped grass beneath a tree a little distance away while they enjoyed a lunch Jennie had prepared for them earlier that day.

After their picnic, the boys played nearby while their parents talked quietly. Jennie, who always kept up with the newspapers, remarked, "We have a new king. George the Fifth is now our Monarch. England seems so far away."

Robert, half dozing with his back against the tree, murmured, "Yes, it is very far away. Would you like to go there someday? I wonder if the royal family have any idea how vast their Canadian colony is?"

"Will they ever visit Canada, do you think?" Jennie asked, then looked at the boys, "Oh, dear, Douglas, come here. Don't sit in that patch of dirt. Play on the grass like your brother, or come into the shade on the blanket with your father and me." The little boy reluctantly abandoned his investigation of an ant hill to join Gordon's game of pick-up sticks.

"Mother, he wrecks everything; he is too little to play," complained his older brother.

"That's enough, Gordon. Douglas, let your brother show you how to play." Robert's soft voice was sufficient to settle the boys to their game.

Robert smiled as he watched his sons, and he and his wife continued their lazy conversation. "We will certainly go to see them if any of the royal family come to Canada, wherever they visit." For a little longer, they enjoyed the silence of the warm afternoon, broken only by the hum of cicadas and the murmur of the two little boys.

"Now, I'm afraid we must go home," Robert spoke reluctantly. "We must have our tea before the boys' bedtime."

Robert left Jennie to pack up their picnic while he readied the horse and buggy. After hoisting basket, blanket, and boys into the buggy, making sure Gordon sat in the front with him, Robert helped Jennie into her seat.

"It has been a fine restful afternoon," he said as they headed back into town. "Next week, I am going to Fort Macleod for a surgical case. I will be away for several days, but I am really looking forward to the journey to the West. The foothills area intrigues me."

Chapter 9
From Prairies to Mountains

Travelling to Fort Macleod, Robert's thoughts turned again to setting up a medical practice of his own. He knew that his surgical skills were equal to any challenge, but he also knew he was one of many medical men in Lethbridge and did not feel that he was getting enough surgical cases. Busy as he was, he chafed at being relegated to a surgical assistant's position in the Galt Hospital.

Lethbridge expanded, and houses and industries spread out into the countryside. As the open landscape he loved so much disappeared, Robert began to quietly investigate other possibilities. Whenever he was called to a town or village outside of Lethbridge to see a patient or consult on a surgical matter, he always extended his time there to look around the town and consider the likelihood of setting up his own practice.

He discussed his journey to Fort Macleod and his thoughts of relocation with his wife as they took their usual walk, enjoying the warmth of the late summer evening.

Jennie listened as Robert confidently set out his ideas for a new medical practice to the West. "There are wide open fields and groves of green trees in the foothills, and, oh, Jennie, you simply must see the mountains rising to the West. The sense of freedom there is so appealing."

Robert abruptly stopped walking and turned to look directly at his wife, who had listened without speaking as he continued to describe his plans.

"The location would have to be far enough from Calgary or Lethbridge that the patients would not call upon the doctors who have already established practices in those centres, Jennie. And yet it must be large enough to ensure a steady income for us."

"Let us continue our walk, Robert. We are blocking the path."

"Oh, yes, of course. What do you think?"

Jennie, who was familiar with the signs of Robert's restlessness, replied a bit wearily, "Robert, we have only been here for six months. The boys are just settling in and making friends. I don't think another move so soon would be good for them."

"Nonsense, they are too young to know the difference. They are just happy to be with us. And I'm not talking about immediately. My practice is going well, but I'm going to continue to look elsewhere." Her husband's voice was firm and his expression resolute.

"And wouldn't there have to be a hospital?" Jennie knew that Robert's pride in his surgical skills required access to a hospital, and she counted on this to limit his choices and keep them in Lethbridge with the Galt Hospital's excellent facilities as the major attraction. "Isn't the Galt planning to open a new sixty-five-bed wing soon? I had heard that Prime Minister Laurier is to be here to officially open it."

Robert was quiet for a moment, carefully considering her words, then nodded his agreement. "As I said, not immediately, but I will soon need the freedom of a new place."

Jennie sighed, both relieved at the postponement and frustrated that the move would happen at all. They had arrived home from their walk by now, and she gazed at the shrubs and flowers surrounding their building where they rented furnished rooms. She quite liked Lethbridge with its tree-lined streets, and they lived near a small park where she walked with the children on paths overlooking the Oldman River.

The Methodist church was nearby, and she attended regularly as did Robert when he was not on a case. Gordon was enrolled there in the Sunday school class. He was a clever little boy and, thanks to his mother's tutoring, was already able to read the Bible stories written for children. Although he was anxious when away from his mother, he enjoyed the games and activities with the other children. Douglas, ever active, played happily with other children his age.

Robert and Jennie sat on the shady veranda and enjoyed their tea and biscuits.

"I've enrolled Gordon in a good school this fall, Robert. This is not the time to move him again." Her husband valued education, but this argument fell on deaf ears.

"There will be schools wherever we go. Gordon is bright. He will be fine. And Douglas is happy wherever he is as long as he can play with others."

Robert was a gentle man but absolutely implacable. If he found a suitable location, they would go despite Jennie's concerns.

"Now, my dear, tell me about the church group you have joined. And what are your plans for the rest of this week?" The subject was closed.

One of the places Robert had been to as a consulting surgeon was Pincher Creek, just to the eastern side of the Crowsnest Pass through the Rockies. He had loved the train trip from Lethbridge, about a three-hour journey through acres of golden grain and pastures where cattle ranged contently. He was thrilled at the sight of cowboys driving a herd across the vast open plain. The Pincher Creek area interested him, but although there was a small surgical clinic there, and plans for a new hospital, he wanted a larger town. And the western mountains beckoned, reminding him of the trees and wilderness of his childhood in Labrador and Northern Ontario.

While he had waited that day in Pincher Creek for the return train to Lethbridge, he had sat for a long time in the dusty shade on the bench in front of the railway station gazing to the West and dreaming of going up into the mountains. "Soon," he had smiled to himself, "soon it will be time."

In the week that followed, he talked to his colleagues in the Galt Hospital about other communities to the west that might need doctors. Several mentions were made of a place called Coleman, in the Crowsnest Pass, about an hour by train west of Pincher Creek. Encouraged by what he heard, he quietly made arrangements to visit this community and informed Jennie of his plans as the weekend approached.

Accordingly, on that Sunday after church, he and Jennie left the boys in the care of one of the student nurses and boarded the train for the little town in the mountains. "We will stay overnight," Robert had told the nurse, "and will return on the afternoon train tomorrow. There is a fine establishment there called the Grand Union Hotel, near the railway station. I've booked a room for myself and Mrs. Ross."

Despite her misgivings about leaving Lethbridge, Jennie felt a tingle of excitement as the train climbed through the foothills and neared the mountains. The great blue wall of rock seemed impenetrable, looming ahead of them as the train pushed westward.

As they entered the Pass, the afternoon sun threw long shadows, and the huge trees rose dark on either side of the train. Robert's excitement was clearly evident, and he smiled as they caught glimpses of the track winding its way through the mountains ahead.

"This is a coal mining area. The rail line was built to carry coal to the East and grain to the Pacific Ocean. Look there, to our west on the slope. Do you see that opening to a mine?"

Jennie peered out the window, searching for and finding the dark opening in the steep and rocky slope.

"So it will be like Lethbridge, dependent on coal?"

"Much smaller, of course, but yes. The coal mines are the major employer."

"And a hospital for your surgery?"

Robert smiled, knowing he held the final card. "They have just built a fine new fifteen-bed hospital, and I know they have an excellent physician in charge, but they need surgeons," was his triumphant reply.

Well, what had Jennie expected but this? When her husband was determined to move on, it would happen. And to be truthful, she felt a bit of excitement at the idea of living in the mountains. She began to mentally list all the things she would have to do to move again.

"Tell me more about Coleman. I know they have a church. But what about schools?"

Robert patted her hands encased in fine kid gloves and clasped neatly in her lap. "There are about eight hundred people living in Coleman, my dear. They have churches and schools and everything a small town needs. We will have time to have a good look around this evening and tomorrow morning before we must take the afternoon train home."

Another large black square in the mountainside caught Jennie's eyes. "Look, Robert. Is that also a mine entrance?"

"Yes, that is the McGillivray Creek Coal and Coke Company. Just opened a year ago, and the market for coke is booming. You will see a long line of coke ovens to the south of Coleman. This will be a very prosperous town."

The train had crawled up through the magnificent mountain pass and now slowed to a halt at the station in the valley. Robert and Jennie alighted, and as promised, they found a porter waiting to carry their bags to the nearby hotel, where Robert had booked their rooms for the night.

"Take a deep breath, Jennie. This is cold, fresh mountain air. And just look at those peaks." It was a pretty little town in a spectacularly beautiful location.

By now, it was late afternoon, but after they had their tea, they went for a stroll around the area that contained their hotel, the new hospital, St Paul's United Church, and other small stores. After the wide open spaces of the prairies, Jennie felt enclosed, but rather than the claustrophobia she had been expecting, the little town nestled in the valley between tall mountain slopes felt safe and welcoming. But she was tired now, so she turned to her husband.

"In the morning, we can continue our exploration, but it is very chilly now, and I would like to return to the hotel for our supper."

That night they slept well, both tired after the trip and excitement. In the morning, the desk clerk, who had welcomed them to Coleman the previous afternoon, recommended a bakery not too far away for their breakfast. They chatted as they walked arm in arm in the cool morning, Jennie in her long dark skirt, white blouse, and snug jacket, with a tiny hat perched on her glossy black curls, and Robert in his suit and vest. He tipped his hat, a dark brown homburg, to passersby who smiled and nodded in return.

"Have you been here before, Robert?"

"No, but I like what I see of it."

"Yes, I can tell. It seems a friendly place. The scenery is truly breath-taking. Look, there is already snow on those distant peaks."

"Yes, it is beautiful. And they are building new houses on those slopes to the north and west. And look, Jen, see that new building with the peaked roof and the archway entrance? I believe that is the new hospital."

"It does look quite fine." Despite her earlier misgivings about another move, she found herself smiling at her husband's enthusiasm, enjoying their walk in the brisk mountain air.

"Yes, yes, it does, doesn't it?" Robert replied. "But now, we must catch our train home. Jennie, I'm glad you find it appealing. We'll come back soon for a second look around, and we'll see then if there are any suitable houses available. In the meantime, I'll find out all I can about Coleman, but I like this place."

COLEMAN 1910-1919

Chapter 10
Coleman and a New House

Short weeks after their first trip to Coleman, they had planned a second trip to look at the town and begin their search for a house. To her surprise, Jennie found that on her walks with the children in Lethbridge, she was comparing the heavy heat of late summer there to the fresh mountain air of Coleman and seriously considering the advantages of a move. Their furnished rooms were small, warm, and stuffy.

They had invested in a house in Portage La Prairie during Robert's HBC years, which they hoped to sell, and had managed to build up their savings in Lethbridge. Although they knew most of their money must be used to establish Robert in the new medical practice, Jennie hoped that perhaps a house in Coleman was a possibility.

Robert was also pondering their coming excursion when he met Dr. Mewburn one morning in the upper hall of the hospital. "Come along to my office after surgery, Doctor Ross. I have some news that will interest you." It was, as always with Dr. Mewburn, an order, not a request.

"In some ways," Robert thought, watching the senior physician walk briskly along the hall to the men's ward, "Mewburn is very military in his speech and movement."

The senior doctor certainly liked to issue commands, and Robert, who had answered to no one during his HBC years in Northern Ontario, sometimes found the other doctor's assumption of superiority irritating. However, Dr. Mewburn was in charge.

Robert knew he had learned a great deal about surgery in his time spent at the Galt working with the senior surgeon so merely nodded and continued to the surgical room. He put Mewburn's cryptic command out of his mind to consider after the morning's operations.

"Sit down, Doctor Ross." Dr. Mewburn was at his desk and spoke without lifting his eyes from his paperwork, "I'll be with you in a moment."

Robert said nothing but simply sat and waited. He knew that his ability to sit absolutely still for long periods of time was disconcerting to others, and he enjoyed their discomfiture, especially when they were trying to make him uneasy as he suspected was happening now.

Finally, Dr. Mewburn put down his pen and looked at Robert. "I hear that you have been looking for another situation?"

"Yes."

A long pause, as Mewburn gazed speculatively at Robert. "Well, a Doctor Westwood in Coleman needs a surgeon in the hospital he runs. He is also looking for a partner in his own practice. Would that suit you?"

Robert remained still and did not change his expression, though he was exultant inside. "Yes, very nicely."

"You've been there, I hear. Do you know that the hospital is owned by the Miners Union? And that there is constant tension between the union troublemakers and the mine management? The word is that there are concerns about the way the hospital is run, though they do seem to be financially sound. You do realize you will be giving up the security of a good salaried position when you leave here?"

"Yes, I am aware of that," Robert replied somewhat stiffly.

"Humph! Well, you are a good surgeon and will be missed here, but it is your decision. Your wish to set out on your own is understandable and from what I hear, it would seem that you have already made up your mind."

Then, for the first time in the months Robert had spent working for him, Dr. Mewburn asked a question about Robert's life outside the hospital, "And Mrs. Ross? How does she feel about this? Lovely lady, enjoyed meeting her."

Startled by the question, and knowing it was none of Dr. Mewburn's business, Robert simply answered, "Thank you. We'll be fine. I'll make arrangements to have my patients transferred to the other doctors' care, and we will leave by the end of this month."

"Good. I'll contact Doctor Westwood with my recommendation. You are an excellent surgeon and a fine physician, Robert, and will do well in a more independent role."

Although he loathed the patronizing tone, Robert held back a sharp retort and managed to say, "I appreciate that, Doctor Mewburn. I have learned a great deal here."

Jennie was not surprised to be informed that a second visit to Coleman would not be required. Robert had acquired the financial records of the practice in Coleman, and he and Jennie went over them carefully. All seemed to be in good order. They were moving again.

The necessary arrangements were quickly made at the hospital and medical practice office, and Robert contacted Dr. Westwood to confirm that he would take the offered position based on the financial information he had been sent. He also set about renting furnished rooms in Coleman, to be ready for them on their arrival. Knowing that the move was inevitable, Jennie had already packed what little they had in Lethbridge and arranged for their few boxes and barrels to be stored until they had a new residence in the mountains.

Robert had several reasons for wanting to move from Lethbridge. While he was pleased to think that he would be a partner in a new practice in the small mining town in the Rockies, and glad of the opportunity to be chief surgeon in the Miners Union Hospital, he would have left Lethbridge anyway.

Even if Coleman had not promised to be a successful venture for him, there had been news recently of several cases of typhoid in Lethbridge, and Robert was determined not to expose his family to this terrible disease. His younger brother and sister had almost died from typhoid in 1904, and when Robert was an intern in Montreal in 1908, there had been a typhoid epidemic where more than four hundred children had died in that city.

The Oldman River was the source of their drinking water in Lethbridge, and Robert was convinced that it was also the source of the typhoid. He had no desire to repeat the Montreal experience, he was worried about his wife and children becoming ill, and he was anxious to get to the mountains where there was far less chance of drinking infected water.

The family was soon on the CPR heading across southern Alberta towards the distant mountains. The sun glared down on the train, but Gordon was too excited to care about the heat and dust as the miles of golden prairie slipped by the passenger car's windows. Robert and Jennie enjoyed their elder son's enthusiasm, and his mother felt her earlier worries about another move into an unknown situation fade away. The landscape slowly changed as they traversed the foothills and entered the mountains.

Jennie, as always, had her hands full with Douglas. The little boy had been sick on and off over the past few months but was very active when he was well, and today he was full of energy, alternately insisting on being held on her lap or struggling to get down from his seat beside her to climb up and look out the window with Gordon. Finally, the four-hour journey ended, and they stepped out into the glittering warmth of the late fall afternoon.

As Robert helped Jennie down from the railway car, he spoke to the boys. "This is Coleman, our new home. For now, we will live in that building just down the street. Gordon, see the snow on the peaks and feel how clean the air is. Douglas, hold your brother's hand and stand still. Feel the cool breeze. Now, here is the wagon to carry us and our baggage. Settle down now, boys, it won't be much longer."

Robert helped Jennie into the horse-drawn wagon and set Gordon beside her. He then picked Douglas up and handed him to his tired mother who commented that the little boy felt feverish. "I do hope he is not getting sick again, Robert. He has just recovered from his last bout of stomach problems."

The toddler promptly fell asleep in her arms, dozing as they made their way along the bumpy street to the small furnished rooms that Robert had rented about two blocks from the railway station. Wearily they settled in, but within hours, Douglas was ill again, vomiting almost continuously through the night. Gordon, a much better traveller, was simply very tired and wanted to do nothing but sleep in their small room. Robert had immediately gone to the hospital and to visit Dr. Westwood.

Between the move, travelling, and a constantly sick child, Jennie was exhausted but knew that, tired as she was, she had to find a better place for them to live. She immediately contacted the local Presbyterian Church and, through them, found a vacant house. It was a little distance to the west of the town centre but still within easy walking distance of the hospital and church. They packed their few belongings and within weeks had moved to the house on First Street.

While Robert began his work with Dr. Westwood in the private medical practice and set about making some major changes in the way the hospital was run, Jennie began to establish their new residence. They had left some furniture in storage in Bow Island, and they still had a few pieces stored back East, but none had yet arrived in Coleman. Nevertheless, she had hopes of making a comfortable home and staying in Coleman for a while.

"I think I can make this place fairly cozy, Robert, and I like this town. The people are friendly, Gordon is very happy to be at school, and now that Douglas is feeling somewhat better, I am able to get a little sleep, although I must find a hired girl to help me. It seems that I have had at least one sick child continuously for four years. However, the Presbyterian Congregation at St Paul's United Church is most welcoming, and the women have been very helpful." She looked around at the empty rooms. "I do wish our furniture would arrive."

"It will come, Jen. Meanwhile, you are doing your best as always. The children are quite proud to have rooms of their own, curtains or not. They don't mind sleeping on blankets on the floor."

Jennie sighed again then changed the subject. "Robert, how are you managing with the changes you believe are necessary at the hospital? It was certainly not as originally represented to you, was it?"

"No, it certainly wasn't, my dear, and I am not going to sign the contract until many changes have been made. The matron was not a qualified nurse and knew nothing about the need for antiseptic conditions in the hospital, but I have already hired a graduate nurse from the Western Hospital in Toronto to replace her, and things are improving under her direction. Jennie, I'm afraid also that there have been some very poorly done surgeries, and there is strong feeling against some of the doctors, including Doctor Westwood, but I think I can put that right."

He paused, looking at his wife's worried face. "I'm also afraid the income from the partnership is not as was told to us when I accepted the position here. Like Bow Island, there is lots of work but not much cash. It may not be the sound financial venture we had hoped it would be."

Jennie's expression was one of dismay as she contemplated another winter of scrimping and saving. Robert's HBC pension just barely allowed them to make ends meet and would soon run out. The weather was still fine but already cold, and she knew it would be much colder when the snows came and the mountain winter set in. Fuel was such a huge expense.

"I pray, Robert, that this house will not be as draughty as our rooms were in Bow Island. I am so worried about the children. Douglas is ill again. I must find a girl to help me, but she will have to be paid. What news do we have of the sale of the Portage La Prairie house?"

"Nothing as yet, my dear. I hope we can sell it very soon as I am afraid we won't be able to keep up the mortgage payments if things don't improve here."

Robert, also concerned about the children and the cold, reassured her that the house was much sounder than their Bow Island place and reminded her that if it became too hard to heat, they could always move into the Westwood home as Mrs. Westwood had gone to Victoria for the winter.

He went on to speak more positively about his work, "However, I am now in charge of the hospital, and since the new matron and I are both insisting on a much higher standard of cleanliness throughout, infection rates have dropped, things are generally improving, and most important for our medical reputation, patients are recovering."

Jennie smiled at the good news as Robert went on, "The village has been desperate for a good surgeon, which explains many of the botched operations of previous years. I will be busy cleaning up those messes for months, but I will be able to change the miners' perceptions of poor doctoring. Although there has been bad feeling towards him as well, I like John Westwood. He is a good man and recognizes that he has much to learn about surgery."

Robert pulled his pocket watch out of his vest, knowing he had to return to work. Jennie wearily nodded then stood to go upstairs as Douglas began to cry in the bedroom.

Robert reassured her. "My dear Jen, the money will come. It will take time, but I think we will be all right here. I am already getting more work through the private practice, for which I am finally being paid.

"I have two serious cases right now, and I will insist they both be hospitalized. One young man has acute bronchitis, and I fear it will become pneumonia; another fellow, a farmer, has septicemia from an injury that was too long left untreated. I'm afraid he is beyond hope, but I shall try. I could have saved him if he had been brought to the hospital right away."

Robert also stood up to leave and smiled at his wife. "My first major surgery is scheduled for tomorrow, and I think I have a little surprise for Doctor Westwood. I told you, did I not, about meeting the injured miner, Mike, on my first visit to the hospital and how we established drainage on the infected wound on his leg? Doctor Westwood still feels we must amputate, but I think we can save this man's leg."

"I hope so, Robert. Amputation is a dreadful thing, and it sounds as though there has been far too much of it in Coleman."

"We'll talk about it this evening. I hope Douglas is feeling better and your afternoon is peaceful."

Later that day, after their supper and with both boys abed, Douglas finally sleeping quietly, they sat in the sitting room, sparsely furnished with two old chairs, thanks to the kindness of Mrs. Westwood, and had their tea.

Robert enthusiastically described his plan for the next day's operation on Mike. "Surgery will be required, and I will have to go deeply as I fear the bone of his leg may be involved, though I hope not. I have gone over the procedure with the new matron. She is an excellent operating room nurse and is prepared. I will also ask Doctor Westwood to assist, as he is eager to learn. This kind of wound is all too common with mine injuries. I dealt with it a number of times in Lethbridge, and I'm sure I will be successful tomorrow."

***

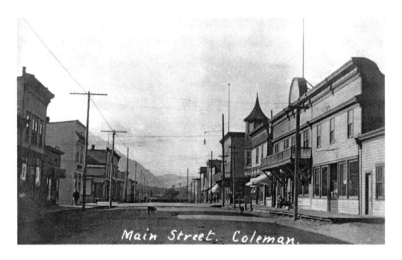

Main Street, Coleman, Alberta, 1912

Jennie was kept busy setting up the house they had rented. It was a one-and-a-half-story building overlooking the valley and Crowsnest River. There were three tiny bedrooms with dormer windows upstairs and a sitting room that opened onto the street on the main floor. Behind the sitting room was a dining room and, behind that, a large kitchen with a pantry.

Through the ladies of the church group she had promptly joined, Jennie had found two young men who were willing to come in and paint through the house under her close supervision. Their furniture was a long time arriving, but she was determined that when it did come the house would be cheerful. To her astonishment, Robert had made a suggestion regarding paint colours.

"Perhaps light colours? Cream or that pale blue you like so much?"

Startled at this intrusion into her domestic realm, Jennie could only nod her agreement.

"I think," Robert continued, "it would be a pleasant change from the darker colours of our Lethbridge rooms."

Now Jennie knew that the only colour her husband really liked was hospital white, but she agreed that cream for the upper part of the walls would be suitable, with mahogany beadboard and white trim.

"I had thought of a dark green for the bedrooms, but the light blue you suggest will be fine."

Robert nodded, glad that his wife was willing to take his suggestions. He had read that darker colours were harmful to someone who suffered from depression, and he knew that the winter nights in the mountains came early, so hoped that light colours in the house would help Jennie with the long dark days and nights to come.

Nell had sent Jennie some cream madras muslin with red and blue flowers for the sheer curtains, and when their household goods had finally arrived from the East, Jennie had also remade the heavy drapes from Dinorwic to fit the windows. Now every window had dark green curtains that were drawn to help keep out the summer's heat and the winter's cold. The carpets arrived and were unrolled, and through the efforts of the church ladies, some old but still comfortable plush chairs for evening conversations were found, and these were set by the small coal-burning fireplace.

Jennie draped their round oak dining room table with a lace cloth and set four chairs around it. The family would take their midday meal together there. With several small side tables and lamps, both gas and electric, the furnishings in the sitting room were at last complete.

Jennie's desk was placed in a bright corner. There she could do the accounts for the family and the medical practice and carry on her own voluminous correspondence. A lamp by her chair supplied a good light for reading. Coleman had enjoyed electricity since 1905, and Jennie was pleased, even on dark days, to be able to read the letters and the medical news she arranged for them to receive everywhere they went. The time she would spend sitting in this room discussing family and medical matters with her busy husband each evening continued to be the happiest part of her day.

The large kitchen was painted white throughout and furnished with a large coal-burning stove, a butcher block counter for cooking and baking, and a table for breakfast and tea. This would become the favourite room in the house for Robert and the boys. The big iron stove meant it was always warm and rich with the scents of Jennie's stews and soups and fresh bread.

As Robert began to earn a little more money, Jennie was able to hire a local girl to help with the children and help her do the work of putting up jars of fruit and vegetables for the coming winter. When the Rosses had first arrived the late autumn markets had been full of the harvest fruits and vegetables, and the women of the village had also generously shared their extra garden produce with the new doctor's family.

There was a partial basement, not large as the house was built on mountain rock, but with enough space for shelves. A large crock of sand was used to store carrots and turnips for use over the fast-approaching winter.

"Next spring, Robert, if we stay here, we will fence the backyard and have our own garden," Jennie announced with satisfaction, looking at the results of her labours. She was exhausted, but the pantry was full, the furniture set in place on the carpets, and she felt she had succeeded in making their new house very homelike.

A trip to the bank to set up their accounts and a trip to the post office to ensure their mail was delivered promptly were two arrangements she had made immediately upon arrival in Coleman. Now, when Robert came home for his noon meal, she left the children with him and walked to the town centre to get their mail. She also stopped by the telegraph office. The important information of the day was posted outside the office for all to read, and even in the most inclement weather, the small figure of Mrs. Ross, well bundled against the cold and snow, could be seen reading the news. Some items would later be published in the *Coleman Bulletin*, but she was impatient. The Canadian government had approved a twenty-four-hour telegraph system across the country from Halifax to Vancouver, and even small towns like Coleman were able to get daily news.

She began to feel at home in this house and this village. Each morning, dressed in ankle-length dark skirt and warm jacket or long coat and cloche hat and wearing her neat black boots, she left Douglas in the care of the new hired girl and walked with Gordon to his school, just a few blocks from their house. All in all, she decided, even though their finances were still very strained, Coleman might be a good place to work and raise a family.

Although the rough, frontier atmosphere of the coal town was not to her liking, the women of the close-knit community, who centred their lives around family and church, made her feel welcome and reminded her somewhat of her home in Mt. Forest in Ontario. Members of the hospital staff soon began to visit the new doctor's house, and Jennie looked forward to tea in the afternoon with the young nurses. At times, especially when the children had tonsillitis or mumps or measles, she desperately missed the support of her family back East and thought longingly of Nell on the West Coast, but she quickly made friends with some of the ladies of the women's group at St Paul's United Church and became involved in church affairs.

Robert was as busy as he could manage, working Monday through Saturday, both at the hospital and in his partnership with Dr. Westwood. He operated many times on miners in Coleman who had been dreadfully injured in accidents at work and was so successful that he became known as "the bone doctor" and was in great demand in other mining towns in the Rockies.

For Robert, being a medical man in Alberta meant many trips by train, horse-drawn buggy, or, one of his great pleasures, riding on horseback to make his calls. Often his journeys took several days as he stayed overnight at farms or small clinics, and each trip was balm to his restless soul. His wife, well used to being left alone with the children, had learned long ago not to worry about his absences. He always came home safely.

Chapter 11
A Hospital, St John Ambulance, and Bones

The Miners Union Hospital was located in the centre of Coleman on the main street, built five years earlier as part of the miners' settlement after a long strike. Although it was very small after Lethbridge's Galt Hospital, Robert believed it could be a fine hospital if it was well run. There were seventeen beds with rooms upstairs for two nurses to stay and for storage.

Robert's initial meeting with John Westwood had been very cordial, and the two men had spent some time discussing the changes Robert had stated must be made immediately if he was to stay in Coleman. He had realized very quickly that the current matron was not a nurse and had no idea of the importance of cleanliness, so within days of his arrival, he had insisted that she be replaced as head nurse by a graduate nurse from Western Hospital in Toronto. The removal of the original matron had created a furor as she had been hired by the Miners Union. But Robert ignored the uproar and was supported by the other physicians and the hospital board in his determination to improve conditions in the hospital. He knew that good nursing care was essential for the patients' welfare, and the other doctors in the hospital would eventually benefit by his efforts.

Robert began to work, ensuring that his instructions regarding aseptic techniques be followed in the operating room, which was scrubbed and scrubbed with a solution of carbolic acid until he was satisfied. Not until then would he perform any surgeries, and before and after every surgery, instruments were scoured and then soaked in a solution of carbolic acid.

The same standards of cleanliness were insisted upon in the rooms and in all aspects of nursing care. Carbolic soap became standard issue for doctors, nurses, and patients.

Once an aseptic environment had been ensured, and not before, Robert was ready to deal with those surgeries that had been awaiting his attentions. A patient named Mike was one of the surgeries that had been held up, and now Robert stood by the side of Mike's hospital bed. Dr. Westwood believed that the young miner needed an amputation of the right leg at the hip joint, but Robert did not.

This would be Robert's first major case in Coleman, and he immediately forgot everything except the man in front of him. It was obvious that Mike was in dreadful pain, though he was very stoic about it. However, he was alarmed at the idea that he would lose his leg and asked Robert, "Doc, can you help me in any way? I have to have two good legs to do my job."

Robert replied, "I can make no promises, Mike, but let's have a look."

The young miner had a discharging sinus, a tunnel wound, about two inches below the head of the hip bone. Robert knew that he had been in the hospital for three weeks under treatment as the staff had tried to draw the infection out of the wound, but it was no better than when first admitted. His leg was swollen and painful, and Robert immediately suspected that an incision would be required to clean it out completely

Dr. Westwood said reluctantly, "We have tried everything and have decided we must amputate." Mike flinched at his words and murmured softly in despair and pain.

Robert smiled reassuringly at both of them. "I think we can improve this situation, but before any kind of surgery can be safely attempted, we must carry out an antiseptic treatment for at least two or three weeks. If nothing else, it will lessen the pain, Mike."

He then turned to Dr. Westwood, "I will operate when the discharge is gone. Let me go now and instruct the nurse in what to do."

The new head nurse listened intently to Robert's instructions, and after ten days of treatment the purulent discharge was considerably lessened, and the operation was scheduled.

When Robert again examined the young miner's leg and found the infection much diminished, he spoke to Dr. Westwood. "I am ready to operate. Would you care to assist me, Doctor Westwood?"

Dr. Westwood responded positively so Robert continued. "Instead of an amputation, I am going to do my best to save this man's leg. I have reviewed the procedure with our new operating room nurse, and she is prepared. Ether anaesthetic will be administered."

Robert made an incision almost down to the bone, commencing about one inch above the discharging sinus and reaching down to the middle of the thigh bone. He then chiseled a trough of about the same length along the incision, and the nurse repeatedly curetted the trough to remove all evidence of infection and diseased tissue. The trough was then packed with a strip of gauze soaked in bismuth paste.

Dr. Westwood asked, "Why are you using that paste, Doctor Ross? I did not think it could be used inside the body?"

Robert continued packing the wound as he answered. "I know from my Montreal experience and my studies at Queen's that this paste is much used by the medical profession to combat infections in many parts of the body, and I used it successfully at Lethbridge." He deftly allowed the end of the long strip of gauze to emerge from one end of the wound, to be withdrawn later, and closed the incision by apposing the muscles with catgut sutures and the skin with silkworm thread.

Dr. Westwood assisted throughout, asking many questions that Robert, who believed in his role as a teacher as well as a surgeon, answered happily. Westwood was much impressed by the surgical abilities of this new surgeon and his obvious willingness to share his knowledge. John Westwood was a good man and greatly relieved to think that through Dr. Ross's skill and knowledge, they might save Mike's leg.

Westwood commented at the end of the operation, "No one likes to amputate, Doctor Ross, and too many miners have lost their arms or legs following horrific accidents, when there is little we can do. I hope and pray that this is a success, and we will be able to save more men's limbs."

In his satisfied conversation with Jennie that evening, Robert said, "Now I can relax somewhat. All went well, and the healing time begins. But I think Mike will be fine, especially now that I know the risk of infection has been minimized by my insistence on cleanliness throughout the hospital and every aspect of treatment. And the Miners Union will be willing to pay for operations when they see the men being well cared for."

Robert visited Mike frequently over the next few weeks and stressed again and again to the nurses how important it was to change the loose dressings and keep the area sterile. There was no question that his determination to revolutionize the way the hospital was run and the treatment patients received was slowly having the wished for effects. He had made it clear that he would not sign a contract with the board unless his orders were carried out.

Mike simply said every day, "Thank you, Doc, I still have my leg and the pain is not so bad and getting less every day."

Three weeks after the operation, the wound was well healed. "We are letting you up out of bed to start walking and strengthening your leg, Mike, and in about a week, you can go home. Come back to see me again a week after that."

"Thank you, thank you, Doctor Ross, I will." The young man could still hardly believe it was all over, and he had not lost his leg. He leaned on his crutches and cheerfully continued to exercise his leg.

As requested, Mike called in to see Robert in his new medical office on the next block over from the hospital, but after that he disappeared. Robert never saw him again.

Upon making inquiries in the town, he was told that Mike had gone back to Ukraine. To Robert's great satisfaction, he learned that Mike had married an old girlfriend there, a young widow who owned a grocery store. Mike was now set for life and need never go into the mines again.

***

Their first winter in Coleman had arrived, and although there was not much snow on the ground, the daylight hours were short, and it was bleak and cold. On a dark evening in November, with the sitting room lit only by the rose-shaded table lamps and the flames from the fire, Robert and Jennie sat by the hearth in their accustomed chairs and discussed an issue that was dear to the doctor's heart.

He had always been a believer in the importance of first aid. Indeed, his original hope in attending Queen's University had been to find out how he could assist "on the spot" those injured in the North woods at a time when most people died before a medical man could be reached.

"How can I encourage the people of Coleman to support the St John Ambulance Association? You know how important I believe first aid to be. Many lives have been saved by the prompt action of knowledgeable persons at the scene of an accident."

Jennie had a sip of her tea and replied thoughtfully. "You are correct, Robert, and it astonishes me that such an organization does not exist here, especially with the frequent accidents in the mines."

"There has been favourable talk about it, but no one has stepped forward as yet to organize it, and right now, I am exceptionally busy with my hospital duties and the new practice."

"What could you find time to do?"

"Well, I could set aside some time to instruct, perhaps one evening a month. Or perhaps every two weeks? What do you think?"

Jennie had the distinctly un-Christian thought that her husband had little enough time to spend with her and the boys but knew better than to question him when he had a project in mind. And he was right. First aid could save lives.

"Would you be able to use the hospital?" she asked, firmly reminding herself that Christian charity took precedence over everything else.

"I know how strongly you believe in Doctor Osler's ideas of clinical practice being the best teacher."

"Hmm, I'm not sure about the hospital. I'm just finally getting it running the way it should and don't want to disrupt the routines. Patient confidentiality is always an issue, and we have very little space. A class would need room to meet and practice."

"Yes, of course," Jennie agreed, "but I think that a space in town would be found if there is a will to set up the organization. How about the council chambers? And what about expenses? Surely, the mining companies would support such an endeavour? They would realize that it would mean the miners would be back on the job sooner."

"Yes, yes, I'm sure they would. And you know, as we've been talking, I've thought of the very person to get this going. Mr. Whiteside. He has already said he was very interested."

"An excellent thought, Robert. He is a good organizer."

"I will speak to him tomorrow and tell him I support what he is trying to do. But, back to my original question, how can I encourage this effort?"

By now, Robert was up and pacing in the small sitting room. He looked at his wife, noting the strands of silver in her wavy black hair, held loosely in a twist at the nape of her neck. She looked terribly tired where she sat well wrapped in a woollen shawl in her chair by the hearth. They had had to let the local hired girl go, but Jennie had found a much more suitable young woman from Lethbridge who now lived with them. Hannah's presence made a big difference, but even though this gave Jennie a bit of a rest in the afternoon, she was always fatigued.

The move and the financial concerns had been a great strain, especially because they had not been able to keep up the mortgage payments on the Portage La Prairie house, so they had lost that large investment. Her rheumatism was always worse when the weather turned cold and the wind blew hard across the mountain snows. And the whole family had just undergone a siege of tonsillitis.

"Well," she watched him pace and replied thoughtfully, "you could write a letter to Mr. Whiteside, encouraging him and showing your strong interest and support for the movement. In the same letter, you could offer your services as a lecturer. Surely having a doctor offer to do this would be a big incentive?"

Robert sat down again and smiled broadly. "You are right. That is just the thing to do. I know that it is late now, but perhaps tomorrow you could draft such a letter for me, and I will deliver it to Mr. Whiteside?"

Jennie smiled, thinking back to the papers they had worked on together at Queen's. "Yes, of course. I'll write it tomorrow morning when I feel stronger. Hannah will look after Douglas, and Gordon is well enough now to go back to school. Even with the electric lights, I prefer daylight for my writing. Now, you have that early appendectomy in Pincher Creek, so you must get your rest."

"Thank you, my dear. I'll bank the fire so it will catch easily in the morning. We will have to be up early as usual. I hope you are not disturbed by Douglas too often in the night. Goodnight."

Humming to himself, Robert made his way up the stairs to bed, while Jennie sat for a little time as the fire died down, enjoying the few moments of quiet and mentally composing the letter she would write in the morning.

In late 1910, the first meeting of the Coleman branch of the St John Ambulance Association was held, and a letter was read from Dr. T. Robert Ross supporting the organization and offering his services as a lecturer. His offer was accepted, and the first class was held in January 1911. Space for the classes was found in the town council chambers and the mining companies contributed substantially for bandages, stretchers, and textbooks.

Five years later, Robert was to send another letter as part of a fundraising effort. This letter, outlining the proven value of the organization, was published in the *Coleman Bulletin*.

> *Since the inauguration of the classes five years ago, we have had a considerable number of accidents in the mines, and in all cases, the value of having well-trained*

*first aid men among the miners has been clearly dem-
onstrated...stopping of hemorrhage, prevention of
movement at the site of the injury...avoidance of sepsis
or blood poisoning...and prevention of shock. I cannot
set too high a value on the services the first aid men
have rendered to their fellow workers. Such a thing as a
man reaching the hospital in an exsanguinated condition, or dying from shock or sepsis...is ancient history
since the ambulance classes started in Coleman.*

Throughout his long career as a medical man, Robert continued
to support the St John Ambulance Association, teaching first aid and
mine rescue courses. But now, the whole family slept as the snow fell
softly throughout the night on their mountain home.

***

About a year after he had operated on Mike, three local miners whose
accents identified them as being originally from Ukraine came in
to Robert's office. They were accompanied by another young man
on crutches.

"Doctor Ross, we are all miners in Coleman now, but originally
we came from Ukraine. You remember Mike? He calls you "the bone
doctor", and he has sent this young man, Josef, for you to operate on
his twisted leg. Mike has paid for everything, and he will pay for the
operation as well." The three men spoke quite good English and had to
speak for Josef because he had no English at all. Through them, Robert
was able to get the story.

The large windows of his office afforded good light as he examined
the young man's leg and discovered a posterior dislocation of the lower
half of the knee joint. The upper end of the tibia, the main bone of
the lower leg, lay behind the lower end of the femur, the main bone
of the upper leg. This overlap was the result of an accident in a mine
in Ukraine nine years ago when Josef was seventeen. According to
his friends, as well as Robert could understand, Josef's leg had been

caught under a falling beam. When the injury, which must have been extensive, healed, the leg was twisted at what would have been the knee joint and was now much shorter than the other. Josef had been on crutches and in pain for the intervening nine years.

The three men interpreted as Robert asked Josef, "Can you raise your leg off the floor?"

Josef, who was sitting in a chair, seized his leg around the calf muscles with both hands and lifted the leg, which was rigid.

"Do that again without using your hands."

Josef could not, and he could not, of course, bend the leg at the knee.

Robert sat and thought for several minutes. He felt a surge of excitement as he realized that here seated in front of him was a young man who, on the word of a previous patient, had come halfway around the world to see him. Josef had sailed from Europe over the Atlantic Ocean and then travelled more than three thousand miles across Canada to Coleman to get "the bone doctor" to fix his useless leg.

Honoured by Mike's faith in his abilities, Robert thought, "This surely is a surgical challenge that Mike has set me, and I don't propose to sidestep it." To the three miners he said, "Can you arrange for Josef's admittance to the Miners Union Hospital? If so, I will operate as soon as he is admitted and I can get my assistant."

Josef was duly admitted, and Robert arranged for an assistant in the person of Mr. E.C. Crawford. Crawford was currently a medical student at Queen's University and was very interested in becoming a surgeon. He spent his summers working in the office of one of the mining companies in Coleman, his hometown.

Crawford was a very serious young man who had become interested in medicine when he took a course in first aid taught by Robert, and each summer Robert arranged for him to work in the mine office and assist with surgery. In 1914, two years after he assisted Robert in this particular operation, Crawford, who was then in his final year at Queen's, went to war with the University Military Hospital. He was sent with them to the Dardanelles where his experience with Dr. Ross during his summer vacations meant that he was appointed warrant officer for the Military Hospital. He was also allowed to complete his final year of medical training at the British Egyptian Medical College in Cairo. Crawford was honoured to meet Dr. William Osler at Oxford University, and after the war the young doctor spent a year as a surgical assistant in a London hospital.

However, that was all ahead for him, and right now, he listened intently as he assisted "the bone doctor" in his operation on the young man from Ukraine.

"We can't give him back a flexible knee," Robert remarked as the ether was administered and they prepared to operate, "but we can certainly give him back the use of his leg and lessen his pain."

The operation consisted of exposing, by a transverse incision across the front of the knee joint, the lower end of the femur and the upper end of the tibia. Robert then sawed about half an inch off the ends of both bones, which was sufficient to allow them to come into close apposition at what had been the knee joint.

In order to ensure that the upper end of the tibia would not slip back into its now accustomed place behind the lower end of the femur, Robert took two sterilized, squared four-inch nails and drove them through the upper end of the tibia and into the lower end of the femur. The heads of these nails rested under the skin about two inches below the sawed-off margin of the tibia. The tendons surrounding the joint, which had been severed when the joint was opened, were sutured into place using catgut to lengthen them, and the incision was then closed with silkworm gut sutures.

Robert grinned across the operating table at Crawford who had been a steady hand throughout. "We've done what we can, and we've done it well. Now we wait." And with that, they stepped back from the operating table while the nurses carefully applied a cast to immobilize the leg.

The wound healed well, and eight days later, Robert removed the sutures. Although he could not speak a word of English, Josef's gratitude was evident as he looked at his now straight leg.

Robert told him, again through the interpretive efforts of his friends who came daily to check on his progress, "You are getting along nicely. A few more weeks of healing, and then we will get you up and about."

The weeks passed, and Josef was helped out of bed and moved about the hospital with the nurses' assistance. Soon he was ready to be discharged, and Robert happily handed him a walking cane and wished him luck as the young man left the hospital with the cane as his only support.

Assuming Josef would go back to Ukraine, Robert did not expect to see him again, but about three years later, a tall man walked into his office. The stranger walked confidently but had a stiff knee. He spoke to Robert in very good English, "You don't remember me, but I am Josef, the man whose leg you fixed three years ago."

Robert was delighted with Josef's progress, both physically and in his mastery of English. "Of course I remember you. Where have you been keeping yourself since the operation? What happened? How did you learn to speak English so well, and have you encountered any problems with the leg?"

"The day I left the hospital, I travelled to Saskatchewan where I had relatives whom I knew would look after me while I got my strength back. Then I found employment on the railroad where I learned to speak English. I earned enough money to bring my girlfriend out from Ukraine, and we were married. We now have a young baby. None of this would have happened if you had not saved Mike's leg and mine. Thank you." As Robert smiled at the happy story, Josef continued, "My leg is fine, but on cold days, there are two points just below the knee joint that become very painful, right here."

Robert chuckled and asked, "Can you come with me to the hospital? Those are the nail heads, and I will remove them for you." Under local anaesthetic, he made two small incisions and drew out the nails.

"These are for you," he said handing them to the amazed Josef. "That should take care of the pain in cold weather."

"And this is for you, Doctor." Josef replied, handing Robert a fifty dollar bill. "It is all I have now, but someday I will come back with another fifty dollars for you."

Dr. Ross never again saw Josef or the other fifty dollars, but he had helped a man walk again without pain and knew he had met the challenge posed to him by Mike. He was content with his surgical accomplishments and with his life in Coleman.

Chapter 12
A Stubborn Grandmother

As had happened in Lethbridge, Dr. Ross had become known as an excellent baby doctor. It was customary for expectant mothers to be cared for by midwives until near their due dates, but Robert was always aware and kept a close eye on any mother-to-be who showed signs of any difficulty. Problems were rare, and in the three years he had practiced in the small mining town, he had delivered many healthy babies.

Except in those cases where there was a complication, the births took place at home, which often entailed the doctor travelling by horseback to farmhouses or miner's homes. A full night's sleep and time with his own family were often casualties of his obstetrics practice, but for Robert, the joy of a new baby made it all worth it. And, of course, the newest citizens of Coleman and the surrounding area would be brought by their proud parents to see Dr. Ross for checkups and sometimes just to show them off as they grew and thrived.

This night, Robert was awakened just after midnight by the sound of a loud knock on his door. There were no births expected, and, concerned, he quietly murmured, "I hope all is well at the mines." Sleepily, he donned his robe and opened the front door to see a frantic looking young miner, whose wife Robert knew had come to join him from Latvia shortly before the birth of their baby.

"Please, Doctor Ross. You must come. The baby is sick; he keeps crying and twisting."

Robert was puzzled because he had seen their baby for a routine exam just the day before. The infant he had seen was a well-nourished, healthy boy of about six months old. He was teething and a bit miserable as a result but was perfectly normal and well otherwise. The young mother had not been in Coleman as long as her husband, and her own mother had come from Latvia to visit when the baby was born. This was the couple's first child, and they were very proud of him.

The father could understand and speak English fairly well and had come with his wife when they brought the baby into the office the day before. He had answered all of Robert's questions throughout the exam with no evident concern. However, he did remark, "He cries a lot and keeps us all awake. We are worried about the crying."

Following the exam, Robert pronounced the baby well, reassured them that the crying was a normal part of teething, and gave them some teething tablets with directions for their use. "I will look in on the baby tomorrow," he had promised, yet here was the agitated father rousing Robert from a warm bed in the middle of the night and insisting that he come right away.

"Baby is screaming and trying to be sick. He is having what you call convulsions. He is red and cannot breathe properly and keeps passing out."

Robert dressed quickly and hurried back through the sleeping town to see the child. It was very warm in the miner's small shack with a weak glow from the electric bulb, so Robert immediately asked if they had some lanterns to augment the light. They complied and Robert laid the writhing child on blankets on a small table. It was obvious that something was terribly amiss, but until he could determine what it was, all he could do was apply the usual treatments for convulsions. As he examined the baby, Robert asked the parents, "Has this baby had anything to eat? Did he nurse as usual? He was perfectly well when I saw him yesterday afternoon."

Glancing at his mother-in-law, the father immediately replied, "No, he was too fussy from teething to be interested in nursing. He's had nothing to eat for hours. Nothing at all."

Robert was too focused on the baby to give much thought to the deference the young father seemed to pay the grandmother. He knew he had to stop the baby's convulsions as quickly as possible. "Fill a basin with fairly warm water," he instructed and tried immersing the child in the water. No results, except the baby began screaming again and then lapsed into unconsciousness.

Sweat running down his face and arms from the heat and the steam, Robert desperately tried every method he had ever heard of to stop convulsions, even tiny whiffs of chloroform. Occasionally, the writhing and retching would stop for a few moments, and in this brief respite, the exhausted baby would lapse into a semiconscious state. Almost immediately, however, he would rouse, and the convulsions would begin again as he strained to vomit. By this time, Robert was thoroughly alarmed, and he began to fear for the baby's life.

"What is this? I have never seen anything like this." Robert's thoughts raced, and he barked at the parents, "This baby needs to go to the hospital right now. I cannot understand why nothing I have tried is working. I know you said he has not eaten anything, but I believe he is struggling to get rid of something in his stomach and needs to be hospitalized. Look here. Do you see how his stomach bulges out in this hard knot when he tries to vomit? I can feel a mass, right here, at this spot. That's what he's trying to get rid of."

The grandmother glared at Robert, and the baby's parents once more loudly denied that Baby had eaten anything and flatly refused to heed Robert's pleas to take their child to the hospital. Robert was left with no option but to continue his efforts to ease the child's distress. But he could find no other reason for the terrible retching.

"Are you absolutely certain that he has had nothing by mouth?" he asked yet again. "Have you given him anything to eat, anything at all?"

"Nothing, no, nothing to eat," they insisted.

The grandmother, who had been a silent presence in the room shook her head as well, and uttered an emphatic "Nē!"

"Could he have put something in his mouth and swallowed it without you knowing?"

"No, nothing, we watch him all the time."

Robert looked directly at the old woman as he asked the father again, "You're absolutely sure? Nothing by mouth?"

"Nothing, nothing! Make it stop!" The terrified father shouted in response to Robert's questions, "Doctor, please, you must help him!"

The distraught parents still maintained that the baby had had nothing to eat and refused to give Robert permission to take him to the hospital. As the baby's condition worsened, Robert beseeched them, "Please, listen to me. This baby needs to go to the hospital, or he will die."

Again, the parents looked to the grandmother.

"No, no, Doctor, no hospital," screamed the young mother. "No hospital!"

The grandmother nodded her head firmly and said, "Nē!"

Try as he might, Robert could not convince the parents that their baby needed to be hospitalized. Furious at their unwillingness to listen to him, and the grandmother's intransigent refusal to let her daughter and son-in-law take their baby to the hospital, and hopeful that perhaps they would listen to someone they were more familiar with, he left the little shack and rushed to the Miners Union Hospital. There he awoke Matron and told her about the baby's desperate condition.

"I'm sure that they have given him something to eat, and he cannot digest it, nor can he throw it up. Please go right away. Perhaps you can convince them where I could not. They must allow you to bring the child to the hospital. Surgery may be required. Get another doctor to go with you if necessary. They simply won't listen to me. Especially the grandmother."

"I'll go right away, Doctor Ross. I know the young woman. Maybe I can persuade them to ignore the grandmother and bring the child to the hospital."

Matron dressed quickly, and Robert took her to the miner's house. He did not go back inside with her, fearing that his presence would hamper her efforts to help the baby.

Knowing that there was nothing more he could do and realizing that dawn would come soon, he slowly made his way back home. As he walked, he went over and over in his mind the sad and frustrating events of the past few hours. Finally, needing some relief from these anguished thoughts, he turned his mind to a meeting scheduled later that day with another doctor in Michel, British Columbia, regarding a very ill patient who required immediate surgery. He knew that he had to be on the eight o'clock train in just a few hours to get to Michel in time for the scheduled operation. Far too upset to sleep, he sat quietly in the darkened kitchen of his home and waited for dawn.

As he was striding toward the train station, he heard a shout. "Doctor Ross, wait, you must wait."

He recognized Matron's voice and stopped to wait for her as she ran to catch him. Reaching his side, she gasped out the terrible words, "The baby is dead!"

"Dead?" He stopped and spun around to face the breathless woman, "What do you mean, dead? Did they refuse to listen to you as well? I told them and told them how serious it was. That baby needed to be in the hospital. And they knew it. Why wouldn't they listen to us? Why on earth would that old woman refuse to let us save her grandchild?"

Matron spoke shakily, "I don't know. It seems like I was there forever, trying to convince them. I just know that no matter what I said, they refused to listen, and they wouldn't hear of another doctor coming either. Just like they refused to listen to you." Wearily, tears running down her face, Matron said, "The baby died, the parents are numb with shock, and the grandmother is hysterical and shouting in Latvian that you killed the boy."

"I killed the boy? Rubbish!" shouted Robert, who could hardly believe her words. "I did everything I could think of to save that child, and I begged them to let me take him to the hospital."

The nurse, who was also very angry, agreed, "I know you did, Doctor Ross. I asked the father to interpret, and he said the grandmother was screaming that you killed the child. I said to the father,

'You don't believe that, do you?' and he replied 'Grandmother is always right.'"

Robert stood, momentarily frozen with shock and anger under the pale blue morning sky. The sun was coming up now over the mountains, and he struggled to understand this tragedy.

Terribly upset, Matron pleaded, "Doctor Ross, you must take action against the old woman for saying that."

"Matron, I don't care what ignorant people say. I did everything I could to save that child's life. I am sorry for the poor parents, but that old woman is wrong."

Just as he turned to step aboard the waiting train, the RCMP constable who was in charge of the local detachment stepped off.

Robert spoke to him, "Constable Brown, I spent the night, as did Matron, trying to save the life of a baby who has just died. The family lives in that miner's shack just over there. Matron has just reported to me that the parents and grandmother are now saying that I killed the child. I am requesting that you make an immediate investigation, and if necessary call for a Coroner's Inquest and an autopsy to discover cause of death. I am just on my way to Michel for an operation on a seriously ill patient, but I will be back on the nine o'clock train tonight."

"Of course, Doctor Ross. I will look into it right away."

Travelling back home through the mountains that evening, Robert went over and over the events of the previous night. "What could I have done differently? Nothing. How could I have made them take the baby to the hospital? Could I have called the police? For what? I'm certain surgery would have saved him. That grandmother is a she-devil."

When Robert arrived in Coleman, he was met at the station by the constable. "The Inquest is in session, and they are waiting for you to give your evidence, Doctor Ross."

Robert, who had now been up since midnight, went immediately to the courtroom and gave his evidence regarding the baby's distress and convulsions of the night before.

Matron then spoke, "Doctor Ross was with the baby all night. He sent me over there when he was unable to convince the parents to take the child to the hospital for treatment. I, too, was unable to persuade them, and the baby died about an hour after my arrival."

The doctor who had performed the autopsy was then called.

"I removed this from the baby's stomach," he said, as he held up a ball of raw dough about the size of a hen's egg. "This was the cause of the child's death. Surgery would have saved him."

The heartbroken father of the child was then placed in the witness box and, under oath, was questioned by Constable Brown.

"Grandmother fed Baby a paste of flour mixed with butter and water to stop him from crying. The convulsions came on shortly after Baby had swallowed the mixture."

Listening to this testimony, Robert became enraged, thinking of all the times he had asked if the baby had been fed anything. He then turned to the coroner and spoke, his voice tight with suppressed anger, "The parents insisted that their baby had not had anything by mouth," he spoke through clenched teeth, "I was fairly certain that the cause of the child's convulsions was indeed something in his stomach, and I told them this, over and over again. I was very clear about that and also about the need to get the child to the hospital as quickly as possible. Despite this, they refused permission. Had they agreed, I would have rushed the baby to the hospital and used a stomach pump or made a tiny incision into the stomach to remove the lump. But the old woman never left the room and wouldn't let them tell the truth about what she had done. They lied to me every time I asked them if the baby had been fed anything by mouth." By now, Robert's voice was trembling with his anger. "Excuse me, sir, but I must leave before I say any more."

Completely wretched at the unnecessary death of a healthy baby, he walked home in the darkness, bitterly considering the price the child and his parents had paid for an old woman's ignorance.

Chapter 13
Visitors, a Mining Disaster, and World War I

Gordon and Douglas, still panting and sweaty from their exertions, stood on the back porch and gazed triumphantly at the tent they had just erected on the fresh green grass in their backyard.

"Father helped, but I did most of it," ten-year-old Gordon stated proudly to his mother.

"I helped, too." Douglas announced.

"Yes, of course you did, Son." Robert laughed. "Now, get your bedrolls into the tent, and then get yourselves cleaned up. We need to meet the train from Bow Island in an hour, so move quickly now."

Reluctantly, torn between pride in their tent and excitement at the impending arrival of Miss Emma and her husband, Mr. Ludtke, with their daughter, Ora, and Miss Mercilla, now Mrs. Murray, the boys left the backyard and hurried to wash.

However busy and active they were in their new life in Coleman, they never stopped missing the two former nurses who had cared for them on the trip across Canada and for the months they had lived in the rooms above the little hospital in Bow Island. Even Douglas, who had been just a toddler, had a deep attachment to Miss Emma and memories of her gentle voice.

The family had returned to Bow Island for Emma's wedding to Mr. Ludtke in 1910, and Jennie had rejoiced when Emma gave birth to a daughter, Ora, sending a beautiful lace gown for the baby's christening ceremony.

They had gone again to Bow Island in 1913 when Mercilla married Mr. Howard Murray, but now, the Bow Island families were coming to stay with them in Coleman for two weeks, and the Ross household had been caught up in feverish preparations for days.

Miss Emma and Miss Mercilla, as Gordon and Douglas continued to call them, would stay in the boys' bedroom with little Ora, hence the tent in the backyard; Mr. Ludtke, whom Robert called "EC," would sleep in the newly added screened sleeping porch at the back of the house. All was in readiness.

While Hannah and Jennie completed preparations for lunch, Robert and the boys, now washed and brushed to shining cleanliness, set out in the carriage to meet the train. Robert had hired a wagon to transport the visitors' baggage to the house, and the boys, after enthusiastically greeting the Bow Island families, gleefully clambered onto the baggage wagon to ride back to the house, getting thoroughly dusty again in the process.

Jennie stood on the front veranda to greet their guests on their arrival, and, happy to be reunited, the whole group sat down to a magnificent welcoming lunch.

The two weeks passed quickly. Robert and EC spent hours discussing business and world news, while Jennie and the two sisters exchanged news of all the happenings of friends and families in Bow Island and eastern Canada. Regular walks through Coleman were the order of the day, and the boys spent many happy hours in their tent. Several afternoons while Hannah supervised, little Ora was invited to have tea with them in the tent, which delighted the little girl and made the boys feel very grown-up indeed.

Happily, the weather remained fine, and Gordon and Douglas were in heaven sleeping out in their tent every night, giggling to themselves at the sound of Mr. Ludtke's sonorous snoring on the screened porch. On two momentous occasions, Gordon and Douglas were permitted by their father to miss a school day in order to accompany the men on horseback fishing expeditions in the mountains. Both boys were good riders and Douglas's sturdy pony easily kept pace with the horses on the mountain trails. The fishermen were rewarded with good catches of mountain trout that they cleaned and cooked for lunch over an open fire while Robert reminisced about his time as a young man in the wilds of Ontario.

Another day, much to Douglas's chagrin, Gordon accompanied the two men on a shooting expedition. At six, Douglas was deemed too young to go hunting and had to attend school instead while his older brother left him behind. Gordon was already a good shot, and his father was very proud of him, but Douglas was somewhat mollified when Miss Emma walked him to school and Miss Mercilla came to walk him home when school was dismissed for the day.

Dinner table conversation was always lively, covering topics from advances in medicine to the growing prosperity of the West, concerns about the availability of water on the farms, and the slump in coal prices.

Robert spoke about the recently developed electrocardiogram machine and its value in predicting and thus perhaps someday preventing heart attacks. The former nurses relayed information about the clinic that Robert had founded and how busy it remained with injuries and new babies. They also spoke worriedly about a baffling paralytic disease called infantile paralysis that seemed to strike small children. There had only been two cases of this mysterious affliction, but it was a tragedy no one understood. Robert shook his head. He had never heard of it. He glanced at Jennie with a question in his eyes, and she shook her head indicating that she had no knowledge of the ailment. He knew that she would find out what she could for him.

EC Ludtke was a businessman and had owned an insurance company and a land agency among other interests, so he was up to date on the current rate of settlement in the West and very interested in the coal industry in the Crowsnest Pass and the impact that Prime Minister Laurier's defeat in parliament might have on coal prices.

"And does anyone know anything about this new fellow, Borden? How is he likely to treat our western concerns?"

Much to the delight of the two boys and to Robert's obvious interest, EC also told them of a motorcar, a 1909 Oaks, that he owned. He was planning to open a dealership in Bow Island to sell these motorcars.

Gordon and Douglas listened intently as Mr. Ludtke described the motorcar, looking hopefully at their father. They were entranced by the description — Gordon more interested in the way it looked and Douglas asking many questions about the mechanical side of this wonder.

"What exactly is an epicyclic gearbox, sir? And does twenty horse-power mean it could pull as much weight as a team of twenty horses? How fast can it go? Do the roads have to be smooth?"

EC smiled at Douglas's questions, and realizing the boy's interest was genuine, patiently explained that in the gearbox a large outside wheel turned slowly, its interior cogs meshing with cogs on a smaller inside wheel to give the motorcar two speeds forward. In no time at all, he was borrowing paper and pencil from Jennie to draw a diagram of the motorcar's inner workings. He also had a photograph taken in 1911 to show the boys who sighed with longing at the sight of such a wondrous machine.

Discussion turned to the charity and church work that both sisters were doing in the town of Bow Island. Jennie was most supportive of their efforts as they mirrored her own efforts as a member of the church board and school board and her Sunday school teaching. The boys were sent off to bed in their tent as talk moved to the Scott and Amundsen expeditions to the South Pole and the rumours of war in Europe.

All in all, it was a happy two weeks, and everyone was sad when the visit ended and the tent came down.

They could not know as they said their goodbyes at the train station that, within a month, Coleman would suffer a massive disaster, and before the year was out, Canada would be drawn into a terrible war in Europe.

***

Coleman had now been their home for three years, and the Ross family was content with their lives in the small mountain town. The house was comfortably situated so that the westerly breeze, which was almost constant, blew the coal dust and smuts away from their area, and it seemed everything they needed was within walking distance.

Robert had a good-sized practice in his own right with his private medical office about two blocks from the Miners Union Hospital where he was chief surgeon. Both of the boys were in school. Douglas, who was six, delighted in his new friends and everything he was learning. He had been very lonely when Gordon went off to school, and he was happy to be in the younger children's class. Gordon, in his last year with "the babies," as he called Douglas' class, was looking forward to moving up to the senior class in the autumn. His mathematical ability was a continuing source of pride to both Robert and Jennie.

It was just after nine-thirty on a beautiful summer morning, on June 19, 1914, and Robert was enjoying the walk from his office to the hospital. As he made his way, he was pleased that a light rain through the night had settled the dust on the roads and that the air was fresh and cool. He smiled at women with their baskets setting out to shop and tipped his hat to the store owners who were opening for the day. And as he did so often, he thought what a good decision it had been to come to Coleman.

Nearing the hospital, he was alarmed by the sound of panicked shouting and the unusual sight of hospital staff milling about outside in the street. He immediately feared that there had been a mine accident. A hospital orderly spotted Robert and rushed over to tell him the dreadful news.

"We've just had a phone call, Doctor, you must come at once. The mine has blown! It's terrible."

"Which mine? Where? Calm down, young man."

"Hillcrest, sir, she's blown up. The rescue teams are already there, but you must come! Chief Ford will take you in his motorcar."

As Police Chief Superintendent Ford picked Robert up and they swung onto the road that would carry them the ten miles west to

Hillcrest, they saw Dr. Connelly and other medical personnel coming out of the hospital carrying their medical bags and heading for the hastily harnessed horses and buggies.

Dr. Westwood, who was in charge of the hospital, called to Robert. "I'll stay here, Doctor Ross. We have a patient in surgery now who cannot be left alone, and I will get everything ready for the rescued miners when they arrive. There are two nurses remaining here to assist me. I have sent the rest of the staff to render first aid at the mine."

Robert shouted "Yes," in reply, and turned to Chief Ford to ask what information was available.

"Nothing more than what you just heard. We don't know much, but what we know sounds bad, really bad."

Robert, glad he had his medical bag with him, hung on as the motorcar careened along the rough mountain road to the mouth of the mine. They would learn all too soon of the terrible tragedy that had befallen the miners.

Oddly enough, when they arrived at the site, very few people in Hillcrest knew what had happened, and there were only about ten people at the opening of the mine. The first few miners who had escaped by way of Number 2 slope had just emerged, and they were followed by a very few more survivors. The news was worse, far worse than anything the community had dealt with before. Robert had heard rumours in the last few days that the miners at Hillcrest were concerned about a buildup of coal damp, creating methane gas that was often implicated in mine explosions, but they were only rumours. Accidents were an all-too-common part of his medical practice, as the miners' job was extremely dangerous with long days spent underground and mining companies that were reluctant to spend money on anything but what was needed to get the coal out of the ground. Safety, despite the efforts of the miners' unions, was often considered a frill. The Hillcrest pay of $145.00 per year was good for the times, so the men put up with difficult and often unsafe work places. Conditions such as these bred exhaustion as the miners struggled in the dark, sometimes lying on their backs and sides to extract the black gold from the seams beneath the earth.

But no one had any idea that morning of the magnitude of the disaster. Two hundred and thirty-seven miners had gone down into the mine at Hillcrest that morning. One hundred and ninety-five of them had died, either poisoned in the initial gas explosion or crushed by tons of rock when the mine caved in on top of them. Death had come to the Crowsnest with a terrible vengeance.

Of those who were rescued, only a few survived their terrible burns or their crushed and twisted bones and the poison gas and heat that had seared their lungs. The disaster left behind one hundred and thirty-nine widows, and four hundred fatherless children, and a shattered community. In the nightmare of the ensuing days, Robert and all the medical people in the surrounding areas spent long, gruelling hours at the hospital attempting to treat crushed bones, ruined lungs, and devastating burns, but in reality, little could be done for the survivors. There was never a satisfactory explanation of what had happened, but for the survivors and their families, it made little difference. Blame would not bring back fathers, husbands, and sons.

When Robert finally came home in the evenings, he could do nothing but sit in a state of exhausted despair, overcome by the loss of many friends and overwhelmed with the anguish of realizing that nothing he could do as a doctor would ever return these men to their families. Jennie and the boys left him to mourn in silence.

On Sunday, June 21, 1914, one hundred and ninety-six miners were laid to rest in a mass funeral, and the darkness of grief and loss gripped the towns of the Crowsnest Pass.

***

Nine days after the explosion, on June 28, an Austrian Archduke was assassinated in Sarajevo, and on August 4, after a long, uneasy summer, Britain declared war on Germany. Canada, a member of the Empire, was thus automatically at war and offered troops on August 6.

The Crowsnest Pass area, reeling from the Hillcrest explosion and the terrible loss of life, nevertheless saw their young men volunteer to join the Canadian Expeditionary Force. Those remaining in the little mountain town watched solemnly as these brave men left for Europe. Coleman was now a sombre place of older men, women, and children.

Robert could not go overseas with the CEF. He was now forty-four years old, and to Jennie's great relief, the decision was made at the hospital that his services as a doctor were needed more in the Crowsnest area than in Europe as other, younger doctors left for the Front.

Jennie and the ladies of all the church groups did everything possible to help the grief-stricken and bereft families, along with whatever they were called upon to do for the war effort. They also prayed that the war, so far away, would end soon.

For a time, it seemed as though it might, but Christmas 1914 came and went, and still the war raged on. The Ross family tried to celebrate Christmas, but it was a solemn affair. The boys loaded their sleds with boxes of food and other goods that had been collected by the churches and delivered these to families whose men had either died in the mine explosion or had gone overseas.

Jennie and Robert continued their daily routine of talking about Canadian and world affairs every evening when Robert came home from his office hours. They also discussed medical matters and, in particular, advances being made in field hospitals. One of the outcomes of battlefield medicine was an accelerated rate of development of new medicines and surgical techniques, and Robert knew that, horrible though the war was, this new knowledge would also be valuable to doctors on the home front.

Both Robert and Jennie were terribly worried by the European conflict and the toll it was taking on the young men of the country and on the families left behind. They could also see that Coleman was no longer the prosperous thriving community it had been before the war, and perhaps it never would be again.

Jennie, much as she sympathized with the sadness in the town, was also concerned about her family. "I know that you are still busy here,

Robert, but I am concerned about the children's schooling. I don't think the population will sustain a larger school and better teachers, and Gordon is simply not being challenged enough."

"I am also concerned, Jennie, but you know I agreed to remain here for the duration of the war. And Gordon is not working as hard at his studies as he could. Perhaps we should investigate the possibility of a tutor to help him focus?"

"Yes, Robert, thank you, that is a fine idea. I will begin the search for a suitable tutor immediately." Jennie paused then spoke again. "Surely the war will be over soon. I heard many people saying that by next Christmas, the Germans will be defeated and the soldiers will come home."

"One hopes so, my dear, one hopes so."

The telephone rang, which at this hour of the evening almost certainly meant a maternity case. Robert told the midwife he would be there soon, and as the patient's house outside of town was well off the road, he saddled his horse and set off in the cold mountain night. It had been nine months since the soldiers set off to war, and many babies were now arriving, keeping the local midwives busy.

For the next two years, as everyone coped as best they could with their changed lives, Robert quietly investigated the possibility of moving elsewhere. Unlike Jennie, he was not interested in relocating to one of the larger centres, such as Calgary or Edmonton. He much preferred a smaller place, somewhere with open country and room to establish his own medical practice.

"For now," he thought, "we must remain in Coleman, but I will keep looking for opportunities to move elsewhere when this terrible war ends."

Chapter 14
A Birthday and a Dog Bite

A fine May afternoon found Jennie and Robert strolling along the boardwalks through the town centre. They were a handsome couple. Robert, at nearly six feet, was almost a foot taller than his petite wife. He wore his Sunday best, a dark suit with a vest, and Jennie was in her finest skirt and jacket of maroon wool and high-necked white lawn blouse with her birthday present from Robert, a beautiful cameo, at her throat.

Her large black straw hat shaded her face from the welcome warmth of the spring sun as they walked along the village streets.

The birthday stroll this Sunday was made even more special by Hannah's gift to Mrs. Ross. Though the housekeeper usually had Sunday afternoon off, she had offered to take the boys visiting with her as her present for Jennie.

"I think Hannah may have a young man, Robert. Do you know anything of him? I hear he is a farmer's son and a fine young person."

"Yes, I know the family, and he is a hard worker and a good man. He was invalided out when a shell blew his left hand off, and he is now classified as essential labour on his father's farm. He did not go back overseas, which I know he found hard to bear, but someone has to grow food for the troops. As this dreadful war continues, I think he may be one of the lucky ones, though he probably does not agree."

As they strolled along, Robert's thoughts turned to Hannah who had been with them since Douglas was a toddler. She was a kind, plain-faced, hardworking young woman, who had given them very good service and was now an integral part of their family. Douglas adored her and would miss her if she left, but it was no doubt time for her to have a home of her own. Robert shrugged away his concerns about how Hannah's departure would affect Douglas; the boy was at school now. Jennie would find someone else. There were always young women looking for work.

Their steps led them westward, and as they greeted other couples out for a Sunday stroll after church, Robert looked up at the mountains and suddenly felt a great wave of restlessness sweep over him. He stopped abruptly and gazed longingly at the mountain pass ahead.

"What is it? Why are we stopping? Are you all right?"

"Oh, it's nothing, really nothing. I just realized that we have been in Coleman now for five years. They have been good years, haven't they?" He smiled at his trim little wife who was looking at him in some alarm with questions leaping in her dark blue eyes.

"No, no, Jennie," he answered her unasked question, "we are not moving anywhere, this is our home, and we are very happy here." He paused thoughtfully then went on, "And, of course, we must remain in Coleman until the end of this wretched war."

Jennie, who had been praying daily for the end of the war, experienced a sudden conflict of emotions. She was happy in Coleman, especially now that Gordon was doing so well with his tutor, and the implications of Robert's remark made her uneasy. Must they move again?

Firmly, she changed the subject. "Let us walk on, Robert. You have been looking for a larger space for your medical practice. Have you found a suitable building?"

"Not yet, but I will. Yes, we will walk a little further, but we will have to go home soon. Remember Hannah and the boys have planned a birthday tea for you, and we must not be late. Have I told you how lovely you look today? The cameo is particularly fine and suits you."

He had another niggling concern that had been awakened by Jennie's remark about Hannah and that was Gordon's teasing of his younger brother. "I suppose it's normal," he silently considered, "but I must speak to him and to Jennie. It is a little on the cruel side sometimes. I don't like that."

He did not want to spoil the birthday so said nothing. He also pushed away the unpleasant realization that his wife often ignored Gordon's behaviours towards Douglas and that she had never shown the same affection for her younger son as she lavished on Gordon. However, they had almost reached home by this time, and he knew that now was not the time for such a discussion. Time enough for that after Jennie's special day.

Within a few months, the new office space was found. It was a well-lit, recently vacated shoe store that fronted a dusty downtown street, and Robert moved his busy practice and settled in for the duration of the war. But his need to move on had been reawakened.

Time passed, and whenever he had a few moments for reflection in his busy life, Robert thought about the possibility of moving elsewhere. He liked Coleman very much and was completely involved in the life of the town, but the urge to move on grew more insistent.

He knew that when the time came, Jennie would prefer a larger centre, such as Edmonton or Calgary with their colleges and universities, but that was not for him.

He had spent some time in Michel, a little mountain village a few hours to the west, consulting on surgical cases, and the British Columbia location was tempting but still too small. A return to Lethbridge was not an option as that city had endured more typhoid epidemics. Also, though the fresh mountain air and clean water of Coleman had initially drawn him away from the prairies, he loved the open plains and wanted to return to them in the future.

He had heard of a town to the north and east of Coleman called Drumheller, also a coal mining and farming town that was growing rapidly. Its population was increasing as miners, ranchers, and farmers continued to head west, even as the war in Europe dragged on. He found Drumheller quite appealing, and its size and increasing prosperity boded well for him.

Jennie, who was torn between her desire to stay in the mountain town and her worries about the lack of educational opportunities for Gordon in Coleman, was mollified when Robert told her again that nothing would happen until the war was over.

"And before we move anywhere, Jen," he continued, "if we move, and that is not certain yet, we will take the train back East to visit our families. I know you were deeply grieved when your father died, and you could not go home to comfort your step-mother."

With that, she had to be content. What neither of them imagined was that it would be over two long years before the Armistice of November 1918.

**

Surgery at the Miners Union Hospital and other hospitals in the Pass area formed the larger part of Robert's medical practice, but the usual illnesses and injuries meant he was always busy at his office. This snowy January morning in 1916, after dealing with a boy who had suffered a severe dog bite, Robert strode rapidly home from his office to warn his family about the dangers posed by these feral animals.

There were few people in the streets; it was very cold, and the shoppers and townsfolk were keeping home because a pack of wild dogs had been running through the town almost every day for the last week. The town doctors had been cleaning and dressing bites on a regular basis, and the *Coleman Bulletin* was calling for action from the police.

Robert stamped the snow off his boots as he entered the warm kitchen and hung his coat on the drying rack by the stove. "Where are the boys, Hannah?"

"Riding their sleds on the hill, Doctor, the one just at the end of the street."

"Why are they not in school?"

"Boiler's not working again, sir."

"Please call them home right away, and where is Mrs. Ross?"

"I'll get the boys, sir. And Mrs. Ross has gone with Miss Yuill to her regular church accounts meeting. The ladies will be home for lunch in about an hour."

Robert was pleased to hear that his wife had ventured out this morning. Jennie found it difficult to cope with her aching joints, and her black moods increased during the dark days and long nights of January. Going to the meetings at the church was essential, both for the walk and for the social time it afforded her. Her position as unofficial bookkeeper also kept her mind engaged, and her financial skills were much appreciated.

"Thank you, Hannah, please call the boys. I'll have my meal later with Miss Yuill and Mrs. Ross."

Hannah hastily donned her galoshes and warm coat and headed up the street, returning in minutes with two rosy-cheeked youngsters pulling their sleds and grumbling just a bit about having to come home early.

Their questions tumbled out at the sight of their father standing in the kitchen where a small fire in the black iron stove kept the room warm. Surprised and pleased to see him home this early in the day, they looked at him expectantly as they peeled off their coats and mittens and handed them to Hannah to be hung to dry, talking all the time.

"Hello Father. Why are you home so early? And why did we have to come home? It's not time for lunch yet. Is Mother all right?"

"Your mother is fine, boys. Come sit here by the fire with me. I need to talk to you about the dogs in town."

"Yes, sir, we have seen them, sir." Gordon blurted. "Have they bitten someone else?"

"Wait a moment, Douglas," Robert held up his hand as his younger son began to ask a question.

"Gordon," Robert looked steadily at his son. "Someone else? You know about this? Then you must know that they are not pets, and you must not go near them."

"Yes, sir," Douglas interrupted, "Billy Scott was bitten last week. Doctor Connelly fixed it. Billy showed us. It really looked sore."

"Well," Robert stated, "I have just had to 'fix' a very severe bite, and there have been too many attacks. I am surprised that you have not mentioned this to me." At this, the boys looked at one another, their glance revealing their worries that their outdoor activities might be curtailed as their father continued, "I want you to be very careful, and come home immediately if you see any sign of these animals again."

"Yes, sir," Gordon was eager to get back to his friends on the snowy hillside and looked longingly at Hannah, hoping for an early lunch, but dutifully continued, "We'll be careful. May we eat our lunches now? Do you think Mother would mind?"

Douglas, always eager to know the details of his father's medical matters, asked. "How did you fix it, sir? Was there a lot of blood? I bet it hurt."

Robert turned to the eight-year-old and shook his head but smiled as he answered. "We'll talk about this later, Douglas. This evening. I promise I'll tell you all about it. For now, Hannah will give you your lunches, and you may go back outside. But be careful. And Gordon, look after your brother."

He then pulled on his overcoat and boots and spoke to Hannah. "I am going to meet Mrs. Ross and Miss Yuill and walk back with them. We will have our meal when we return."

Later that evening, true to his promise, Robert described the event and how he had dealt with it to Douglas. The boys by now knew who had been bitten. News of the incident had travelled like wildfire through the town and was the talk of the snowy hill where all the children had been sledding that afternoon.

Gordon was not interested in his father's medical practice but sat at the table working on a mathematical problem with his mother, who listened to her husband as she helped her older son.

"As you know, the young fellow was running errands for his mother. Just near the bank, he was set upon by two dogs. A man who saw the attack beat the dogs off with his stout cane and then brought the lad to my office."

Eager for details, Douglas sat in the other chair by the fire across from his father, "What did it look like, sir? Was there lots of blood? Was he, I mean, did he cry? Gosh, I bet it hurt."

Robert, always happy to teach his sons, continued, "There was some blood, Douglas, but most of it was soaked up by his woollen trouser leg, and, no, he did not cry, though it was painful. The body has a mechanism called shock that prevents feeling pain at first, and he was obviously in a state of shock."

"Then what, sir, what did you do?"

"First, the nurse and I cut off his trouser leg above his knee. The bites were just below the knee, and his pant leg was badly torn and very grubby."

"You cut his trousers? Won't his mother be angry?"

Robert chuckled. "Of course not, Douglas. She knew I had to do that. And you do know, don't you, how very important it is that wounds are kept clean?"

Douglas nodded vigorously, "Were they real wounds? Like a soldier's? Gosh."

"Douglas!"

"Sorry, Mother."

Behind his mother's back, Gordon muttered, "Silly baby," and smirked at his younger brother, who had fallen silent at the reprimand and now looked warily at his mother. Robert, who saw the smirk and noticed Douglas's instant silence, looked over at his wife and shook his head slightly, indicating his displeasure at the interruption. "I really must talk to Jennie this evening about this teasing," he thought as he smiled reassuringly at Douglas.

"It's all right to ask your questions, Son. I'll tell you the rest." He continued, describing the process of cleaning and dressing the bites with enough details to satisfy the boy's curiosity.

Gordon, listening despite himself, shuddered, but Douglas urged his father on, "Oh, that must have hurt! Then what, sir, what next? Did you stitch it up?"

"Yes, and I used loose stitches to allow the wound to heal without pulling. Remember that, Douglas, loose, not tight, stitches. A doctor's job is always to help the body heal itself."

"Yes, sir. Then what?"

"The other punctures from the dog's teeth were too small to need stitches. We put sterile dressings on the wounds to keep them clean. He is young and healthy and will heal in a week or so."

Douglas sat considering the story for a moment, then, "How about his trousers, sir?"

Robert laughed out loud. "By this time, the lad's mother had arrived with a pair of his older brother's trousers, which he pulled on before limping out of the office. He was sleepy from the stress and shock, but I know his mother will look after him, and he will be fine. I gave her some aspirin tablets to give to the boy because his leg will be sore for the next few days."

Jennie looked up from her work with Gordon. She did not approve of Robert encouraging Douglas's interest in medicine but agreed that the boys needed to know how serious a dog bite could be. "I hope your father's words have made you both aware of the danger, and you will be very watchful."

"Yes, Mother," the boys chorused. Douglas mournfully realized that his own dream of owning a puppy was probably not going to come true.

"What are the police going to do about these wild dogs?" his mother asked.

"Probably shoot them, Jennie. There have been too many dog bites lately. No one has claimed the dogs, and the animals are starving. So far, we have been fortunate that the bites have not been too serious, but sooner or later someone is going to be badly mauled by this pack. It is worrisome."

Robert ruffled his younger son's hair, thick and black and curly, just like his mother's. He nodded more formally to Gordon, who at twelve had decided he was too old for displays of parental affection.

"Time for bed, boys. Your mother and I have matters to discuss."

The boys gathered up their homework and trudged upstairs to bed. Hannah brought more tea for Robert and Jennie, and they settled into their chairs by the fire.

The first matter that Jennie wished to discuss was the recent passage of a bill giving women the right to vote in Alberta. She had been firmly in favour of its passage but knew that most of the men in Coleman, and many of their wives, had not. She wanted to talk to Robert about any implications her public support for the legislation might have for his practice. Before she could speak, though, Robert pulled a telegram from his pocket.

"Oh no, Robert. What is it?" A telegram rarely meant good news in these years, so Jennie clasped her hands tightly together and braced against the possibility of sorrow.

"It is from my brother, George, in London, in regard to the Shackleton mission. He was to go as a dog driver, on loan from the Hudson's Bay Company, but it seems he will not be going to the South Pole after all. Instead, he is going to France, I assume as an Army surgeon. I fear his chances of survival might have been better in Antarctica."

"Why is he not going with Shackleton? What does the telegram say?"

Robert silently handed her the creased yellow paper.

"Plans changed. Not wanted on the voyage. France instead. George."

As they sat in bemused silence, the telephone rang, and Hannah came into the room to let the doctor know he was needed at the hospital, so any discussion about voting and about Gordon's teasing and Douglas's increasing silences would have to wait.

By the time Robert had walked through the snow to the hospital, his thoughts had already turned from his brother and his sons to the patient who waited for him.

Chapter 15
The Halifax Explosion

When Robert arrived home from work late on a snowy afternoon in December 1917, he found his wife sitting silently by the fire, her face a mask of grief and shock.

"What is it? Has something happened to the boys? Jennie, what's the matter?"

Jennie raised her tear-streaked face to her husband and whispered, "No, the boys are fine. They are in the kitchen with Hannah, but, Robert, the news from Halifax? Have you not heard?"

"What news from Halifax? I've been busy all day and have heard nothing. Tell me."

In a monotone, Jennie described what she had heard several hours ago at the telegraph office. "Robert, there has been a terrible explosion in Halifax. We did not hear about it right away because the telegraph lines have been so badly damaged by the fire that only relatives of those killed were informed right away. But it is desperately bad news for thousands of families across this country. Over sixteen hundred people are dead, Robert. Two ships collided in the harbour, they exploded, the city is almost destroyed, homes gone, fires, terrible burn victims! Oh, those poor, poor people."

Robert called to Hannah, "Bring us more hot tea and put extra sugar in Mrs. Ross's cup and more wood for the fire." He quickly wrapped a shawl around his wife who was shivering, though the room was warm. He remembered how upset she had been when news of the sinking of the Titanic had reached them in 1912. "Jennie, you are suffering from shock. How long have you been sitting here like this? You know you must not get cold. When did you hear about it? What a dreadful thing."

He shrugged off his coat and built up the fire talking all the time. "I will telephone the editor of the *Bulletin* to see whether more news has come in on the wire service. I am sure there will be a relief fund, and we will contribute. Now, are you feeling any warmer?"

Jennie assured him. "Yes, I am starting to feel a little warmer. Hannah brought me tea and built up the fire earlier when I arrived home, but I was too distressed to talk about this with her. I have been sitting here for the past few hours, struggling to understand how this could happen. I did not notice how much time had passed, nor did I realize how cold I had become."

"This horrible news has shaken you badly, my dear. Perhaps Miss Yuill would come over for supper with us, and you could pray together?" Robert paused, considered this and spoke again, "And we need to talk to the boys about what has happened. It will be all over the town very shortly, and they should hear from it first from us. Gordon especially is already too worried about war and death."

Jennie's good friend from church arrived, the women prayed together, and then the rest of the evening was passed in sombre discussion of the tragic events in Halifax. Both boys were very quiet as they examined the map to find far-off Halifax and listened to the adults' sad conversation.

"Could it happen here?" Douglas asked his brother as they went up to their beds.

"No, silly, we don't have a harbour or boats."

"But there was a big explosion in the mines when I was six. I remember that. Lots of people were killed, and Dad and Mother were very sad."

"Yes, but we don't go down the mines. Go to sleep, or Dad will hear us."

But both boys lay awake for a long time worrying about the explosion and all the people who had died.

***

Through the winter months of 1917, Jennie and Robert continued their evening routine of discussing Canadian and world affairs when Robert came home from his office hours. They also discussed medical matters as Robert, with Jennie's assistance, continued to study everything new in medicine. This evening, their medical discussion centred around a discovery made by a Dr. Alex Carrel. He had found that irrigation of wounds using a solution of hypochlorite ensured that sterilization of the injury was achieved with a minimum of disturbance of the healing process.

"I will be able to use that technique for mining injuries, Jennie. What else have you discovered in your reading of medical news?"

Jennie looked through the papers in her lap.

"A Doctor Winnett Orr has developed a therapeutic technique where he uses Vaseline and loose bandaging to coat a surgical incision. Shall I see if I can learn more about this method for you?"

"That would also be most useful, thank you."

Even with the tutor they had hired for Gordon, Jennie continued to worry about her older son's education, putting his increasing irritability and rebellious behaviour down to boredom. As they talked about the war, she realized she had begun to seriously consider moving to a larger centre as Robert had suggested some time ago.

"I know that your practice is still busy, Robert, but I am concerned about Gordon's schooling. I don't think the population here will sustain a larger school and better teachers, and even with his tutor, Gordon is still not being challenged enough. Could we not move to a bigger place when the war is over, somewhere there will be more educational opportunities for the boys?"

Her husband, surprised at her suggestion, did not answer for a moment as he considered his own worries about Gordon. He, too, had noticed an increasing lethargy and irritability about his older son, and it seemed the teasing of Douglas was getting worse, no matter how often he reprimanded Gordon.

"I am also concerned, but you know I must remain here for now. And Gordon is not working as hard at his studies as he could, even with the tutor."

"Robert, I know you have been thinking about moving elsewhere. I heard on the wireless again that by next Christmas the war will be finished."

"One hopes so, my dear, one hopes so. But on the matter of Gordon's behaviour..."

Before the discussion could go any further, the telephone rang, and Jennie overheard Robert telling the midwife that he would be on his way immediately. Worries about Gordon and a possible move were over for now. War or no war, babies were still arriving.

Over the next months, Robert, pleased to know that his wife was not as reluctant to move from Coleman as he had feared, intensified his efforts to find a suitable community to set up a new medical practice.

Chapter 16
A Pandemic

Before the longed-for peace arrived, however, another disaster struck the Crowsnest Pass area, and indeed the whole of Canada and much of Europe. In the fall of 1918 when the dreaded Spanish 'Flu epidemic broke out in the other towns in the Pass area, the town fathers of Coleman made every effort to keep the sickness at bay. Acting on the advice of the medical personnel at the Miners Union Hospital, the councilmen decided to try to keep the epidemic out by placing the town under a strict quarantine. Travellers getting off the train were told that the town was under quarantine and were escorted back onto the train from which they had just disembarked.

Robert also made plans for his family's welfare. "Jennie, the boys must not go to school, and no one else is to come to the house. You must get in supplies for at least two weeks, preferably a month or more. Fortunately, we have all the goods you and Hannah have put up in jars over the summer."

"Let us pray that the town escapes, Robert, and also pray for all those families in the world who have been struck by this vicious plague. I have heard that the influenza has killed more soldiers than are dying on the battlefield. Could that be true?"

"I don't know, Jennie, but I know it is terrible."

All surgery from out of town was cancelled, and for two weeks the town quarantine worked well. While neighbouring towns were in the clutches of the epidemic, Coleman remained healthy.

Then one Sunday morning, a man who worked in the Coleman mines and lived on the edge of town, decided to go and visit a relative in Burmis, a village about fifteen miles to the east of Coleman. He took the early morning train and spent the day with his friends and relatives. When he returned to Coleman that evening, the police tried to get him back on the train, but he explained that he was from Coleman and lived on the outskirts of town, in an area called Bushtown. The police allowed him to disembark.

The miner went to work early the next morning and put in his full shift then, feeling desperately ill, returned to his home. In the middle of that same afternoon, Robert received a telephone call he had been dreading for a month. It was the miner's wife, and when she described her husband's symptoms, Robert feared that the epidemic may have finally arrived in Coleman.

Knowing that he must act quickly to contain the disease if it was indeed the 'flu, Robert rushed to the miner's shack. Once there, he was left with little doubt that it was Spanish Influenza.

Robert made the miner as comfortable as possible and told the man's wife, "Your husband is very ill. No one, including the children, must leave the house. Give him water and these quinine and aspirin tablets and use cold cloths to try to reduce the fever. I will call in to see him tomorrow."

Robert immediately went home to warn his own wife of the danger. "Jennie, it has come. It is even more important now that no one goes out. Keep the house warm, we have a good supply of firewood, and be sure everyone continues to eat well. The boys can go outside to play in the backyard, but no one, I must repeat, no one, may visit here."

Jennie understood what was happening but felt that she should be able to assist through the work of the church.

Robert, who rarely had to raise his voice, did so now. "Jennie, your job is to look after our household. It is truly a matter of life or death.

This is so serious. You know this influenza is a killer. Do not leave the house, and do not let any of our household leave. Am I understood?"

Jennie, shaken by her husband's unusual vehemence, nodded silently.

"Good," Robert said, reassured. "I must go now to the hospital to let everyone else know."

The next morning, Robert returned to the miner's home and knocked. A thin voice came from inside the shack, "Everybody is sick. We can't leave our beds."

The family consisted of the miner, his wife, and his six children, and when Robert let himself in, he found that truly they were all so sick that no one was able to get up to keep the fire going. It was late autumn in the mountains, snow covered the ground, and the house was terribly cold. There was plenty of wood on hand, and Robert went to work building a good fire then left a pile of wood inside the house within easy reach.

"Here are more quinine and aspirin tablets for each of you. As soon as I can, I will send someone with broth to leave outside your door. The first person who is well enough to get up must feed everyone else."

Suddenly, there was a hammering on the door. Another miner's boy stood there, shivering in the cold. "Doctor, you must come right away. My pa worked with Bill here, and he is sick, terrible sick. So is Mr. Dark from Pa's shift."

Robert realized his efforts to contain the epidemic had failed. He found both these men and their families suffering from the same illness. "Keep the house warm and drink lots of fluids. Here are quinine and aspirin tablets for every patient." He wished he could offer more, but there was nothing else he could do.

Within the next few hours, Robert visited a dozen families who had caught the disease in that same mine. He returned to the hospital to pick up more tablets and found that all of the doctors and nurses were also out tending to people who had succumbed. In three days, there were so many patients that no one could keep track of the numbers. The most severe patients were admitted to the hospital, but there was little that could be done for them. The death toll mounted, but there was no time to spare for the dead. Bodies were stacked in sheds where they would remain frozen until they could be buried.

The days blurred together as the horror continued. Early one morning at about two o'clock, the phone rang in Robert's home. Under normal circumstances, Jennie would say nothing, but these were not normal times.

"Must you go? You have been home for only an hour, and you are so tired. I am afraid you will also catch the 'flu."

"Nevertheless, Jennie, go I must. This is a maternity patient of mine, and since it is her first baby, I fear it may be a long and difficult labour."

Such was the case, and it was close to nine o'clock the following night when Robert returned home. To his dismay, there were nearly fifty people waiting for his return on the sidewalk in front of his house. Robert knew that Dr. Westwood and all of the other medical personnel in the town were equally busy.

"I must wash and eat, and then I will help as many as I can," he promised as he entered his house.

Hannah had his meal ready, and Jennie and the two boys watched silently as their father ate and left again.

Most of Robert's patients were pathetically grateful for whatever he and the others were able to do to help them, but there was one patient, a miner, who, when Robert first saw him, was already so ill that he had begun to bleed from the lungs. Though Robert was working steadily with many patients, going from home to home to hospital, he made a point of seeing this particular patient every day. Finally, the man showed definite signs of recovery and, because there were other patients whose needs were far greater, Robert chose not to see him as often.

When the doctor failed to visit this miner for two days in a row, the man sent his boy to Robert's home at eleven o'clock at night. Robert, exhausted, had just returned from another hospital visit and had hoped for a meal and a short rest.

"My father is worse and wants you to call at once," announced the boy.

Robert's horse had already been unharnessed from the buggy, but he put the animal back in the traces. "Get in, lad, I will take you with me," Robert said to the boy, and they went to make the call.

When they arrived at the house, the boy's father was partially sitting up in bed, leaning on his elbow, and obviously much improved. He whined at Robert, "You haven't been here for two days. Are you going to let me lie here and die like a dog?"

Robert looked at him in silence while he recovered from his own surprise. Then the accumulated weariness of the past weeks caught up to the doctor, and he snarled, "Yes, you can lie there and die like a dog, and go to hell after you are dead."

He then turned around and walked out the door, ignoring the frantic apologies of the miner's wife.

When he reached the sidewalk, he met the minister who was on his way to make a call next door. Robert wearily told Reverend Arthurs of his reception by the miner and what he had said to the man. "What would you have done in those circumstances, Reverend?"

"I would have liked to say exactly that, Doctor Ross, but probably would not have dared. It might have had a different effect coming from a man of the cloth. But good for you to do so."

The men smiled tired smiles and went on their way to the next patients who required their help.

It was weeks after the epidemic had ended before Robert heard from that miner again. The ungrateful fellow sent his boy to Robert to apologize for the way he had spoken on the doctor's last visit. Realizing that the boy could not be held responsible for the behaviour of his father, the doctor looked down at him and said, "Tell your father that I have been too busy to think about his rudeness. In any event, I believe I evened the matter up by telling him to go to Hell." Then with a smile for the worried youngster, he continued, "Tell him I have changed my mind; he needn't go."

At the height of the epidemic, the night trips had been the worst for Robert who had often found it impossible to stay awake. Fortunately for him, his horse would stop when the reins went slack, and the doctor, slightly refreshed, would waken and continue to the patient.

It had become necessary to hospitalize a number of patients who had no one to look after them, so the schoolhouse had been fitted out as a hospital, and the school teachers, who had no students since the schools were closed, had been asked to assist in the nursing under the supervision of a graduate nurse. All the teachers had volunteered except for one who had said she was afraid to catch the disease. Strange to say she was the only one among them who caught the 'flu and had to be brought to the hospital as a patient herself.

During the epidemic, Robert had purchased his first motorcar, an old Ford touring model. "Jennie," he had said, "I badly need a driver, but he must be a teetotaller, as I have to be able to trust that he will get me safely to my night calls without drinking."

Alcohol was considered by some to be an antidote to the influenza, and the powers that controlled its sale during Prohibition had relaxed their rules considerably on the distribution of liquor in towns struck by influenza. Many people, believing it would save them from the ravages of the 'flu took frequent preventative nips, some spending most of their days and nights quite soused, and Robert could not risk a drunken driver on his calls.

After several phone calls to members of her church group, Jennie had found him a first-class driver who was, like Robert, a teetotaller

"Thank you, my dear, you have found me a fine reliable fellow. He takes me where I have to go, and I can sleep in the back of the car and trust him to drive safely and awaken me when I get there."

Jennie, more and more concerned about her husband, was happy to have done something to make his days and nights a little easier. "You're welcome, Robert. He is an excellent man, and as you know he is also the town undertaker." She had smiled. "I am pleased that he will be driving you and thus ensuring that you do not become one of his customers."

As always in times of extreme danger, a little humour, however dark, often saved the day.

Frequently, there had been considerable difficulty in getting the patients to the hospital, so Robert and the hospital orderlies had obtained a stretcher and laid it across the two seats in the back of the car. The motorcar was of the type that allowed the top to be let down on the back end. When Robert and the attendants picked up a patient who needed hospital care, they were able to load him or her into the car through the open top and rush the person to the nearest available bed.

The 'flu was deadly to pregnant women, especially in their fourth to six months. One day, Robert and the attendants had been called to the Italian section of the miners' town to see a sick young woman who was pregnant and had the 'flu.

Loading her onto the stretcher and into the car, they had heard a frantic voice calling from across the street. "Doctor, you must come here. My wife is expecting a baby. She is very sick with the 'flu. Please help."

It was agony to make these decisions, but Robert had replied. "We can only carry one at a time, but we will return immediately after taking this woman to the hospital."

They had driven away hearing the miner's sad pleas behind them.

As soon as the first woman had been placed in her cot at the school house hospital, they had returned to pick up the second patient, who had been taken to the same building and placed alongside her neighbour. Sadly, both of them had miscarried and died a few hours after being admitted, within minutes of one another.

Beyond exhaustion, all the medical people of the Crowsnest Pass had continued to do their best for the sick and dying as the 'flu claimed victim after victim, including nurses and doctors.

"Pray for all of us, Jennie; pray that this will end soon." Robert had asked his wife when he stumbled home and into his bed after another night of sickness and death.

***

Late one evening a week later, as the number of patients seemed to be lessening, Robert arrived home hoping for a meal and a brief rest only to find a man leaning heavily on the gate.

"Don't get out of your motorcar, Doctor. I need you to come to my house at once. My wife is having a baby. We live about two miles from town, and our midwife now has the 'flu. There is no one at home, and my wife is having really bad birthing pains."

Robert sighed wearily but did not hesitate. "Just let me get what I need, and we will be on our way. Can you drive? If so, I will not send for my driver."

"Well, I can drive a tractor, Doc. A motorcar can't be so different," the farmer replied.

Robert instructed the man to keep the car idling so it would not have to be cranked again then hurried into his house, gathered his instruments, told his worried wife where he was going, and hastened back to the automobile.

"I think I'd better drive," Robert said, having considered the remark about the tractor. "Just keep me awake, and tell me how to get there."

They travelled as fast as the gravel roads and rough trails allowed to find on their arrival that the wife's pains had stopped and she was asleep. The one-room shack was very hot, and after examining the woman, Robert sat on a chair, rested his arms and head on top of the only table in the place, and immediately fell fast asleep.

When he was awakened a short while later by the intense heat of the fire, he saw that the expectant father was sitting as close to the stove as he could without burning himself. "Why are you hugging the stove?" Robert asked sleepily.

"I have been cold all day, Doctor, and I have begun to feel really poorly."

Sadly, knowing what was coming, Robert said, "Let me examine you, man. I think you have the 'flu."

Robert looked at the young mother-to-be, now deeply asleep, and made a difficult decision, knowing the man's illness was a great danger to her and the unborn child. "You are a sick man, sir. I will have to get you to the hospital. I don't want you here when the baby is born. We must go right away so I can be back quickly to help your wife."

By now, feeling too ill to protest, the father allowed Robert to bundle him into the motorcar, and they left, taking care not to disturb the sleeping woman.

Robert took the farmer to the hospital and drove back as fast as the roads allowed. When he returned, he found that the woman had awakened in his absence, very frightened to find herself alone and once again in the grip of labour pains. He resumed his place by her bedside, speaking reassuringly to her. "Rest as much as you can. Your husband has the 'flu, but he is being cared for, and I am here when you need me."

The pains subsided, and Robert fell asleep once more. He was awakened three hours later by the cries of the young mother.

"You are fine, and your baby will arrive soon. Just push when I tell you to, and relax as much as you can in between pains."

It was an easy birth after all the drama of the night, and the baby was born safely just before six in the morning. Robert had to melt snow on the stove for hot water to give the newborn his first bath, but all was well. When the baby boy and his mother were comfortably settled, the problem became finding someone who was able to stay with them and provide care while the father was in the hospital. This was no easy task, as so many were not yet well enough to leave their own beds.

"Mrs. Chalmers," Robert thought, "she had the 'flu early on, as did all of her children, and they are all quite recovered. I will ask her to come." Robert knew also that Mrs. Chalmers had lost her husband in the Hillcrest mining disaster some years earlier, and that she had proven herself to be a strong and resilient woman after that sad event.

He drove back to town, explained the situation to the widow, and asked for her help. Her answer was most heartening. "Of course,

Doctor Ross. Bessie is fifteen now and can look after the younger children. Just let me get some things together, and I will come with you to care for the new mother and baby."

As soon as she had joined Robert, he turned the automobile around and headed back for a third journey to the farmer's home and then once more back into town.

That evening, when Robert was finally able to eat and rest, he recounted the events of the past few days to Jennie. And a few weeks later, he was happy to tell her "All is going well with that family now, Jen. The farmer recovered within a week and went home, mother and baby are doing well, and the new father tells me that Mrs. Chalmers made a splendid nurse. Thank goodness, there is some happy news in this terrible time."

Robert made a point of seeking Mrs. Chalmers out as soon as he had time. "Thank you for your splendid services. I would like to pay you for what you have done."

"No, Doctor, you did not charge me for looking after my children when they were all ill with the 'flu. This is my small way to repay you for that kindness, and I will be godmother to the baby boy. It is good that there is new life in the midst of all this dying."

November arrived, and those who had survived took a collective breath of relief, counted their dead, supported fellow survivors, and hoped that the dreadful epidemic had finally passed.

Then it was November 11, 1918, and the news everyone had been longing for finally came. The war was over.

Chapter 17
Drumheller via Toronto

Although the Armistice had been signed and the European conflict had finally dragged itself to a painful, mud-soaked end, the suffering continued. Young men and women, terribly injured both physically and mentally, began arriving back in communities across the country, including Coleman. Robert, John Westwood, and the other medical men who were still grappling with the final throes of the 'flu epidemic now found themselves also dealing with the sad aftermath of the tragedy in Europe.

Everyone suffered in the small town. Those who returned with missing or damaged limbs and war-torn spirits, their wives and daughters, and their mothers and fathers all bore the brunt of the war's devastation. Life would not go on as before.

After the initial euphoria of their return passed, it was evident that many of these dazed and wounded young people would be incapable of working or supporting families.

The pain of limbs set in field hospitals overseas continued to torment the returning soldiers, or worse, the phantom pain experienced by amputees destroyed lives upon their return home.

One young man who had lost his lower leg to a shell burst came to Robert's office one afternoon seeking some relief from the pain of this "aching leg," but as Robert listened compassionately to his tale, he realized that far more than physical pain tormented the young man.

"I will give you morphia for the pain for the next couple of days, just to let you sleep, but you know it is terribly addicting, and I cannot give it to you for any longer than that. If you become addicted, that will help no one. You have seen what happens to your fellow soldiers when they cannot live without it."

"I know, Doctor Ross, I know, but I can't sleep, and I can't work, and my girl has left me, and...please."

Robert had carefully examined the recently healed stump when the young man first came into the office and concluded that the amputation had been performed by a competent surgeon. The wooden prosthesis was also well crafted, so while he felt that the soldier's pain was very real, he recognized that there was more involved here than phantom pain. "I can give you some salve to rub on your scars where your prosthesis has chafed. It will ease the pain there. But I think there is more to it than you have told me. Why can you not get work in the mines? They are crying out for workers." He knew the work force had been decimated when the young men went to war and again when the 'flu had taken so many lives of older men who had not gone to the Front.

The young soldier sat stoically for a few moments, then to his own horror, broke down, and almost sobbing, wailed, "I cannot go underground, Doctor Ross. I just can't. There was a cave-in when the shell hit my trench, and it took my leg and buried me alive. I just can't go underground again."

Robert knew his pity was not what the soldier required so spoke bracingly. "Get hold of yourself, man. You are young and still strong, and the farms around here are crying out for farmhands. It's hard work, but you'll be out-of-doors, the wages are decent, and your leg will not stop you from working the land. You'll sleep much better with hard labour and fresh air than with morphia. Now, here's the name of a farmer just south of town who is looking for workers. Catch up on your sleep, then see him and tell him I sent you. I'm certain he will hire you, and you need not fear having to work in the mines."

Some months later, Robert passed the man walking along the main street of Coleman, looking fit and healthy and with an attractive young lady on his arm. The ex-soldier tipped his hat politely to the doctor and smiled his thanks.

"Good," thought Robert as he smiled and tipped his hat in return, remembering his own experiences as a young man regaining his health in the woods of northern Ontario. "Fresh air and hard work are good medicine for body and soul. My 'prescription' has done its job."

Accidents in the mines and on the farms continued to occur as 1918 slowly became 1919. The doctors were very busy. Morning surgery was usually spent caring for the needs of the returning soldiers as well as the usual accidents and ills of the townsfolk, and the afternoon and evening clinics were similarly well attended.

"Too well attended, really." Robert said to Dr. Westwood. "We need at least another doctor and more nurses." But he knew they were hard to find just now. "Perhaps when the nursing sisters have all returned from overseas, we will be able to hire some for Coleman."

Robert was very aware of the returning doctors as he had continued to look and think about moving to a new place. He knew he would have to make his decision soon. For some time, he had been quietly investigating the possibilities offered by a small town called Drumheller, located about two hundred miles northeast of Coleman.

Robert was ready to move again. As always, his restless spirit drove him on, and they had been nearly ten years in Coleman. He doubted that the town would prosper as the war's end meant the country no longer required coke in huge quantities. As the town's main source of revenue, this would have significant economic impact on the area. He also knew that the government of Alberta had decided to fund the building of a Municipal Hospital in Drumheller, locating it there because of the high incidence of mining injuries in the area. For Robert, this would be an excellent opportunity to use the surgical skills honed in Lethbridge and Coleman, and it also presented him with the opportunity to be instrumental in setting up a new hospital in a much larger region.

He knew that despite her own concerns about Gordon's schooling and what she saw as his need for a more challenging curriculum, Jennie would still be reluctant to leave Coleman. She had settled into life there, made some good friends, and was very active in St Paul's United Church, where she and the other ladies had contributed to the war effort and continued to support the community.

In truth, both boys were doing very well in school. They were bright lads. Gordon was fascinated by numbers and, ever his mother's favourite, was considered by her to be absolutely brilliant. She was anxious about getting him even more tutoring, and Robert was hopeful that she would see this move as an opportunity for educational advancement for Gordon. He knew her preference would be Edmonton, a university town, but he hoped that the idea of relocating to a rapidly growing centre, such as Drumheller, would soften the blow of another move. And he had no desire to live in a big city, such as Edmonton or Calgary. Having made his decision, he began to plan.

Douglas was also an excellent student, although his interests lay more in the mechanical area. He was forever constructing something in their yard. His mother called these projects "Douglas's messes," but Robert encouraged him in his engineering efforts. Douglas also continued to evidence keen interest in what his father did, and Robert quietly and patiently answered his questions about the medical practice, taking great joy in his younger son's inquiring mind.

Gordon's erratic behaviour was worrying his father more and more. Although Jennie put the boy's increasing irritability and bouts of lethargy down to his brilliance and his age, Robert was now convinced that there was an underlying physical reason. Sadly, he believed he knew what it was. There was no gentle way to say it, although Robert understood that it would be a huge blow to his wife.

"My dear, we need to discuss Gordon's health. I'm afraid he may be developing childhood diabetes, and the only thing we can do to slow down the progression of the disease is to carefully control what he eats and be sure he gets sufficient rest and exercise. The boy's diet needs to be strictly controlled and a very strict regimen established for his sleeping and periods of rest."

It was a terribly frightening idea, and Jennie at first refused to accept it. "No, Robert, you can't be correct. He is only a boy going through a stage. He'll grow out of it. Please say you are mistaken."

Robert's own heart was breaking as he thought about the death sentence diabetes mellitus posed for his boy, but he kept his voice steady as he continued, "Jennie, I'm a doctor. This condition is unusual in one so young but not unknown. I've seen it in hospitals in the East and treated it in Montreal at the Children's Hospital at McGill, and Gordon has all the symptoms of the early stages of this disease."

Jennie wept, then rallied. She rarely defied Robert, always deferring to his position of authority as her husband and to his medical knowledge, but this time, she wanted desperately for him to be wrong. "I think you are mistaken, Robert. However, if you think his behaviour is caused by this disease, rather than just his age, we'll take him to the East and seek a second opinion. I refuse to believe it's diabetes."

But Jennie had been a doctor's wife for many years, and as such, had done her own research on many conditions, including this one. Unwilling to recognize the symptoms she had been observing in her own child, once Robert had spoken, she could no longer ignore the possibility. Although she had challenged Robert's diagnosis, her own fears now came to the surface. "Please, Robert, say he'll be all right," she pleaded. "Please, Robert, please. I have to have some hope."

"My dear, of course we can certainly take him to the University Hospital in Toronto and see what the doctors there have to say, but meanwhile you must control his diet, especially his sugar consumption."

Gordon, at fifteen already an indulged and rebellious youngster, resisted all efforts to follow the regime his mother devised. Sugar made him feel better, if only temporarily, and he certainly didn't want to go to bed when Douglas did. He did not understand what was happening to him and was very angry at his bouts of illness and the unfairness of it all.

A trip to Ontario before they moved to Drumheller was planned for the beginning of September, and the family spent the summer months packing their belongings in preparation for the move. Robert had made several journeys to Drumheller already. He had found a house there for them to rent and had met a Dr. McGregor who was looking for a partner. On one of his journeys to see their new town, he took both of the boys with him, and he made sure the trip coincided with the date of the first Drumheller Stampede. The three of them had a wonderful time, and both boys reported gleefully to their mother on their return.

Douglas immediately threw himself into every book on dinosaurs he could find in the little Coleman Library and questioned Jennie about the subject nonstop. Gordon's interests lay more in the number of motorcars they had seen on the streets of the town, and he began talking wisely about miles per gallon and which would be the best motorcar to buy. Robert had already decided to buy a used Ford similar to the one he had in Coleman but said no more on the subject now. He made arrangements to have their household goods moved to their rental home in Drumheller while they were on their journey to the East.

Hannah had decided to marry her young man and would remain in Coleman, so Robert had obtained the services of a new housekeeper-cook to meet them on their arrival in Drumheller.

Jennie had initially resisted the move to another prairie town of dust and heat. She hated the idea of leaving her friends and the life she had constructed for herself and family in Coleman. But she was now so distraught by her concern for Gordon that she acquiesced to the plans with little discussion.

She knew this would be a quick trip East so Gordon could be examined by the doctors in Toronto and then back west so that Robert could begin his new medical practice before the end of September. However, she was also eager to go to Ontario to see her remaining family, and Robert agreed that this was important.

The diagnosis in Toronto confirmed what Robert and Jennie already knew. It was diabetes, and the treatment was as Robert had prescribed. Little could be done beyond careful diet and rest, but again, Jennie's medical research, plus Robert's inquiring mind and his well-maintained network of medical colleagues led them to explore the work of a brilliant doctor-scientist named Frederick Banting at the University of Toronto. Banting and his colleague, Dr. Best, were working towards a possible treatment for diabetes.

This information gave Robert and Jennie some hope for their son's future, though they would have to wait for Banting and Best to make more progress in their research before any real help for Gordon and others like him would be available. To further ease their anxiety and to help Jennie cope with the distressing confirmation of their fears about Gordon, they planned to stop in Sudbury on their way home so that Jennie could visit with those of her cousins who still lived there.

After their stay in Sudbury, Robert had scheduled a stop in Sault Ste Marie to attend the Grand Opening of the Welland Canal, where they would view His Royal Highness The Prince of Wales and the Canadian Prime Minister, Sir Robert Borden.

The visit to Sudbury lasted too long for Robert. The plight of the post-war city was a shock. His memories of 1908 were of a small bustling city with new immigrants arriving by train and a mining industry promising wealth for all. By 1919, those same industries had stripped the surrounding areas of trees for fuel resulting in a near total loss of natural vegetation. The streets of the town were scarred with gaping vacant storefronts, and the pink and grey granite rocky outcroppings of his youth were now stained a permanent black from pollution carried by the rain.

The surrounding lakes of his boyhood memories were devoid of fish, and the demand for copper and nickel during the war meant Sudbury was now a grimy industrial town dominated by towering stacks of smelters. Coleman also had coke ovens but nothing on the scale of those in Sudbury.

There was also a sense of desperation in the city as the realization that the end of the war signalled the end of the demand for copper and nickel that had brought prosperity to the area. Miners and merchants alike knew that the booming economic times were over.

And there was a seemingly permanent drizzle, washing the city in tones of grey. Robert had planned to take his sons with him into the surrounding countryside while Jennie visited her relatives. He had thought they might perhaps revisit his old home at Whitefish Lake, but fearing that he would find the place similarly blackened, he decided instead to get them out of the house by simply taking them for long walks.

There were still trees in the residential areas, though they, too, struggled with the grimy air. The gardens were well cared for, and he did find the house of a family he had known as a young man, but the Howeys were not at home. He and the boys continued to trudge along the dreary streets in silence, until finally the day came when they could board the train to continue their trip west to Sault Ste Marie.

Feeling ill and out of sorts most of the time now, Gordon was so angry to be afflicted by this strange disease that he had little interest in the trip to the Welland Canal. Douglas, now eleven, was absolutely delighted to see all the machinery and peered excitedly out of the portholes of the ship in which they travelled down the canals. He marvelled at the huge cranes towering over the shipyards and chatted animatedly with his father, who thoroughly enjoyed the boy's enthusiasm and the time they spent together on the journey.

Jennie had spent most of the train trip East in a torment of worry about her older son. The same behaviour was repeated on the boat ride down the canals where she remained in her cabin, sleeping or sitting in grim silence. It saddened Robert to see his wife's once glossy black hair now heavily streaked with grey and her face lined with care and worry.

Burdened by fear for Gordon's health and worried about Jennie, Robert could hardly wait to leave Ontario on the train journey that would take his family to their new home in Drumheller.

DRUMHELLER 1919-1929

Chapter 18
The Valley, the Pilot, and Manslaughter

In sharp contrast to their journey up into the Crowsnest Pass and Coleman, this train trip from Sudbury to Drumheller crossed several thousand miles of prairie and then dipped down along the Red River Valley. Unlike the green-tree-clad mountain slopes, these low hills on either side of the train tracks rose in layers of brown and grey and black, sere and stark under the brilliant blue sky.

Even Jennie was roused out of her grief to comment at the sight of this prehistoric geography. The hills on either side appeared to be the oldest land she had ever seen, even more ancient and desolate than the black rocks of the Canadian Shield they had left behind in Ontario. Gordon, whose diet and rest had been strictly controlled on the trip, was feeling somewhat better and watched with great interest as the train moved along the riverside. Douglas, wide-eyed, talked excitedly about dinosaurs. He had been reading about the 1884 discoveries of fossils in the valley and was delighted to see the ancient landscape appear before his eyes.

The trees lining the riverbank were changing from summer green to autumn's red and gold in the valley when the train finally crossed the wide brown river on the wooden railway bridge. Both boys stared down at the water below and waited eagerly for their first sight of the town.

They were all glad to arrive at the station and disembark into the late afternoon sunshine of a crisp fall day. As Robert had arranged, they were met by a horse-drawn surrey followed by a team pulling a wagon into which their baggage and goods were loaded. The surrey was driven by a smiling young man who doffed his cap to Mrs. Ross and announced that he would take them to their new home.

Douglas immediately began asking the driver questions as the boys clambered into the buggy, followed more sedately by their parents. They set off at a steady pace to the house they would be renting while their new home was being built, passing neat residences with carefully landscaped yards and young trees planted in hopes of shade in years to come. Horses clip-clopped along the dusty roads and across the two main streets, and Robert commented on the apparent affluence of the town, noting the raised boardwalks in front of the stores and the tie railings for the horses. There were also several motorcars among the buggies, and the boys were very taken by them, questioning their father about how soon he would buy one.

"All in good time, boys, all in good time. We've only just arrived."

Jennie was by now quite interested in the town. "Everyone seems to be very busy, Robert. Look at the number of people. Are they farm families or miners, do you think?"

"Probably both. This is the business centre for the entire region. You would have to travel as far as Calgary to find anything larger. That is why the new hospital was built here. And this could be a market day as well."

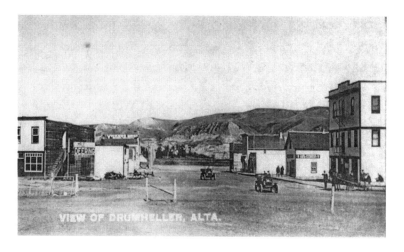

Drumheller, Alberta, 1919

Many men tipped their hats and smiled at the newcomers in the surrey. Jennie shyly nodded in return, and the boys waved politely at their father's urging. Gordon looked around with some energy and interest. The fifteen-year-old had been thoroughly reprimanded for his stubbornness by the doctors they had seen in Toronto and seemed to have accepted, at least for now, that he was old enough to take some responsibility for managing his affliction.

"Look, Mother," he whispered, "that man on horseback has a gun in a holster, but he is not in uniform. Do you think he is a soldier back from the war?"

Robert knew that many enlisted men had brought their service revolvers home from the war as souvenirs but did not want to alarm his wife. "Probably an off-duty policeman," he answered quietly. "Douglas, sit down, please. Don't bother the driver."

The eleven-year-old was asking rapid-fire questions of the young man in the high seat ahead of them, and the driver was happy to reply, but Douglas sat down quickly at his father's request and passed on the information he had gleaned to his older brother. "Dinosaurs, Gordon, there really were dinosaurs here, just as Mr. Tyrrell said in his book. Let's go digging for them as soon as we're allowed. Can we, I mean, may we, Mother?"

Happy at the interest Gordon was showing, Jennie smiled and nodded her head to the boys and then said to her husband, "This seems to be a very prosperous community, very tidy and busy. I like the gardens and trees in this part of town and the beautiful river drive we are following. Oh, there is the new hospital. Will we live close by? I know you always like to be able to walk to work."

"Yes, I think we will do very well here, Jennie. The house is just along here."

Robert chose not to tell his wife that Drumheller was in reality still a very rough and tough town, without nearly enough policing. He envisioned much "patching up" of fighting injuries as part of his practice. He was used to that and also used to playing a semi judicial role and working with the police. But for now, that needn't be mentioned.

"Ah, look, that is where we will live while our new home is being built, and see, the new housekeeper is waiting for us."

Martha Klaussen was a young woman who had grown up on a nearby farm and had been working as an orderly in the new hospital. When she heard of the new doctor and his young family moving to town, she immediately applied for the position of cook-housekeeper. Jennie was pleased with the recommendations from the matron of the Drumheller Hospital, and Martha would prove to be a most fortuitous choice for everyone. She was an excellent plain cook and very quickly grew to admire the doctor and his dainty lady wife and soon came to adore the boys.

The family settled in, the boys were registered at their schools, although they would be a little late starting, Jennie and Martha unpacked, and the routine of daily life was established.

Robert had quickly set about establishing his new practice with his associate, Dr. McGregor, and met the other doctors in town. Robert applied for and was granted staff privileges at the new hospital, which he announced to Jennie was, "Very fine, indeed," and gave careful thought to the interest expressed in his new private practice by the other town doctors.

It soon became clear to him that the rapidly growing town would need more doctors, and a larger medical practice had great appeal.

He also quickly realized that such a growing practice would require the services of a full-time bookkeeper and accountant. Dr. McGregor already employed a capable fellow as a part-time bookkeeper, and the man was looking for more work. Doctors were paid directly by their patients or by other agencies, such as the mining companies or the railroads, which meant the accounting tasks could become quite complex.

Since their Hudson's Bay days, and during his time in Bow Island, Lethbridge, and Coleman, Jennie had always been Robert's bookkeeper and in many ways his business partner as well as his wife. He knew she was proud of her role, so he foresaw that asking her to give this up would be a thorny issue for them. He also knew if she had to go to work in the medical office, rather than at home, it would be seen as taking a job away from a man who needed it to support his family. Besides, Robert agreed with the prevalent idea that women of a certain status, such as a doctor's wife, simply should not need to work outside the home.

As always, having made a decision, Robert was direct in his approach. He discussed his plans with Dr. McGregor who was amenable both to enlarging the practice and to hiring the full-time bookkeeper. When that discussion reached a satisfactory conclusion, Robert made his way back to their rental house for tea. Upon his arrival, he instructed Martha to give the boys their tea in the kitchen and asked Jennie to join him in the small sitting room.

"Jennie, leave the unpacking until later. We have something important to discuss."

Jennie removed her large apron and sat quietly, hands in her lap, waiting for Robert to speak.

"My dear, I have always valued your contribution to our financial well-being. You have managed the medical practice accounts very successfully for the past ten years. Our present financial security is in great part due to your meticulous accounting. But, in this new situation, things will have to change. I intend to make this practice much larger with several more doctors, and Doctor McGregor and I have decided to hire a full-time bookkeeper and accountant. Surely, you can understand this must happen."

Jennie had been expecting something of this sort, and in truth, felt some relief as she knew that convention would not allow her to be seen as a working woman. "I do understand; of course I do. It is clear that you must proceed as convention demands in order to build the medical practice here in Drumheller." But she was surprised at the sorrow she felt as her role in Robert's daily life was reduced. "You do know, Robert, being your bookkeeper and silent partner has been a source of pleasure for me. I truly believed that I was contributing in no small measure to our family's welfare."

As she spoke, the realization of what this would mean became clear. She flushed bright red as a wave of fury overwhelmed her as she considered the diminishment of her role in Robert's professional life. She struggled to keep her voice steady and hide her hurt and anger as she said, "So we must discuss my household allowance as I assume I will still manage the household accounts? It's considered right and proper for a woman to do that?"

Startled by this outburst, Robert was silent for a moment then asserted his authority as her husband and head of the house. "Jennie, that is unfair. I have never been one for convention, but surely you have more than enough to do to keep you busy setting up our new home and caring for the boys, especially Gordon. We will also be expected to entertain more formally once the new house is ready, and you will soon be involved with the church. I know you will be busy. Now, I need to have my tea before I go back to the new office. The matter is settled."

Robert was relieved that this unpleasantness had been dealt with, and his wife had accepted the change in her role. No more needed to be said, although he, too, felt a small twinge of regret that they would no longer share this aspect of his business.

Between the long hours he spent on his medical practice and her concerns for Gordon, the closeness they had shared in the early days of their marriage seemed to have disappeared. However, there was nothing he could do about it, and he was also secretly relieved that she no longer controlled all the finances. There had been times when he would have liked to have had more freedom in his spending, without discussion with Jennie.

"No," he thought, "that's unkind." Jennie had always been an excellent manager, and he had always spent as he chose. At any rate, it was done. Jennie would get her household and clothing allowance. He would, of course, be generous, and the rest of his earnings would be deposited in his account.

One of his first large financial decisions was to donate, along with Dr. Gibson, another Drumheller physician, over two thousand dollars in medical equipment to the new hospital. This magnanimity cemented his growing reputation as an excellent, caring doctor and a philanthropist with the welfare of the citizens of Drumheller at heart.

Jennie recognized this and supported the expansive gift to the community but quietly worried that sometimes Robert ignored his Scot's thriftiness in favour of the grand gesture. However, Robert was a fine provider who worked long, hard hours to ensure that she and the boys wanted for nothing. Control of the family finances was no longer in her hands.

***

Their move to Drumheller at the end of September coincided with the much-anticipated arrival of the first aeroplane to land in the area. For many people, this was the first aircraft they had ever seen, so excitement ran high in the small prairie town. Eagerly, the Ross family set out early in the morning to Audy's farm field east of Drumheller to see this wonderful machine, a Curtiss Jenny, flown from Calgary by the World War I Air Ace, Captain Fred McCall, RAF.

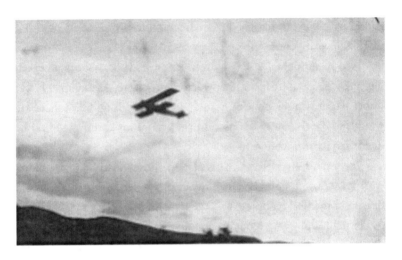

The Curtis Jennie in flight, Drumheller, Alberta, 1919

When their buggy arrived, there were already several hundred people gathered around the edges of the field watching the pale blue skies to the east and hoping to be the first to see this marvel. Of course, it was a youngster whose sharp eyes saw the tiny speck and raised the cry, "Look, look, there she is. Look over there! Gollee!"

Heads swivelled, and sure enough the speck got bigger, and soon the distinctive grumble and growl of the engine could be heard. The bi-plane, looking as fragile as a dragonfly, landed with a few bumps and hops on the brown stubble of the field, and the pilot climbed out of his cockpit to the welcoming cheers of the crowd. A long lineup snaked back from the farmer's shed that had been pressed into service as a booth where tickets were being purchased for rides in this marvellous machine. Business was brisk at the entrance to the field.

Jennie, terrified at the idea of flying, decreed that it would not do for either the new doctor to risk his life or for Gordon to chance feeling even sicker than usual. Robert, remembering the excitement of his canoe trips over the raging rivers of Ontario in his HBC days, longed to fly away in the bi-plane but reluctantly agreed to stay on the ground. He knew his wife would not allow their older son to go for a ride, but he happily purchased a $15.00 ticket for eleven-year-old Douglas to go for a flight over the Badlands.

Gordon truly did not feel well enough to go up in the plane but resented his younger brother doing something he could not.

Douglas could not believe his good luck and, once back on the ground, raced over to hug his father animatedly describing the plane's cockpit and the soaring flight. "It was really noisy. You couldn't hear anything but the engine and the wind. It's all held together with wires, and the propeller is just a blur. And, Dad, you could see everything from up there, all the fields and valleys, even the mountains. I am going to be a pilot when I grow up. It was so neat; I love flying."

Jennie frowned at this public display of affection, but Robert kept his arm close around his younger son, savouring the boy's enthusiasm. The other townspeople smiled at the youngster's joy, and many came over to introduce themselves to Robert and Jennie. The first couple were Mr. and Mrs. E. A. "Bert" Toshach. Robert had been on one of his walks through town and had gone into the Toshach's Department store on Centre Street, so he already knew E.A. The two men had quickly become good friends.

They nodded at one another as Bert introduced his wife, Muriel. It seemed the women had something in common as they both came from Ontario, and very soon Muriel was telling Jennie some of the history of Drumheller. She had lived in the valley for five years and described the rapid growth. Robert and Bert also talked about the changes in the town and opportunities for business. Soon other townspeople joined the group, and it was quickly evident that, as it had been in Bow Island and Coleman, the prairie welcome was warm and supportive of the new family.

Gordon, now taller than his mother, stayed with the adults, but Douglas received his father's permission to join a group of boys his own age who called him over and eagerly questioned him about the experience of flying.

Invitations to tea and promises to get together soon were exchanged by the adults, and the memorable day finally came to a close. Tired after the excitement but buoyed up by new friends, the Ross family climbed into their buggy and headed home.

Then it was school for the boys, church and library groups for Jennie, and a rapidly growing medical practice for Robert.

A basic tenet of Robert's medical belief system was that many injuries and illnesses could be prevented. This was most clearly shown in his ongoing passionate support for first aid classes, especially for the miners who made up the bulk of the work force in Drumheller as they had in Coleman. Within months of the family's arrival, he had volunteered his time and medical expertise to instruct first aid classes, following the model he had used with such success in Coleman.

Weekly classes were organized in one of the cottage schools, and each course lasted for ten weeks. Robert also travelled to neighbouring coal-mining villages, such as Midland and Rosebud, to teach. He was involved many evenings each week and often on Saturday afternoons, and he and another doctor not only taught but also acted as doctor examiners to certify the men upon completion of the course. A separate course was taught to women, as Robert never underestimated the importance of the women's roles in first aid.

As in Coleman, Robert insisted that first aid saved lives and made it clear to all that his foundation instructions, clearing of airways, stopping of hemorrhage, prevention of movement at the accident site until bones could be stabilized, cleanliness to avoid blood poisoning and sepsis, and preventing men dying from blood loss or shock, all contributed to saving men's lives long before they reached the hospital.

By 1923, there would be a dedicated mine rescue car in Drumheller. This would be a railway car, converted with volunteer labour from the miners and railroad workers, and available to be taken by a yard engine to the site of mining or railway accidents. The car itself would be donated by the railways and local merchants, and mine owners would provide money for necessary materials.

But that wouldn't come about for another three years. For now, the doctors volunteered their time, and the men they taught were eager to learn the skills necessary to save lives. A First Aid Certificate was also a requirement in order to be trained as a mine rescue worker, which enhanced job-finding prospects for the miners.

Upon his return from one of these classes, Robert remarked to Jennie, "I'm really pleased with how well the lessons are going. Everyone in town has embraced the importance of first aid." He paused and thought about another issue that was dear to his heart. "I haven't been nearly so successful in my efforts to convince people of the link between water, sanitation, and health. Although the medical people in town continue to press for an effective chlorination system for our water, something has to be done at the provincial level as well to augment our local efforts."

He settled into his chair and accepted a cup of tea from their housekeeper. "Thank you, Martha."

"Hm-mm-m," Jennie was thoughtful. "Well, Robert, most people don't understand waterborne diseases, and many still believe that any imposed rules threaten their individual and property rights. It is also hard to convince people that putting a poison, such as chlorine, in their drinking water makes it safer."

"It is not just that, Jennie. You know how hard it is to persuade people to have their children vaccinated. I am delighted when a scientist discovers something that will save a child's life and prevent epidemics. The Good Lord knows I saw epidemics destroy the native people's lives when the Europeans came with their infectious diseases. And even isolation wards such as we had at Queen's can only help prevent the disease from spreading to others. What news do you have for me tonight that might give me more hope?"

"There is some promising work being done in Germany on a vaccine for diphtheria, Robert. But it is still several years away, and many trials are required. It will possibly be available by nineteen twenty-three. And then you will have to persuade people to use it, since I also read that some children in the States died after being injected with the anti-toxin. You can understand people's fears when that happens. Again, you are correct, a healthy population and a clean way of life, including clean water, is the best protection we have. I will let you know, of course, if I find any more information about other vaccines."

"Thank you, my dear. Now I think I will have another cup of tea and sit for a while. Tomorrow after church, we need to visit the builders at the new house. They will not be able to work on the outside once the snows come, so I hope they have made enough progress to get something done on the inside through the winter. Are you going up to bed? You look very tired, and I can see that the cold weather is making your rheumatism worse. This place is quite comfortable and warm, but it will be good to have our own home."

For a moment, Jennie sat quietly. She had been thinking that she would like to leave the prairies for a month each winter when the cold was at its worst but decided that now was not the time to speak of this to her husband. She nodded her assent to his suggestion and went to her warm bed. She had a church meeting tomorrow after the morning service, and her joints were aching, but looking at the building site was important to Robert so she would make time. It also seemed to take his mind off his worries about his patients, and although it had snowed and was very cold, the days had been sunny and bright so an outing would be good for them all. She would simply bundle up against the chill.

***

The autumn days of 1919 passed quickly into winter. Robert became a well-known figure as he walked to work, often stopping to talk to the merchants and other townsfolk he met on his walks. Dr. and Mrs. Ross joined the congregation of the soon-to-become Knox United Church; Jennie joined a church fundraising group, and her mathematical strengths became evident as she volunteered to organize money matters for the group.

Robert gradually built up his practice, and more and more people turned to the new doctor when they fell ill. He loved his surgery in the hospital and enjoyed his work in the medical office, but most of all, he revelled in his journeys by buggy or on horseback and, once the snow fell, by sleigh to the mines and out to the surrounding farms.

All of his surgical cases were challenging, but one of his cases that first winter had medical and legal implications that would disturb him for years.

He received a phone call about ten o'clock on a cold February night upon his return from evening office hours. The call came from a man who identified himself as a country doctor with his practice in a farming area about an hour by train from Drumheller.

"Can you come to the farm, Doctor Ross? I am dealing with a case of acute appendicitis with abscess formation, and I believe the case is too far gone for me to risk sending the patient to the hospital. I am quite sure that in order to save this man's life I will have to operate at the patient's farmhouse. I'm a doctor, but I have heard that you are a surgical graduate, and I am asking you to come and assist me. It is an opportunity for you to extend your practice."

Robert agreed and asked, "How do I get to the farm, especially at this hour of the night? Shall I bring a nurse? What else do you need?"

The country doctor, more confident now that he had secured Robert's agreement to his request, said, "I will make all the necessary arrangements. There will be a yard engine available as soon as you can get to the train station. Yes, bring a nurse and the required instruments for an abdominal section. Get off the yard engine at the way station I will specify to the engineer. You'll be met by a man with a sleigh to transport you to the patient's home. Hurry."

Robert was a bit puzzled by the request for surgical instruments, wondering what the doctor was about if he did not already have what was required, but he quickly packed the necessary instruments and anything else he thought might be needed and phoned a graduate nurse. She agreed to be at the station immediately, and the two of them met and climbed into the warm cab of the waiting yard engine.

They hurtled through the dark and the snow until the engine puffed to a stop at the way station. It was nothing more than a small shack at the side of the tracks in the midst of acres of snow-covered fields, but they climbed off and into the waiting sleigh with its team of horses, whose breath smoked in the cold wind.

The engineer, used to such emergency calls on the services of the yard engine, shouted to them as they wrapped themselves in blankets and buffalo robes and set out through the night, "Good luck. Remember to call if you need me. I'm only an hour away. I'll come right back."

The nurse, well known to Robert from the high quality of her work at the hospital, said, "I hope we are in time, Doctor Ross. This sounds very serious, and it has already been over an hour since the doctor called you."

Robert just nodded in agreement, his mind already caught up in what they might find at their destination, another five miles across the windblown fields. It was dreadfully cold, and as the snow fall increased, they huddled in their blankets and robes, trying to protect their faces from the wind and the icy flakes that stuck to any exposed skin. Robert, thinking of the surgery ahead, yelled through his scarf, "Keep your hands warm; we must keep our hands warm."

There was nothing so welcome as the lights of the farmhouse and then the warmth within. The farmer's wife took their outerwear and led them to the kitchen, expressing her deep gratitude to them for coming out this far distance on such a dreadful night. It was clear also that she was terribly worried about her husband. Robert was relieved to see that, despite her obvious distress, she had attempted to prepare for the visit. There was plenty of boiling water on the stove to sterilize the instruments he and the nurse had brought with them, and the kitchen was warm.

The room had been prepared as an operating room with as many lamps as possible pressed into service, and the table, which was to be used for the surgery, was covered with clean white linen, upon which the patient lay, also draped with clean white cloths.

With the country doctor hovering over him, Robert examined the farmer and confirmed the diagnosis of acute appendicitis. However, much to the presiding doctor's annoyance, Robert strongly advised him not to operate. "A condition such as this requires special treatment and aftercare, best obtained in a hospital. If an incision is made immediately and drainage established as a first step in treatment now, a few hours delay in taking this patient to the Drumheller hospital will not lessen and will probably improve his chances of recovery."

Robert was not used to having his advice as a surgeon ignored so was quite taken aback when the doctor replied angrily, "I was called by this man's wife. I have looked after the family for years, and I am in charge, not you. I called you to assist, not take over. I am ready to operate, and I believe that if I do not operate immediately, this man will die. Nurse, help me get the patient ready."

Somewhat reluctantly, the nurse complied, looking sideways at Doctor Ross whom she knew and respected as a fine surgeon. However, she also knew that she had to follow the instructions of the doctor in charge.

The patient's wife had been listening carefully to this exchange, and while the country doctor and the nurse prepared the man for surgery, the wife called Robert into the sitting room, lit only by a few candles. There, her family and friends, wrapped in their overcoats, were huddled together around the small fireplace, many praying by candlelight.

"Doctor Ross," the wife spoke urgently, "I have heard of your skills as a surgeon, and it was me who suggested that our doctor call you as his assistant. Now, having heard what you said, I want you to take charge of the case and do the operation."

Robert replied, "Yes, I would be glad to do so, but you would have to tell that to the presiding doctor. He called me to assist him, and I cannot take over the case without his consent."

The woman was obviously not willing to do as Robert asked, perhaps fearing that she might need the services of the country doctor in the future and could be refused if she had Robert take over now. Her friends also counselled her against it, saying the country doctor had looked after them all very well for years and would be angry if Doctor. Ross, a newcomer from town, took over the case.

At this point, the country doctor, who had apparently overheard some of the sitting room conversations, shouted for Robert to come into the kitchen again and shut the door to the sitting room. "I want you to administer the ether, Doctor Ross. The nurse, not you, will assist me with the operation."

Robert was very annoyed but knew that short of trying to physically restrain the doctor, he could do nothing without the wife's permission. "Let me offer one final caution about the danger of a massive infection." He tried again, although he knew now that the other doctor would likely not heed his words of warning.

As expected, the doctor pointedly ignored him, and Robert agreed to act as anaesthesiologist rather than as surgical assistant as had been originally requested. He offered his sterilized instruments for the surgery as he soon realized the doctor had nothing as good.

The doctor began to operate, but when he opened the abdomen and inserted his fingers to search for the inflamed appendix, he instead broke into a walled off abscess. Try as he might, he could not locate the appendix.

Robert, extremely anxious now, advised firmly, "You must put in drainage tubes right away and close the abdomen for the present. Let me stress that this is a much safer procedure than to continue to hunt for the appendix in an already infected area. The infection will spread if you carry on in this fashion." Robert continued, quietly but insistently. "If you close up now with the drainage tubes in place and leave the appendix, it will probably slough out. But, even if it doesn't, it is far safer to operate later and remove it. At that point, the infection, which is now presenting a serious threat to the life of the patient, will have subsided. Remember we can have the yard engine here within the hour to transport him to the hospital."

To the dismay of Robert and the nurse, the doctor again refused Robert's advice and stubbornly insisted, "I'll get that appendix out if it takes me all night."

He continued with the operation and, in his hunt for the appendix, started to remove the bowels. By the time he eventually located the appendix and brought it out of the man's abdomen, there was a great mass of intestines lying on top of the patient. To add to the horror of the scene, the intestines distended when they came into contact with the air of the room.

Robert was furious, but remained calm as he continued to administer the anaesthetic. The nurse was frantic, but there was little they could do now. It took them over an hour to force the intestines back into the cavity and then get the muscles approximated and the skin sutured. Angry and distressed about the procedure and desperately concerned about the patient in her care, the nurse did her job, teeth clenched in rage. Nothing Robert had said had made any difference, so they just did their best to lessen the damage.

After the hours spent in surgery, Robert and the nurse were greatly relieved that the patient was still alive, although now dreadfully ill and burning with fever. They made him as comfortable as possible before leaving the man in the care of the country doctor. The farmer's wife and family were now sure they would lose their husband and father.

Robert and the nurse returned home, and although few words passed between them as they retraced their route through the bitterly cold light of a winter dawn, both were shaken to the core by the terrible events of the night.

The man's death was inevitable and after three days of agony, he died, a life sacrificed to the willful ignorance and stubborn pride of a country practitioner who thought he was a surgeon. Robert especially struggled with the realization that by obeying the rules of professional courtesy, he may have taken an active part in what might be construed as an act of manslaughter. He felt sure the man's life could have been saved or, at the very least, spared such a painful death.

The incident haunted him for weeks. He could not even discuss it with Jennie for many days, and as he went about his daily rounds in the hospital or visited his own patients in their homes, he kept going over and over in his mind the events of that night. Although he was still new to Drumheller and working hard to build his own practice, he vowed that such a travesty of good medical practice would never happen again with his knowledge, no matter who or what he offended.

When he was finally able to talk about it to his wife, she listened to his story and shared his anger and grief and firmly supported his resolve. "Professional courtesy and the goodwill of your medical colleagues is important, Robert, but I am sure every one of them would support your determination to ensure that this doesn't happen again. Now, you must try to let it be."

She moved the conversation on to a discussion of the worrisome rumours of a possible miners strike. Unrest in the mines and the possibility of strikes was a constant concern for the Rosses, especially since a portion of Robert's income came from the mining companies, who paid a flat fee per miner for their care. However, their fears would come to naught. The miners did indeed go out on strike within weeks of their conversation but only for a short time.

On the same subject, though, a topic that troubled her a great deal was the ongoing labour turmoil resulting from the Winnipeg General Strike.

"Robert, this unrest will spread to the mines here. You saw what happened in Coleman. Does the news from Winnipeg not worry you?"

"Of course it does. But my larger concern is with the shameful actions of our government and the police. The inhuman treatment of the strikers in Winnipeg will only inflame the workers, and the unrest will spread. And I have always been suspicious of unlimited power for the police."

"But surely the miners here in Drumheller are better treated?"

"No, I fear not. I have already seen the results of poor safety standards and the terrible injuries that occur. I had to amputate a man's toes the other day, and the accident was purely the result of the rushed timbering of a new mine shaft."

Jennie never asked the names of Robert's patients. She would know soon enough as word spread rapidly in a small town. However, she silently promised herself to be sure the church groups, no matter what faith, helped to take care of the miner's family if assistance was required. Her deep Methodist faith meant that quietly doing good for others was the largest part of her life. She knew that the miners looked after their own, but sometimes a little extra made a big difference.

The boys were long abed by this time, and Robert was nodding in his chair, so the fire was dampened, the lamps extinguished, and they retired, each with their own hopes and worries about the days to come.

Chapter 19
A Necessary Appendectomy and Frederick Banting

When the winter of 1920 finally came to an end and the snow had melted sufficiently to allow outside work to begin again, construction proceeded rapidly on the promised house. By the end of May, the family moved in to their home.

It was the largest dwelling they had ever owned, and they were all delighted to be settled in such a fine space. The main floor, with a glassed-in front porch, consisted of a large front room entered from the main hallway, with a dining room under a wide archway at one end, and a large kitchen at the rear. A hallway, with stairs on the right that went up to the second floor, ran from the front entry to the back of the house, where the large, brightly lit kitchen, with its cozy room for the housekeeper, was located. The back windows filled the entire wall and overlooked a spacious yard, where Jennie's vegetable garden would be planted when the ground was fully thawed. And on the second floor, four bedrooms gave each family member their own room.

There was a bathroom with a large hand basin and a five foot long tub standing on ornate feet. Hot water was piped up to the room from the coal boiler in the basement, and heat from the pipes warmed the towels in the linen cupboard. There was even an indoor water closet, the very latest in design.

The house was built on a slope so that when viewed from the front it appeared to have only two stories, but when seen from the back, it actually had three. The basement level included ample storage space for a cool cellar to store vegetables and eggs over the winter. Robert, whose medical practice had become extremely busy, thought longingly of the day when he would have time to make one of these basement rooms his own study.

Jennie furnished the front room with blue velvet chairs and mahogany furniture, lace curtains and heavy draperies to help insulate against the cold, and fringed blinds that could be lowered to keep out the heat of the prairie summer. The dining room was splendid with its large oak table and glass-fronted cabinets for her china, long packed but now lovingly displayed. A desk and sewing machine at the side window overlooking the porch completed the furnishings.

Jennie sat at her desk now on a lovely June evening, watching Robert and the boys at the dining room table where they were busy constructing a wireless radio from a kit Douglas had ordered by mail, diligently following the building instructions in the Boy Scout Handbook. The family already owned a receiver from Horne's Department Store in Pittsburgh, and both boys were wildly enthusiastic about putting on headphones and listening to news from Calgary and, on repeaters, from across the country. And music! A Mr. Conrad who worked for Westinghouse had begun transmitting music from his collection of gramophone records, and all over North America the idea of recorded music coming through the air to everyone who had a receiver was a revelation. There seemed to be no end to what could happen with this new technology.

"Perhaps," Robert chuckled, "we will someday have live concerts sent over the radio. I do miss live music."

Building their own radio set was a challenge they could not resist. Gordon was feeling well enough to be completely involved, and Douglas's engineering abilities shone as the three of them worked intently at the table.

"I hope," Jennie thought to herself at this rare undisturbed scene of family contentment, "I hope the phone doesn't ring."

***

Jennie sat in silence at her desk, gazing out the window at the first heavy snowfall of the winter of 1921. It was December, and the last few months had been bitterly cold. The ground was frozen hard. Today, the sky was lowering, and the grey clouds seemed to be touching the hills surrounding the valley. Finally, a true snowfall had arrived.

Jennie had promised herself that she would ignore the dark sky and spend the time until noon reviewing the latest medical news from the University of Toronto that Robert had brought home from the office last evening. She also planned to look over the accounts from the fundraising efforts for the new church building.

Her husband had left for the hospital at eight o'clock for two scheduled surgeries and morning rounds to be followed by a brief hospital board meeting before he returned home for the midday meal.

The boys were both at school. Gordon continued to do well, especially in mathematics, but his health was increasingly precarious. He was unhappy and tired very easily. Douglas enjoyed all his schoolwork, loved to read, and excelled in anything he found interesting. Jennie's younger son was a healthy, active, even mischievous boy who would be thirteen in a week.

But her thoughts kept returning to her older son as Jennie read and re-read the news from Toronto concerning the work of Drs. Frederick Banting and Charles Best and their astonishing experiments with insulin. The church papers on her desk were forgotten as Jennie's thoughts focused on Gordon's illness.

"How long until Banting and Best will be ready to treat humans?" she wondered. "I know Gordon's condition is getting worse. He is more and more tired and irritable, and his thirst and cravings for sugar increase daily, no matter how we try to control his diet." Her attention was caught by a delivery wagon passing on the street. The horse was straining to pull the wagon through the rapidly accumulating snow. "At least," Jennie murmured to herself, "the snow means the frozen mud ruts will be filled and this snow is heavy enough to last. Everyone will be able to travel by sleds again." Her reverie was broken by a quiet voice from the kitchen doorway.

"Mrs. Ross, it is nearly ten o'clock. Would you like your tea and perhaps a biscuit?"

"Yes, please, Martha. I will have tea but nothing to eat, thank you. I will have lunch with Doctor Ross when he returns."

"Shall I put more coal on the fire? I have a full scuttle in the kitchen."

"No, thank you. The room is quite warm, and I have my shawl. I even have the writing gloves I knitted for myself to wear if my hands become chilled. The miners will be glad of the cold, won't they? It means more shifts for them, poor souls. They don't get much work in the summer." Jennie drank her tea and made herself settle to the church accounts for the next few hours as the snow continued to fall.

Shortly past noon, the kitchen door slammed open and Douglas's voice was heard as he shook off the snow and yanked off his boots and coat, leaving them in a pile by the door. "Hello, Martha. That soup smells good. Boy, I'm hungry. I'll wash up and come to the table. Did you know it was snowing? I'll bet there will be enough to go sledding this weekend, but those sure are little hills compared to Coleman."

As he entered the dining room, his voice became subdued, and he walked neatly to the table and sat down, squirming a little to get comfortable. "Good afternoon, Mother."

"Good afternoon, Douglas. Don't fidget."

Gordon, as befitted his older brother status, made a more dignified entrance a few moments later, kissed his mother on the cheek, and sat down at the table across from Douglas. Both boys waited quietly for their father.

"Good afternoon, my dear. Good afternoon, boys. A prayer of thanks, and then Martha will serve our food."

The family lowered their heads over clasped hands as Robert recited the Grace and then quietly ate their hearty soup and cheese and biscuits. There was no conversation until all the meal had been consumed.

"What did you learn in school today, Gordon?"

"Nothing new, Father. I know more about numbers than they do. I can hardly wait to finish school."

"I'm sorry you learned nothing, Gordon. I think there is always something to learn. And you, Douglas?"

"My teacher in science told me about a doctor in Toronto who is doing some experiments with dogs. Is that true, Father? Will it hurt the dogs?"

"Your teacher is remarkably well informed, Douglas, and I rather think it helps the animals."

Robert caught Jennie's eye. "Your mother and I have some things to discuss. Excuse yourselves from the table and say thank you to Martha for the excellent food. We will talk further this evening about your interesting science lesson, Douglas."

The boys bundled up in coats and scarves and boots and mittens to return to school and thumped out the door while Martha cleared the table and served Robert and Jennie their tea.

"Yes, Jennie," Robert began, "I know that Banting has made great strides, and I have already sent a telegram to the University of Toronto to ascertain when the insulin will be ready for human use. It is promising, but you must try not to get your hopes too high."

Jennie sighed deeply but said nothing, although her sadness and frustration at the delay was evident as her agonized worry about Gordon overshadowed everything in her life.

Robert spoke, "The man is a brilliant scientist as is his partner, Charles Best, but isolating the islets of Langerhans and preventing the digestive juices of the pancreas from destroying the hormone is only part of their work. They have been successfully experimenting with dogs as Douglas noted," Robert paused, smiling as he thought of the bright and curious mind of his younger son, and then continued, "but they have yet to maintain consistency in the dosage, and they must do that before they can use a human subject. I know how hard it is. I, too, pray for their success. It could change Gordon's life and the lives of many other young people afflicted by this terrible disease." Silently, Robert said a prayer to the Great Creator, hoping it was not already too late for his son. Jennie also bowed her head and clenched her hands in fear as she thought of her boy.

Robert continued, "Now, I shall have a short rest before I return to the office. Please be sure I am not disturbed."

That evening, Robert spent some more time talking to the boys about Banting's exciting discovery and his experiments with dogs. After Gordon and Douglas had gone upstairs, Jennie and Robert discussed the subject further, but there was little to do but wait for news.

Aware that, although promising, the talk of Banting and Best had brought Jennie's always present anxiety back to the surface, Robert attempted to distract her with an interesting anecdote. He hoped telling her the story would take her mind off her distress about Gordon for a few moments before bed "Shall I tell you about the appendectomy patient whom I finally discharged today? I think you will find aspects of it quite amusing. I know you agree with me about some of these so-called 'cures.'"

Although he still depended on her for much of the latest in medical news, Robert spent far less time talking over his work with Jennie now that he and his partners in the clinic devoted an afternoon each week to reviewing all their current cases, but as they settled comfortably for the evening, he decided to share this case with her.

"You will remember, my dear, that this began about a month ago when Matron phoned me at my office regarding a patient she had just admitted for me, whom we will call Doctor Penny. This patient insisted that he was a graduate doctor and did not want another doctor's advice or prescriptions. He just wanted to be in the hospital and would take charge of his own care."

It was evident from Jennie's puzzled expression that she could not understand why anyone would request admittance to a hospital and then refuse the medical care offered, but she nodded to Robert to go on with the story.

"It really is not surprising that a doctor would ask to be admitted under his own care, Jennie. Many medical men have given up their careers in tough times and taken up other occupations, such as farming or working for hire, but you're right, this fellow was particularly stubborn.

"Matron told me that she had explained to Doctor Penny that under our hospital rules, he could not be admitted unless he was under the care of a member of the hospital medical staff. He reluctantly chose my name at random from the list she gave him. She said he was not happy about having to do that, but he was in pain and needed to be in care."

"Was it you in particular, or just having to choose any doctor?" Jennie asked.

Robert answered, "I think he was unhappy about having to be under the care of any doctor. He was still annoyed when I called in to see him that afternoon and told me that he did not need my services; he was a doctor and much preferred to treat himself.

"I wasn't much bothered by his attitude. I asked him what his self-diagnosis was, and all he would say was that he was suffering from abdominal pain. I stated firmly that his diagnosis was much too vague and not acceptable either to the hospital management or to me, telling him that he had been admitted under my name and my care, which meant I would be held responsible for his treatment, and that I must examine him."

"And did he accept that, Robert? Surely he must have allowed you to examine him?"

"Yes, Jennie, but very grudgingly. Doctor Penny permitted me to examine him, muttering throughout about how unnecessary it was, but flinching in pain whenever I touched his abdomen. I knew immediately that he was suffering an attack of appendicitis, so told him that I advised an immediate operation or his condition would get much worse. His reply to me was that I was talking nonsense and that he did not believe in surgery for appendicitis. Further, he told me that the disease could be treated safely without surgery."

Jennie, knowing full well how Robert would have responded to such a remark, asked, "What did you say, Robert? How could he have questioned your medical advice?"

Robert was pleased that his wife was totally engaged in the story and carried on. "Of course, I told him that the pain might ease temporarily, as it sometimes does with chronic appendicitis, but it is very rarely the case that an acutely inflamed appendix 'cures' itself. I also told him, as politely as I could, that he was well on the way to acute appendicitis, and the best and safest treatment for acute appendicitis is removal of the appendix. Further, I stressed that delay in the performance of the operation would endanger his life.

"I must admit, my dear, that I was angered when he ignored my words again, saying that he just needed nursing care and bed rest, telling me that he could cure himself and that he did not need an operation, nor would he consent to one."

"What a foolish person," Jennie commented, recalling the tragic outcome of the country doctor's botched farmhouse appendectomy. "How did you respond, Robert?"

"By this time, I was more than a little annoyed by the man's stubborn foolishness and his obvious lack of medical knowledge. In an effort to discover exactly what his qualifications were, I calmly asked him some questions that soon confirmed my suspicions, such as, are you a medical doctor? Do you have surgical experience?"

"And did he, Robert? Was he a real doctor or just one of those 'doctors-by-mail' we hear about?"

"You are correct, Jennie. I wasn't surprised when he told me that he was a naturopath physician with no real medical training or qualifications. He had not been trained as a surgeon, and furthermore, he didn't even believe in surgery. He told me again to just leave him alone, and he would get better. He was somewhat rude, although I put that down to his anxiety and increasing pain.

"I wasn't pleased about the situation, but I told him that if he insisted, I would leave him alone, and he could go ahead and cure himself. I also told him that I would be interested to see how he did it and would not interfere with his treatment. However, I made it clear that I reserved the right to examine him daily to see how he was faring."

Jennie smiled, completely engaged in the story. "Of course, Robert. He sounds a very stubborn man, and he must have been in considerable pain by then."

"Yes, he was, but with that, I left him and continued on my rounds to visit my other patients in the hospital. I must admit I smiled to myself, though, as I could predict with great accuracy how Doctor Penny would be feeling over the next twenty-four hours. Sure enough, when I examined my reluctant patient the next day, I found that his temperature had risen, his pulse was faster, and the rigidity and tenderness of his abdomen were worse than they had been the day before. In Matron's presence, I told him again in no uncertain terms what I believed, speaking very clearly so that there could be no misunderstanding and telling him that it was evident that his self-treatment was not having the desired effect, and advising him, once again, that he was endangering his own life with his foolishness and should consent to the operation. It was obvious that he continued to be in a great deal of pain. Still stubborn, he insisted that he would get better, saying it would just take more time, and repeated his request to be left alone. I noted, though, that this was all said through clenched teeth."

Recalling the moment, Robert smiled ruefully at Jennie, "I knew he was hurting but obviously not yet in enough pain to change his mind about surgery. But by now, I was too busy to try to persuade him again. I had other patients in the hospital who needed my attention. So I left him alone as requested. I did tell him, though, that it was on record that he had twice refused the correct plan to save him.

"With that, I left the room. The nurse informed me that the other patients in the ward had looked askance at the man, and some had tried to persuade him to do as Doctor Ross suggested, all to no avail."

Jennie shook her head, dismayed at this obstinate man, becoming a bit anxious about the outcome.

Her husband continued. "When I saw him the next afternoon, his symptoms were no worse but also no better. Now he told me that he wanted to leave the hospital. He said he was not getting enough good care and felt that he might as well be on his own. He insisted that he be discharged. This struck me as extreme foolishness, given the pain he was in, but by now nothing this patient said or did surprised me. So, I signed him off, knowing there was no possible way I could do anything without the patient's consent. Doctor Penny left the hospital, and I had to let him go, knowing that while there have been miracles, I didn't expect to see him alive again and that he may well suffer a painful death."

"Oh, Robert, tell me he didn't die. Poor soul. So foolish."

"No, he didn't die, Jennie, remember I said I discharged him this morning? But it was a near thing. About a week after he left the hospital for the first time, I received a telephone call at four o'clock in the morning from a farmer saying that Doctor Penny was being brought in to the hospital and could I arrange for an emergency operation? Doctor Penny was working as a farmhand at the time. His fellow farm workers were bringing him to the hospital and told me that they expected to arrive at about six o'clock in the morning.

"I telephoned the hospital and asked them to have the operating room prepared for Doctor Penny's arrival in two hours and asked Matron to notify me as soon as he arrived and was prepared for surgery. I then promptly fell asleep again, as you know I always do, certain that the telephone would waken me. I was somewhat surprised to wake at my usual seven o'clock without a telephone call. I immediately called the hospital and was told that Doctor Penny had not yet arrived.

"Matron and I surmised their trip may have been slower than planned. The recent heavy snowfall had made many roads impassable, and they had a long way to travel. I said that I would come along to the hospital as soon as I had breakfasted, and we could only hope that Doctor Penny would be there by then. Of course by this time, Jennie, I was worried about the delay as I had begun to fear a ruptured appendix.

"Matron told me that everything was ready as I had requested, and since we had all of Doctor Penny's information from his previous admittance, he would go straight to the operating room as soon as he arrived.

"I made my way to the hospital, getting there just in time to meet the farm workers and Doctor Penny. While the orderlies transferred my returning patient into the hospital, I learned that it had been necessary to haul him half a mile on a stone boat across the fields to reach the road into town. There he had been placed in a motorcar that was waiting for him, but the road was so slick with ice and snow that the vehicle kept sliding into the ditches. The farm workers told me that they were forced to borrow a team of horses from a nearby farm and hitch them to the car to haul it the final ten miles to the hospital. The men were very concerned about Doctor Penny, but they were still heartily amused by this journey, telling me that there was nothing like a good team and laughing at the whole ridiculous trip.

"I told the men that they had done their job to help their friend. I thanked them for their efforts, paid them, and sent them, complete with horses and car, on their way."

By this time, Jennie was chuckling at the picture Robert had painted of the horseless carriage being pulled through the snow by horses.

Glad to see that his wife was completely distracted by this tale, Robert went on, "I walked into the operating room and, without a hint of a smile, greeted Doctor Penny and told him that I was glad to see that he had come to his senses before it was too late. At least, I hoped it was not too late. He was in agony by this time, and although he could barely speak, he still had enough spirit to tell me not to rub it in but to get this surgery over with and get him out of his misery as soon as possible.

"In the event, the operation took place. Fortunately, the appendix had not yet burst and was still easily removed, but it was a close run thing. I established drainage to clean up any infection that may have spread into the abdominal cavity as a result of the delay and left him in the excellent care of the nurses.

"Matron was on hand, and I thanked her as the nurses transferred Doctor Penny to his bed, and I told her that I was hopeful he would make an uninterrupted recovery. She was not as relaxed as I was and still very annoyed about the man's behaviour but said nothing. We both knew that he was a fortunate devil, and if he had waited any longer and the appendix had burst, the outcome could have been much different."

Jennie laughed, "I'm sure you were smiling then, Robert. Poor foolish man and his 'cures.'"

Robert agreed and told her the rest of the story, "During his convalescence, which lasted about three weeks, Doctor Penny and I had several friendly conversations. I asked him where he had taken his medical training as a naturopath physician, and he told me that he had taken the course by mail. I then inquired whether he had any actual training with patients. He told me he had none and that he had taken the examination and received his diploma in the mail as well. I smiled at him and asked if he had ever treated any patients since receiving his diploma, and he sheepishly admitted that he himself was the only patient he had ever treated and that he had now lost all faith in the treatment.

"At this, I laughed out loud as it was obvious the man had learned the hard way that some conditions simply require surgery, and acute appendicitis is one of them. Doctor Penny also laughed along with me but then told me, very firmly, that I was not to call him 'doctor'. He didn't want to ever be called by that title again as long as he lived. He just wanted to forget the whole thing."

Jennie knew that her husband had told her the tale in an attempt to ease her anxiety about Gordon's illness, and she was grateful for his thoughtfulness. She stood and, as she walked to the stairs, turned and smiled, "Thank you for that story, Robert. I'm glad it had a successful outcome, and it made me laugh at human foolishness. I think I will sleep now."

Robert sat for a while longer, his own nagging worries about Gordon coming to the fore in the quiet. "There is nothing I can do for him beyond what we are doing now," he thought, "my other patients need me to concentrate completely on them. I, too, must sleep."

***

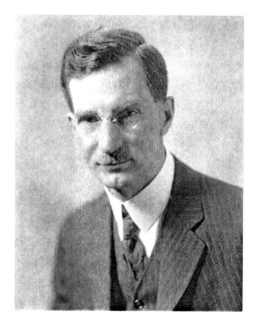

Robert, Drumheller, 1920's

Three months later, in February 1922, news of the successful trial of insulin on a severely ill diabetic patient reached Robert and Jennie. Within days, Robert had arranged care for his patients, had sent a telegram to the University of Toronto, and was on his way to the East to meet with Banting.

While he normally enjoyed every minute of his travels, this train trip across the plains found his emotions alternating between soaring hope at the possibility of a real treatment for diabetes and deep fear that the long-awaited insulin might not prove to be the lifesaving solution that his son so desperately needed. Well aware that Gordon's health was deteriorating quickly, Robert was desperately impatient at the time it took to get to his destination at the university where Banting had his laboratory.

Robert was not alone in his pursuit of insulin; many of his colleagues from the medical schools of eastern Canada were also meeting with Banting and his partner, Charles Best, to learn more about this wonderful discovery. Robert was, however, one of the few doctors to make the trip from the new western provinces. Although other parents had brought their diabetic children to the university in the hopes of treatment, it was not yet ready for, or even available to, the public. Clinical trials were still underway. However, the research team was amenable to Robert's plan to take insulin back to Alberta and to volunteer his own son as a trial subject. Since Robert was a doctor, had shown interest in the research since its inception, and would monitor the experiment with great care, they knew that his observations would be a valuable addition to their own work in their race to save the lives of those afflicted with diabetes, especially children.

Within the month, Robert arrived back in Drumheller with the precious insulin packed in a chest of ice that he had renewed constantly from the train's supplies. He had also made arrangements for a steady supply of insulin to be shipped to Drumheller, both for Gordon and his other diabetic patients, once the required trials in Toronto were completed.

The difference in how Gordon felt once he began the treatment was dramatic, and for some months, it seemed as though the dark shadow that had lain over the house for so long had been lifted. Jennie smiled again, Robert was pleased that not only his son but also other patients could benefit from this discovery, and Douglas was glad his brother was no longer so tired and irritable.

For nearly a year, Gordon took his daily injections faithfully and followed the controlled regimen of diet and rest that his parents had designed for him. If the eighteen-year-old had continued to accept and take on the necessary responsibility of his eating and behaviour, he might also have continued to enjoy a happy life. However, as more years went by, no matter how often his parents reminded him of the importance of this regimen to his continuing health, he grudgingly took the daily injections but angrily insisted that the insulin should be enough to cure him. He began once again to indulge more and more often in his craving for sweets.

Further, despite prohibition of alcohol, both familial and legal, his father suspected Gordon was now drinking with his friends. Douglas, whose relationship with his older brother over the years since insulin had changed their lives — going from hopeful to awkward to almost hostile as he watched Gordon self-destruct and once again cause his parents such grief — was quite sure that his brother was drinking.

Jennie, who had initially held such high hopes for the insulin and who had been overjoyed with the initial results of the injections, despaired at her older son's intransigence and was convinced that the "rough" crowd Gordon was spending so much time with was leading him astray.

Witnessing his older son's stubborn refusal to accept the reality of his disease, Robert was not so sure others could be blamed. Although he understood how very difficult it was for any eighteen-year-old to accept the necessary restrictions that came with living with diabetes, he knew only too well that Gordon must begin to exert more self-discipline if he was to control this disease.

Chapter 20
A Goiter, Mumps, and Three Killers

Even though he was relieved by the improvement the insulin had made, Robert knew he could do no more to help Gordon. Despite his ongoing anxiety about his older boy and Jennie's depression, he was determined to enjoy, as much as he could, his own increasing involvement in the affairs of the growing community. Settled into life as a family man and doctor in Drumheller, Robert rarely spent evenings at home now. After his evening office hours were done, he met with like-minded friends to talk about ways to organize events for the town.

Always interested in sports, Robert encouraged the development of a local hockey team, was a member of the Masons, and did his part for the new United Church. His restless spirit and his complete lack of any sense of time when he was intrigued by an idea or medical challenge meant he would go anywhere any time to explore his interests.

A year after his trip to Toronto to obtain Gordon's insulin, Robert heard of a new treatment for goiter being used by a surgeon in Cleveland. In what Robert considered to be a happy coincidence, one of his patients was suffering from the results of a large goiter, and Robert blithely informed Jennie that he was going to Cleveland with this patient to find out about the new surgery.

"I have decided to accompany my patient for the operation. We leave within the week. I have referred all of my cases to Doctor McGregor and a new young medical man who has just joined our practice."

Jennie shook her head, not in disbelief, but in resignation. "Of course, Robert, Martha will pack for you. Do you have any idea how long you will be gone?"

"No, I will stay there for the surgery and postoperative period and will return with my patient when he is strong enough to travel."

"Will you visit Sybil and Tarn?"

"Of course. My sister's last letter said that Tarn was quite ill, but she didn't go into details. I hope his illness is not serious. It took Sybil years to recover from the baby's death, and losing her husband now would be another dreadful blow for her."

Jennie's face was bleak as she recalled her own deep sorrow when she had learned that she could never have another child, but at least her two babies had survived. "Yes, no woman ever recovers from losing a baby. But Tarn is quite young. Surely it can't be that serious?"

"Yes, he's just in his forties. I don't know what the problem is, but I will certainly visit while I am there."

"Will your mother be there also?"

There was a little silence, and then Robert replied. "I don't know, Jennie," he paused then asked his wife to have Martha to prepare his things for the journey. "I will leave on the morning train three days from now. That will give us ample time to get to Cleveland for an appointment."

Robert sat in quiet thought for a moment, pondering the series of events that had led up to his somewhat cavalier decision to go to Cleveland.

It had begun a few days earlier, when a patient who was having trouble swallowing had come to see him for help. Ivan Petrov had submitted to a thorough examination of the large growth at the base of his throat.

"What you have is called an exophthalmic goiter, Ivan. It's curable, and I could deal with it, but it would be wiser to let a specialist handle the matter. I know of just such a doctor. He has a clinic in Cleveland that specializes in this condition. I would like to refer you to him as soon as possible. When could you be ready to travel?"

Ivan's voice was hoarse, and he was having difficulty swallowing as the goiter was large enough to cause pressure on his esophagus and trachea. "I could make the trip as soon as you got an appointment for me, Doc, but are you sure that I need to go? Do you think I need surgery? Why can't you do it here in Drumheller?"

"The clinic I have in mind specializes in this condition, and, yes, I think it will probably require surgery. However, these doctors have the experience to know if an operation is necessary, and I don't. They may also pursue other treatments."

"What caused this...what did you call it? A goiter?"

"Yes. Goiter. My first thought is that it was caused by an absence of iodine in your diet. It is only recently that iodine has been added to table salt, and we are now seeing far fewer of these thyroid problems since iodized salt has become available to everyone. For now, your goiter is large enough to cause you problems that will get worse without treatment, and the Cleveland clinic offers the best options for you."

Although Ivan was somewhat alarmed at the idea of surgery on his throat and the journey itself, he had complete confidence in Robert's counsel. "All right, I'll go."

"Good man. Now, there will be an initial consultation and then some tests before we even know if surgery is required. That will likely take the better part of a week. Then, if surgery is deemed necessary, a further two weeks is probable, so you should plan on at least a month away. It's a major undertaking."

By now, quite overwhelmed at the daunting prospect of a month spent alone in a large and unknown city, Ivan began to look very glum indeed and was obviously rethinking his original decision to go. Robert, never one to miss an opportunity to travel, offered a solution.

Clapping Ivan on the shoulder reassuringly, Robert announced, "I'll come with you."

"What? Come with me? Why?"

"Well, I'm very interested in learning how the medical men there will deal with this, and it means that you will have me with you on the return journey, especially important if you have surgery."

Ivan looked at his doctor in stunned amazement for a moment, then, "Right, we'll do it. Thanks, Doc."

Robert smiled happily as they shook hands, and he had his nurse call the Cleveland clinic to book Ivan's first appointment with the specialist for the following week. The nurse then sent in Robert's next patient, and his busy afternoon continued.

Jennie's voice recalled him abruptly to the present. "Robert, you do realize that you will be gone for at least a month, do you not?"

Robert was always pleased to have another journey in the offing and to learn something new, but he understood that Jennie was not always happy with his frequent travels.

"Yes, my dear, it will be a longer journey than most, but remember, that will allow me extra time to visit with Sybil and Tarn. And this is also the opportunity I have been waiting for to enrol for my American Surgical Certificate."

Three days later, doctor and patient boarded the train for Cleveland. In the event, it was determined that surgery was required, and Robert was a welcome and keen observer.

While Ivan recuperated, Robert visited his sister, Sybil, and her husband, Tarn, who was very ill. Robert was glad he had made this time to see him. Maggie McKenzie, Sybil and Robert's mother, was also there. When Maggie's second husband, Peter, had died, she had moved to Cleveland to live with Sybil and Tarn, and Robert was pleased for the opportunity to visit with his mother as well. Under normal circumstances, having her brother Robert stay in her home would have made Sybil very happy, but with Tarn so ill, it was hard to enjoy it fully.

Robert also used his time in the city to enrol in an extramural course in the latest techniques in surgery, with a view to gaining his American Specialization in Surgery within the next few years.

When Ivan was declared ready to go home under Robert's care, the two men boarded the train for Drumheller. It was a quiet journey, with Ivan not yet able to speak for very long and Robert's thoughts turning often to Maggie, Sybil, and Tarn. Ivan was still astonished and grateful that Robert had accompanied him on this journey and thought long and hard about ways to show his gratitude to the doctor.

"Doctor Ross, you have given me time that I thought I wouldn't have. How can I thank you?" he whispered hoarsely.

"It was my pleasure, Ivan. I learned a great deal from observing your surgery that will be of value to me in my practice back home. It also gave me an opportunity to visit with my family, and I love to travel. Just be sure to take the iodine supplements as prescribed and see me regularly for checkups."

Several months later, a beautiful long-case grandfather clock arrived at the Ross home, a gift of time from a grateful patient.

***

It seemed that every March, whether in Coleman or Drumheller, along with the slow disappearance of the snow and the very faint first signs of spring's return, all of the doctors had to deal with the mumps. Thus, Robert was not surprised by the symptoms the miner's wife described when the phone rang on a cold Sunday afternoon.

"My husband has a swelling on the side of his face, Doctor Ross. He has been complaining of a headache all weekend and has been very tired for some time now. Didn't even go to work Friday night shift; he is that sick. Slept all day today, and nothing I cook can tempt him. He's afraid he won't be able to go the mine tomorrow. And, Doctor, he seems to be very angry with me. That is not like him; he is a good man and a good father. Can you come?"

Robert donned his heavy coat and scarf, put on his warm hat and boots, and prepared to set out into the gloom of the late afternoon. "Keep my dinner warm, Martha. Jennie, I'm afraid you will have to go to evening service without me. Be sure to dress warmly. Do you want me to harness the horse and sled for you before I leave?"

"No, Robert, you needn't do that. It is only a short walk, and I'm feeling well today and would enjoy the outing. I'll go along with Mrs. Ewing next door. She had planned to accompany us anyway."

"All right, my dear, but beware of the icy paths. You know a fall would be disastrous, so walk arm in arm with Mrs. Ewing. I don't have far to go for this call, and I'll try to get to the church before the service ends."

With that, Robert, also choosing to walk, trudged the short distance along the darkening streets to the Rozzani's home. "The exercise will do me good," he thought, "it's only a few blocks, and it would be a shame to get the horse out for such a short distance. Thank goodness there is no wind tonight."

The frozen snow, now dirty from the winter's traffic and piled in grimy heaps along the roads and sidewalks, glittered in the warm light from houses along the way. These lights grew less frequent and less bright as Robert approached the streets where the miners' cottages were huddled close together, each in their own scrap of yard.

"It may be almost spring," he grumbled to himself, "but warmth seems to be many months away."

Mrs. Rozzani, a short, plump woman, her husband, and their large family had arrived in Drumheller several years ago. Mr. Rozzani, whom Robert knew to be a fine chap, worked in Nacmine. His wife welcomed the doctor to their small but tidy home and told Robert that all of the children had already had the mumps. This was good news, but Robert was still concerned about Mr. Rozzani. He knew the hardships for a family if the breadwinner had to miss even a day's work, so he was aware of how any illness could make a man very angry.

"He is in the back room, Doctor. He won't let me or the children near him. I've told him that we all had the mumps, but he keeps telling me to leave him alone."

Robert smiled reassuringly as he walked past the silent children, pushed back the heavy drape, and entered the dark back room. He could see the shape of the miner lying on his side on the bed, facing the wall. There was no electricity in the shack, but Mrs. Rozzani had given him a lantern, and he set this down on the small table by the bed. "Tell me what the problem is, Mr. Rozzani," he said in his best no-nonsense voice, although he already had a pretty fair idea of what was bothering the man, besides his illness.

Rozzani, normally a polite and pleasant fellow, turned his head and glared at the doctor, his expression a mixture of anger, pain, and embarrassment.

"I can't tell her about this, Doctor. I didn't want her to get you, but the pain...it's like I was kicked there by a horse."

He gestured to the blankets covering his lower body, muttering in a mixture of English and Italian, "Mi coglione, Doctor...si, so swollen." Robert moved the lantern to the floor. He had no need to examine the man and cause him further embarrassment.

"You have the mumps, and the infection has spread to your testicles, your coglione. That is what is causing the swelling and the pain. It will go away in a few days. Meanwhile, cold cloths will help reduce the swelling, and I'll give you aspirin for the pain."

"A few days? Cold cloths? But I have to work, and I can't even walk. And what am I going to tell her?"

"First of all, she already knows. Women just know these things, and besides she nursed your sons through this very same illness last spring. She is a good woman, and she will understand. She knows that you need to rest and eat as much of her good food as you can."

"Will the children get it? What about my boys? Can they get it again?"

"No, once you have the mumps, you cannot get them again. Your boys are safe. They have already had the mumps. They cannot catch them from you, and you will be fine in a few days. I'll give you a letter so that your wife can take it to the mine manager explaining why you cannot come to work. He wouldn't want you there spreading this to the other miners anyway."

"Doctor...," there was a long pause as Mr. Rozzani struggled to ask the question to which he feared the answer, "...Doctor, will I be able to, that is, can I, will this mean...?" He could not say any more.

Robert, knowing full well what the man was attempting to ask and knowing that the chances of sterility were very small, patted him gently on the shoulder and told him, "You will be able to father more children."

Mr. Rozzani heaved a sigh of relief at Robert's reassuring words and called for his wife to come into the room, telling her he was ready to try some of her good cooking. The men smiled at one another, and the doctor quietly took his leave.

When Robert left, chuckling to himself, it was full dark with the winter stars glinting like small ice chips in the black sky, but as he made his way the three blocks to the welcoming lights of the church, he smiled, quite sure that the air was a little warmer and that spring was truly on its way.

***

There were other childhood diseases that the valley doctors dealt with on a regular basis, and many of them were far less benign than the mumps. Three that were often killers were scarlet fever, typhoid fever, and diphtheria.

Scarlet fever usually struck children between the ages of four and eight and could have devastating effects for the survivors, including loss of vision and hearing, severe sinus infections, pneumonia, and meningitis. In these days long before penicillin, kidney infections and rheumatic fever were also consequences of untreated scarlet fever, and these secondary conditions also led to death. Treatment for scarlet fever consisted of little beyond bed rest, nutritious fluids, isolation, and calamine lotion for the rash. In 1924, Robert had begun using a vaccine that reduced the severity of the disease, but mortality was still widespread.

Another killer was diphtheria, often called "the strangler" because of the thick, choking layer of mucous that formed a membrane in the back of the throat. A vaccine had been discovered the year before, but it had not yet been widely accepted by the medical community, many of whom were averse to fighting a toxin with a toxin. Further, this vaccine was expensive, making its use unaffordable for most. Until the vaccine was refined and made both safer and more affordable, treatment was limited to isolation, bed rest, and aspirin to help reduce the swelling of the throat. There were several gargling solutions that claimed to clear the throat, but most did no more than ease the pain. Often, the doctors would scrape away the growths, but this had to be done in the very early stages of the disease before the pseudomembrane caused by proteins and toxins had formed. Once this tenacious grey membrane was present, the only option remaining to the doctors was to remove it surgically. This was rarely successful. Diphtheria was the second highest cause of childhood death after pneumonia with the terrible choking disease carrying off many young children. As always, poor sanitation, personal hygiene, and malnutrition played a major part in spreading the disease, and the children of poor families, often living in cramped and crowded houses, were particularly vulnerable.

Typhoid fever, with its fierce headaches, soaring temperatures, muscle weakness, terrible abdominal pain, and usually fatal diarrhea was another killer of children. As with the other two diseases, mortality was high, and treatment was limited to bed rest, isolation, and fluids. Ice baths were used to bring down the fever and prevent convulsions. Solutions of kaolin were prescribed to relieve the diarrhea, but it was a matter of treating the symptoms and not the disease itself. There had been a vaccine for typhoid fever available since 1914, but the side effects were so severe its use had been discontinued.

There was no doubt in Robert's mind, based on his experiences in Montreal and Lethbridge, that typhoid fever was a waterborne disease. He was adamant in this belief to the extent that he himself would drink only water that had been boiled. And in the years before chlorination of the municipal water supply, he insisted that all members of his household observed the same rule. There was a large copper boiler always simmering on the stove, and the distilled water it produced was kept cool in sterilized glass vessels in the ice box.

"Jennie, why can't people understand what they risk? The river is polluted. How can I tell them more clearly than I already am? Don't drink the water without boiling it first."

Jennie, who faithfully transported distilled water to church suppers and for that matter, everywhere they went, knew that for many people the distilled water was considered a mild eccentricity of the doctor. "Robert, we do all we can. Eventually, the city will chlorinate the supply. I am tired and going to bed. You must try to get some rest as well."

Robert, believing quite correctly that preventing waterborne diseases was easier than curing them, campaigned tirelessly to have the Drumheller water supply chlorinated. When this finally happened, it drastically reduced the number of cases of typhoid fever, although the disease was still a concern for those who chose to swim in the river to escape the summer's heat, often swallowing the water as they did so.

Chapter 21
Battleships and Bushels

"We're going to Vancouver? All of us? That's wonderful, Dad. The West Coast!" Douglas' enthusiasm for the trip his father had just announced was gratifying.

"Yes, I have decided that we should all go to Vancouver to see the arrival of the great British battleship, *HMS Hood*. She will arrive in Vancouver on the twenty-fifth of June."

It was a beautiful day in May 1924, and for once all of the family was together for a light supper, enjoying the warmth of the early evening.

Robert continued. "This will be a wonderful experience for us as a family. Everyone knows that the *Hood* is the greatest battleship in the world. And she's not travelling alone. There are six ships with her. They are not as big, but it will be an impressive sight, nevertheless."

"That would be swell, Dad," an excited Douglas interrupted his father. "We have all been reading about the *Hood's* round-the-world tour in school, but I never imagined that I would actually have a chance to see the fleet in person. Wow!"

Pleased at his son's enthusiastic response, Robert smiled and continued. "Yes, Douglas, we will be there in person for this celebration of the might of the Royal Navy."

Jennie was aware that the medical practice was flourishing and that they could well afford the trip. The pain of her rheumatism had subsided with the advent of warmer weather, and both of their sons had earned a break from their studies. Gordon was watching his diet again and feeling well, and it had been a long time since they had travelled together as a family. Also, it meant that she would be able to have another visit with her cousin, Dr. Helen Ryan, who lived in Victoria. Surely, if they got as far as Vancouver, something could be arranged. Her voice was hopeful as she asked, "The West Coast? Robert, that is very exciting. How long will we be away, and where will we stay?"

"We'll stay at the Sylvia Hotel in Vancouver. It is not far from Stanley Park, and we will be able to walk along the famous seawall and watch the ships come steaming into English Bay. It will be good for you, my dear, especially as you were not able to visit the West Coast last winter. We've heard from Douglas. Now, what do you think, Gordon?"

"This is a wonderful idea, Father." Gordon spoke calmly, but it was evident that he, too, thought the trip was a fine idea. "I am feeling so well now with the insulin, and a trip is just the thing. I can think of it as a celebration, and my friends will be envious."

"And I can see that you have more to say, Douglas. Go ahead."

"I'm really excited about this, Dad. A train trip through the mountains to see great ships on the Pacific? What could be better? How many nights will we sleep on the train? Will we each have our own berths? Wait until I tell Hec and Joe."

"Probably three or four days and nights on the train. Your mother and I will have a private compartment, and, yes, you will each have your own berth."

"I get dibs on the upper berth, Gordon."

"Of course you do; you are younger. I prefer a lower berth anyway."

"We'll discuss this again once I have made all the plans and reservations. Your mother will organize your packing. Jennie, everyone may have something new for the trip. And, yes, we will try to manage a visit with your cousin Nell. I am glad you are all pleased with the idea."

Douglas half rose from his chair as if to dash out to tell his friends but, at a warning glance from his mother, settled again to wait for the conversation to end.

Robert rose from his chair. "Now, I must go into the office for a few hours. I'll be late, my dear. I also have a house call to make, and you must get your rest. You, too, boys. Good night."

The great day finally arrived, and the trip through the mountains was as exciting as they could have hoped. Their first sight of the ocean was stunning, an endless vista of water and sky stretching before them. It was so vast its immensity rivalled the prairie landscapes of their home.

The city itself, curving around the sparkling water of English Bay, was no less impressive. On their way to the hotel, they drove along tree-lined streets and passed lovely old buildings.

Jennie's cousin Nell, who was well used to travelling around the province for her work as an advocate for women's franchise and education, had also booked rooms at the Sylvia Hotel, and the two women spent many hours together. Nell was concerned about Jennie's frail and pallid appearance so quietly discussed her worries with Robert, doctor to doctor.

"She is very thin, Robert. As you requested, I have examined her and can find no physical cause beyond the obvious one of her rheumatism and her incessant worries about Gordon. I agree that the trip has been good for her, if somewhat exhausting. Like many women her age, she spends too much time sitting and, as a result, has poor muscle tone. I know that her rheumatism prevents her from taking vigorous exercise, but, if she were my patient, I would prescribe long walks every day and a good tonic. The difficulty is that all of the popular nostrums contain alcohol, which we both know Jennie will not touch. In addition, I don't think she is eating enough, certainly not enough of the right foods. A good walk each day would help with her appetite. And could your cook not ensure that she had more vegetables, not cooked to mush, please, and a good non-alcoholic tonic of some sort? Perhaps she could make a fruit and vegetable concoction for Jennie? Tea is lovely, but she needs more than that."

Robert, who shared Dr. Ryan's concern, smiled wryly at the thought of Jennie drinking raw vegetable juice. "Perhaps if you prescribed it, Nell, and I tried to enforce it. We'll see. It has already been a tonic for Jennie to see you. Thank you for your advice. Do you think I should take her to a specialist in women's disorders in Calgary when we get home?"

"I think that would be a good idea, Robert. Although I doubt we have missed anything, an opinion from a specialist might impress upon Jennie the need to take her health more seriously."

On the twenty-fifth of June, the whole family, suitably garbed for a misty Vancouver day, joined the exuberant crowds gathered on the seawall ready to cheer the magnificent parade of naval ships as they crossed English Bay. The fog lifted just as the eight hundred and sixty-two foot long Hood led the parade of ships across the water before them. Men and boys shouted, "Huzzah! Three cheers for the King!" and threw hats and caps into the air while the women clapped and smiled. It was a great occasion and would be long remembered by the family from Alberta as the high point of a wonderful journey together.

As their stay in Vancouver drew to a close, the Rosses and Dr. Ryan enjoyed a farewell dinner together. The following day, as the family prepared to board the train for their return trip, the women promised to maintain the correspondence that they had begun when Jennie was a young girl in Mt. Forest. Nell's final worried admonition to Jennie echoed in the cavernous train station. "I hope you will be able to visit me in Victoria next winter when the cold strikes Drumheller. Meanwhile, do as the doctor says, and remember to go for walks often and drink your tonic."

***

The next years flew by. Gordon's health was now more stable, and he was doing well in the extramural accounting course offered through Queen's University, his father's alma mater. Douglas was an active, popular young man in his high-school years, Jennie was deeply involved with the United Church affairs, and Robert's very successful medical practice mirrored the prosperity of the growing town. The

Drumheller Valley was thriving, the coal mines producing over one million tons of coal in 1922, thus pouring six million dollars into the economy of the town.

Throughout the 1920s, Drumheller became known as the fastest growing town in Canada. New businesses came to town and new farm families took up homesteads on the flatlands on all sides of the valley, growing wheat and raising cattle for eastern Canada and European markets. The rains came with regularity, and it began to look as if the flourishing town would have sufficient population to be called a city within the decade.

Always supportive of young people and athletics, Robert's own family background meant he had a personal interest in hockey. His younger brother Art Ross was a well-known figure in the world of professional hockey, and Robert had followed his career with great interest and pride. As an executive member of the Drumheller Miners Hockey team, Robert delighted in offering his services as a doctor and his motorcar as transportation for the team's away games. Many happy days were spent driving the young men to neighbouring towns over rough to nonexistent roads.

Gordon had neither the time nor the energy to participate in hockey but, under his father's tutelage, became an excellent rifle shot, eventually competing at the national level and winning the Dominion Marksmanship medal. Douglas, physically too slight for hockey, also enjoyed shooting but left the competitions to his brother.

Always a sociable fellow, Robert continued his active participation in community affairs. He enjoyed getting together with the men of the town to discuss business, and he had long been an advocate of the work of Rotary International with its mandate of service to the country and the world. When a group of his friends suggested starting a Drumheller Rotary Club, he was pleased to support their efforts. He was a charter member when the club was formed and over the years to come would speak often at the meetings on topics of interest to the members. He also contributed generously to the fundraising efforts of the group and was especially pleased to contribute towards the construction of the Rotary Swimming Pool.

It had become a pleasant part of his daily routine for Robert to take a late afternoon break and join his men friends in the café on the corner across from his office. There, he caught up on the business of the town with the group, many of whom were small business owners. Farmers who had come into town to buy equipment for their rapidly expanding farms or ranches were often part of these afternoon get-togethers.

The quiet hum of conversation in the restaurant paused briefly as Robert entered the café one afternoon in late 1924. He removed his hat and paused briefly at several tables, asking after the health of families or the new baby, and nodded courteously to other townsfolk as he made his way to his usual table in the corner. He was well known and well liked by the community and had seen many of them as patients. There were a few women, store clerks as a rule or farm wives, who had been shopping and were waiting for their husbands to take them home. But most of the café's patrons were men, local merchants pausing for a late afternoon cup of tea or coffee and perhaps a sandwich before returning to their businesses for the evening hours.

"Another good week, then, Howard?" Robert greeted the other men at the table in turn. Howard and Nels Vickers ran a very successful hardware store, and as the homesteaders and miners continued to pour into the valley, their business had continued to grow.

"Couldn't be better, Doc. Delivering lots of babies?"

"Yes, indeed, and I enjoy doing it. How are things at Toshach's, Bert?"

And so the conversation went on, the men enjoying one another's company and happily discussing the glowing future of the town. A sober note was introduced when the topic turned to grain prices, which had been erratic and low this past year.

One of the merchants expressed his worries about the situation. "The farmers are really suffering this year. It costs more to grow a bushel of grain than they get when they sell it. That has to change."

There was agreement all around and more questions asked. "What about this idea of a grain cooperative? This Alberta Wheat Pool? Will it help, do you think?"

Howard had been a farmer for some time, so he spoke with authority. "Well, it will help stabilize grain prices. And prices can only get better. I've heard news of the growing European Market demand for more Canadian wheat. There are already twenty-six thousand prairie farmers in the organization. And we've all heard the talk of building our own grain elevators, which would mean farmers could cut out the middleman. That's a cost saving."

This particular afternoon, the group had been joined by James Holden, the president of the Atlas Coal Mine, one of the biggest mines in the valley. He had been listening intently to the discussion and now spoke. "Good. We're doing so well with the coal; it would be a terrible blow to the town if the farmers couldn't make it."

James was very active in community affairs as were all of the men at the table. He continued, "I can't get enough men for the mines sometimes; the demand for miners is so high. That's why I'm in town today. Some new chaps are registering for work at the post office, and I'm hoping that a few of them will be willing to work in the mines."

The conversation became more general again. "How was the trip to Vancouver, Robert?"

Robert entertained the group with stories of his trip, and the hour passed pleasantly. The café emptied as the men went on their way with talk of getting together the following week. They all went back to work or collected wives and shopping, and the quiet of early evening descended on the town.

Robert mulled over the conversations as he walked the short distance to his office. "I wonder if there might be an opportunity to make a little money on the wheat market. This new cooperative plus the growing demand from Europe might make wheat a good investment. Gordon's extramural course is proving to be more expensive than I planned, and Douglas is talking about the University of Alberta and then McGill in Montreal. I have some money put aside for their education, but maybe I could add to it. And a new motorcar would be just the thing...." He was deep in thought as he entered the waiting room of the clinic, where his receptionist greeted him.

"Good evening, Agnes. Do I have any patients waiting? Ah, yes, please come in, Mr. Newman. That looks like a nasty burn. Dangerous work blacksmithing. You've burned yourself deeply there. Good thing you missed the tendons. Here, I'll give you a shot of morphine to kill the pain before I clean it up. Are your boys available to take you home? Good."

The investment idea was put aside but not forgotten, and over the next few years, Robert began to put a little money into wheat futures each month. These small investments showed great promise as a future source of extra income as long as the price of wheat continued to rise. This it did, steadily and reassuringly, as did the overall fortunes of the small prairie town.

Chapter 22
Drugs and Music

The little blue glass bottle on the bedside table of the young widow reflected the glow of the single kerosene lamp and caught Robert's eye as he stood quietly and looked down at the pale face on the much laundered pillow. It was a scene encountered all too frequently by doctors in any mining community.

He examined the sleeping woman, whom he understood to be in her late twenties, for any injuries but was unsurprised to find none. Her exhausted face was marked by care and grief, and although her nightgown, modestly closed at throat and wrists, had obviously been washed until it was threadbare, it was clean. Her hands were rough and red, and her nails bitten to the quick. Eight children, ranging in age from a boy of perhaps fourteen to a wee girl of three, were lined up solemnly by their mother's bedside, their own eyes red and swollen from their grief at their father's death.

"Your mother is not dead," he reassured the children, "she is sleeping deeply and cannot wake up because she has taken too much of her medicine. When she does wake up, she will need your help," he directed these words to the two women who sat quietly in the corners of the small dark room, "and she must not take any more of this medicine, though she will beg you for it."

The women, both neighbours of the patient, nodded their understanding as Robert continued, "Make sure she eats something, soup and some bread if you have it, and she must drink lots of water but no more of this medicine. Have these children eaten?"

Despite his certain knowledge that the mother would try to continue to take the laudanum to numb her pain and fear at her husband's death, Robert felt a deep sadness for the children and knew he must do what he could. "If you have nothing to make broth, go to my kitchen, and the housekeeper will give you whatever she can."

He looked with pity at the oldest boy, whom he knew would be going into the mines where his father had died. Someone had to earn a livelihood. The youngster could not go below ground until he was sixteen but meanwhile would try to get a lower paying job on the surface. The family, despite the willingness of neighbours who would share what little they had, would need every penny this youngster could bring in to feed them. Both the boy and his next oldest brother after him would eventually have to go down the dark tunnels under the valley.

"Give me the laudanum," Robert ordered, "I'll give you something else that will help her but that's not so dangerous. Mix this syrup with water, about one-half teaspoon per glass, twice a day. It will last about two weeks, and when it is finished, call me and I will come again to see how you are all faring."

Robert put the blue glass bottle of laudanum in his bag. It was an easily obtained powerful mixture of alcohol and opium, the equivalent of almost three hundred milligrams of morphine per ounce. The syrup he left with them in exchange also contained morphine but was much less potent, with about sixty-five milligrams of morphine per ounce. Mixed with water, it would help the young widow sleep but would not be nearly so dangerous or addictive. And, after two weeks, he would wean her off completely. He knew the miners' wives were incredibly hardy, and as long as she was not allowed to kill herself, she would be able to cope with the dreary life ahead of her.

As his car rattled over the dusty buggy tracks and onto the rough roads to town and his office, Robert reflected with a shudder on what could have happened with his own wife and opium.

Jennie had always been physically fragile, and following Douglas's extremely difficult birth and the bitter realization that she could never have more children, she had sunk into a dark ongoing depression from which she never fully recovered. There were any number of preparations available to combat depression and "female conditions." These paregorics were prescribed and sold under various names such as "Mrs. Wilson's Soothing Syrup" and were guaranteed to cure almost any ills. They also claimed to elevate moods, which they no doubt did as they were potent mixtures of alcohol and opium. Heroin was easily available over the counter and was touted as a remedy for asthma, coughs, and pneumonia as well as depression. Many of these so-called soothing syrups were considered indispensable to mothers and child-care workers. These concoctions often contained as much as five hundred and fifty-six milligrams of morphine per fluid ounce and were said to effectively quiet restless infants and small children and to help mothers relax.

Although Robert was well aware that such preparations were commonly used by his patients and his friends, thanks to Jennie's strictures regarding alcohol they were never used in his house. Although her physician had prescribed laudanum to allow her some relief in the early years of her severe depression following Douglas's birth, she had steadfastly refused to take it as soon as she was strong enough to object, and with Robert's assistance, she took nothing stronger than aspirin. She coped with her pain and depression over the years with tea and prayers, good works and good books, and Robert's steady support and understanding.

Jennie's aversion to alcohol in any form was based both on her strict Methodist beliefs and an earlier terrifying experience when she saw her father become addicted to laudanum after his leg was amputated.

In the early years in Drumheller, as in Coleman, Jennie's reticence and strict views on alcohol were seen by many as a character flaw. Her rigid morality was thought to be out of place in a town still governed by an "anything goes" frontier mentality. However, she was never openly judgemental but simply maintained her own beliefs with quiet dignity.

Eventually, her involvement in church groups and her work for the community was recognized as helpful, especially by the women of the town. She was an adherent of the Winnipeg preacher James Shaver Woodsworth and his credo of "social gospel." He taught that it was the duty of a Methodist to improve people's lives and not just preach to them. Jennie believed in her faith and works of mercy, compassionate service and works for God among all of God's human family. Even those who felt she was too strict in her behaviours understood and appreciated her desire to help others. For some reason, the fact that the doctor himself was a teetotaller was accepted without comment, perhaps because Jennie was seen as disapproving while Dr. Ross was seen as a fine fellow despite the fact that he did not partake of alcohol.

Robert's own abstinence from alcohol was founded in his family history and his experience with the terrible toll paid by the native people in Canada when the Europeans, especially the traders, introduced alcohol to their lives. Robert's father, Thomas Barnston Ross, was an alcoholic and would eventually die alone as a result of this disease. More immediately, as a doctor, Robert dealt regularly with the cruel and violent consequences for men who turned to the bottle in an effort to escape their pain and poverty.

The easy availability of alcohol and drugs made it extremely difficult for Robert to prevent his patients, especially the women, from turning to the use of these patent medicines for comfort in times of pain and loss, thus the blue bottles at the bedsides of widows. The Pure Food and Drug Act of 1906 had required manufacturers to list their ingredients, but the various syrups containing opium, cocaine, and morphine continued to be sold. And alcohol, despite all evidence to the contrary, was believed to be a preventative for some diseases.

***

Robert understood very well that he needed his own place at home away from his busy medical practice. Accordingly, he had converted a small area in the basement from a storage area to a home office and music room. His books and papers were on shelves and his desk was prepared with the necessary writing instruments, including a small typewriter.

"Someday, I will write my memoirs from my case notes, but for now this is my music room," he thought happily as he looked at his guitars. Robert had always loved music and was a very good amateur guitarist. He owned several fine instruments, and playing them in the evening was his way to forget all the stress and cares of the day.

The music of Isaac Albeniz was always a favourite, and Robert sat and pensively strummed the haunting chords of *Recuerdos de viaje*. When he was content that his rendition was sure, he carried the guitar up the stairs to the front room where his wife sat reading.

"Do you have some time, my dear? I know that you play this composition on your piano. Perhaps we could play together?"

Jennie, who had heard her husband practicing, smiled her consent.

"Of course, Robert. I'll need a few moments to warm up my fingers, and then I would be pleased to accompany you. It is one of my favourite pieces, also."

"Thank you, Jennie. I will listen as you prepare." Robert settled happily into his chair and smiled contently as Jennie played her warm-up exercises. Her piano had travelled to Drumheller when they moved, and he knew what a comfort it was for his wife to have it there.

"Could you ask Martha to make us tea later, Robert? It would be pleasant to share a pot of tea before we retire for the evening."

"Indeed I will, and we can hope there will be no calls this evening."

They enjoyed an hour or so of music and, while drinking their tea, spoke quietly of the activities of their sons.

"Robert, Gordon is doing exceptionally well in his studies. He is a bright young man, and it was wise of him to choose to take his work by correspondence. It makes it much easier for us to help him to control his illness when he is at home."

"Yes, Jennie, it was a good decision on all our parts, and your help has been invaluable. How is he doing with his practical work at the bank?"

"Very well, Robert, very well."

Douglas was in his final year of high school where he was achieving top marks academically and was also the president of the student council. Both achievements were a source of great pride for his father.

"Douglas is becoming quite fond of young Elizabeth Stevenson, Jennie. She is a clever young woman and plans to become a school teacher. I like her a great deal. And Gordon is interested in young Elsie Gabriel. She has a good head on her shoulders, and I find her a kind young woman."

"Robert, it is far too early to discuss any young women either of the boys may be interested in. They both have their careers ahead of them. I believe that Gordon is being more careful with his activities and friends now, and I am sure he will shine in whatever he chooses to pursue. I wish Douglas would consider a career as an engineer. He loves to build things. This talk of going into medicine is nonsense. Please do not encourage him." Jennie already resented what she saw as Douglas's competition with Gordon in the academic area. She was also fiercely proud of her husband's reputation as a wonderful doctor and was becoming uneasy about the possibility that their younger son might overshadow his father if he, too, went into medicine

Robert, who had thoroughly enjoyed the evening of music and peaceful conversation, sighed but kept his hopes for Douglas and his worries about Gordon to himself. He knew that despite his best efforts and those of his mother, Gordon, who had been taking insulin for four years now, still did not always stick to the diet prescribed for a diabetic. Even during the years of Prohibition, his father was sure that Gordon and his friends were finding alcohol somewhere, but he knew how distressed Jennie became at any such talk so did not pursue the subject.

"Thank you for the pleasant evening, my dear. You must be tired. I'm going down to my music room to practice a little more. Are you going to retire? Sleep well."

Chapter 23
Montreal for a Reo

"An elegant repast, thank you, Martha, no, no more, thank you again. I have eaten very well." Robert smiled at his own little joke. "An elegant sufficiency."

Jennie nodded her head. "Please clear the table now, Martha, it was very good."

The family had enjoyed a special meal together, partly to celebrate how well Gordon was doing in his accountancy studies and partly to celebrate Robert's successful attainment of the American Medical Association Surgical Specialty Degree, which he would receive in Cleveland. Robert was contented as he left the table and spoke to his family. "Gordon, Douglas, please join your mother and me in the living room. We have plans to make for our trip to the East."

"Sure, Dad," Douglas replied, with a quick glance at his brother. Gordon simply walked into the room and sat down, muttering about his own plans for the evening.

Jennie and Robert were travelling to Ontario and Quebec to visit family and would then go on to Cleveland to pick up the Surgical Certificate on the return trip. Their plans included the purchase of a new motorcar while in Montreal, and Robert wanted to hear his sons' opinions about that.

Neither of the young men was able to travel with them, but they both listened politely as their father outlined the travel plans. They were particularly attentive when conversation turned to a happy discussion of new cars.

"What kind of a motorcar will you purchase, Dad?"

"I'm not sure, Douglas, I will have a look at what is available in Montreal. What would you like me to buy?"

"Robert," his wife interjected, "don't encourage him. You are the one making this decision, not the boys."

"Yes, my dear, but I enjoy their opinions. What do you think, Gordon?"

"Something red would be swell, Dad. A red convertible would be just the cat's meow."

Robert laughed at the use of slang, but Jennie frowned. However, she was so pleased at Gordon's enthusiasm that she said nothing.

"Yes," Douglas chimed in, "a red convertible would be super, Father."

"If you had a car, could I drive it sometimes? It would sure liven this town up," asked Gordon, imagining himself impressing all his friends.

Douglas murmured to his brother so quietly that only Gordon could hear. "You'd have to stay away from the giggle water."

Gordon shot him an evil look.

His mother, who was not pleased by the idea of Gordon driving at all, turned the conversation to the necessary arrangements for the boys in their parents' absence.

"Gordon, your father has made arrangements for you to get your insulin from Doctor McGregor each day, and you will seek him out for any medical matters. You know how careful you must be with your diet."

"Please, Mother, I know all too well. I am twenty-two years old after all, and I am the one with the disease."

There was a heavy silence for a moment, and then Jennie turned to her younger son. "Study hard, Douglas. If you have any problems, I am sure you can get help at school."

Douglas, who never had any academic problems, sighed and nodded.

Their father then spoke, "You both will have our itinerary and can always reach us by telegram. Please ensure that you are, as always, respectful of Martha and let her know about any meals you might miss. We will talk further of this as the time comes closer."

Seeing that his wife had all plans well in hand, Robert retreated to his music room to read his most recent medical news. There was information about a new vaccine for pertussis, and he hoped to secure a supply in Montreal. It would be well to vaccinate the children of the town before the winter arrived. He would ask to speak on this topic at the first Rotary meeting when they returned. A report to Rotary plus word to Jennie's church and community groups would spread the news quickly. He also thought of contacting one of the town's newspapers, the *Drumheller Mail*, but that could wait until his return.

Robert also needed to read some information he had received from the Alberta Medical Association. This year would be a good time to offer his services to the provincial organization with its headquarters in Edmonton. Douglas would soon be attending the University of Alberta, also in the provincial capital, as he was to take his pre-medical courses there.

Robert was still not sure that he altogether approved of his younger son's desire to follow in his footsteps, but he knew that Douglas was an extremely bright young man and very keen. Robert chuckled to himself at his own use of slang, glad that Jennie could not read his thoughts.

"If I become a member of the AMA Executive, that will mean frequent trips to Edmonton, and I can spend time with Douglas and share my medical expertise. We would both enjoy that."

He turned to his papers to read more about the new vaccine, but his mind was already on the way to Montreal and the new car. "Hmmm...red? I don't think so, but a swell little Roadster would truly be, as Gordon says, the cat's meow."

***

Robert and Jennie enjoyed their time in Montreal where they were guests of his younger brother Dr. Colin Ross, a surgeon specializing in diagnostic radiology who hoped to travel to Edinburgh someday, to obtain his FRCP. Jennie and Colin's wife, Ethel, had corresponded for years and were pleased to have time together. This visit with his brother and several days spent at McGill University where he would catch up on the latest medical news and developments pleased Robert. He was happy to be able to arrange for a quantity of the new vaccine for pertussis, more commonly known as whooping cough, to be shipped to Drumheller. This ailment plagued the small prairie town every winter. There was also talk at the university of a vaccine for tuberculosis now in development that might be ready the following year. Robert could only pray that this would be so.

The days passed pleasantly as Robert and Colin solemnly discussed medicine and politics, and the two couples visited and dined with other family and friends. Robert was interested in Colin's opinion of what everyone in Montreal thought of this William Lyon Mackenzie King fellow and the current government scandals.

The brothers also spent happy hours at several car dealerships and were delighted when they found a spanking new Reo Roadster for sale. The dealership had a model with the newest innovation, an automatic transmission, so Robert and Colin promptly took one for a test drive up the winding roads to the park on the top of Mount Royal. They sat looking over the view of the city and chatting about their lives before reluctantly heading back downtown, with Robert mulling over which car to buy.

"I think I'd better purchase one with a regular transmission. The parts for the automatic will be too difficult to come by in Alberta, and the roads there are still very rough compared to the macadam surfaces here in Montreal. What do you think, Colin?"

"You are probably wise, but my goodness, this one is fun to drive, isn't it? I especially like not having to change gears going uphill, but you're right. It's good to be practical, and besides, you don't have hills in Alberta, do you?" He grinned at his older brother as he asked, "So you'll be getting a sedan? Not a sporty two-seater like this Roadster? Of course, it is not so practical as a sedan but a lot more fun."

Robert wheeled the Reo around a corner as they drove down the steep hill between tall trees and hedges. He had already lost his heart to the sports model but pretended to be giving the choice serious thought. "Well, Colin, I don't need to use my private vehicle as an ambulance any more, and I usually drive alone or with Jennie. I've decided. I'm going to get the two-seater. In black, however, not red as Gordon and Douglas had hoped."

"I think," Colin laughed heartedly in reply, "I think they really will think this car is the cat's pyjamas! You will certainly be able to 'boogie along' in this automobile."

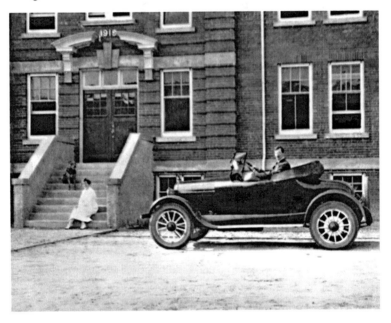

Robert and the REO, Drumheller Hospital, Drumheller, Alberta, 1926

The shiny black Roadster was purchased, and arrangements were made to ship it to Drumheller. Robert was delighted with it and was sorry now that he and Jennie had made other plans to visit while in the East, so he couldn't travel home with the new car.

They left on the trip to Cleveland to pick up Robert's Surgical Certificate and to spend some time with his sister Sybil and her husband, Tarn. Robert's mother, Maggie McKenzie, was still in Cleveland staying with her daughter.

Jennie fell ill while in Cleveland, and although Robert suspected her willingness to be confined to her room had something to do with Maggie's ongoing disapproval of his wife, he said nothing, but was more than ready to leave after a few days of the tension between the two women. He was irked not to have more time to spend with Tarn whose health continued to fail but, after receiving his certificate, knew it was time to move on. They planned to make a short stop in Sudbury to visit the Ryan cousins who still lived in the area.

Travelling to Sudbury, Robert felt restless, his thoughts moving uneasily from Tarn's illness and his sister's worried face, to Jennie's continuing malaise, however feigned it might have been. It was not like her to avoid unpleasantness, usually meeting it head-on, so her pallor concerned him. She was also listless, heavy with fatigue, and unwilling to talk, so much of the train journey north was spent in silence. Robert sighed, remembering the happy days they had spent in Montreal. Though it was never spoken of, he knew that, even now, Jennie would prefer to live in an eastern city.

They travelled up the shores of Lake Erie and Lake Ontario, watching farmland alternate with forests and then travelled inland with Georgian Bay to their left as they approached their destination. Robert was astonished at the growth of towns and cities in Ontario and thought longingly of the emptiness of the Great Plains.

Finally, Sudbury came into view. While the landscape was still a bleak industrial wasteland, the economy was on the upswing. Land had been set aside for parks, there were schools and many churches, and the stone and brick houses announced the growing prosperity of the merchants and mine owners. An effort had been made to plant and nurture trees and shrubs, which greatly improved the look of the residential areas, though the pollution from the mills still poisoned the struggling native vegetation surrounding the town.

Altogether, this was a much more optimistic city than they had seen in 1919, and they both hoped it would be a happier time than their previous visit when Jennie and Robert had been so distressed about Gordon's health.

And so it was. Visiting all the cousins and meeting their growing families was a pleasure for the Drumheller couple. Jennie was beginning to feel much better as they boarded the train again for the long trip home.

Robert, much as he loved to travel, was always glad to get away from big cities. He looked forward to his return to Drumheller where his new automobile would be waiting for him, and he could catch his brother George up on news of the eastern branch of the family. He was well satisfied with their journey but was ready to go home. And Jennie was missing her sons.

"Robert, I need to be home for Gordon. He is doing very well in his practicum at the bank, but he will require my assistance in his final coursework, so I am glad we are returning home. He also needs our firm guidance in his diet."

Gordon was nearing completion of his accounting courses, which he was taking extramurally through Robert's alma mater, Queen's University. Although insulin had made a huge difference to their son's life, Jennie and Robert both continued to worry that Gordon may have strayed off his careful regimen in their absence.

Douglas was in his final year at Drumheller High School and planning to go to the University of Alberta for his arts degree and perhaps on into pre-med.

"Robert, I do wish Douglas was not set upon going into medicine. I don't think he will ever be the doctor you are, and he might be a good engineer. Remember how he enjoyed building that radio?"

"My dear, I have not encouraged him to become a doctor, but if that is his wish, I will support him, and that is the end of it."

Jennie spoke no more of the matter, and her thoughts turned to her involvement in the ladies' church group and other community activities. She had her duties awaiting her. It was time to go home, and to her quiet relief, the trips to visit relatives seemed to be assuaging Robert's restless need to move on, and Drumheller was feeling more and more like a permanent residence.

Chapter 24
A Tragic Epidemic and Measles

Of all the illnesses that afflicted children, the most terrifying was polio-myelitis, called infantile paralysis, so when in the early summer of 1927 Robert sat quietly in his office listening as Mrs. Walkerson described the symptoms her four-year-old son was experiencing, he felt a wave of desolation engulf him. Robert's expression was gentle and kind, but his heart was sinking, and desperate anger swept through him as she spoke. He rarely despaired when faced with illness, but a seriously ill child hurt him deeply, and the cruelty of infantile paralysis left him struggling with the knowledge that he could do little to help.

"He is so tired all the time, Doctor Ross. He says he hurts all over. I thought at first it might be the 'flu again, just like nearly killed my husband after the war, but Little Sam keeps talking about bad pains in his legs, and he is so sick to his stomach..." her voice trailed off as she held her little boy in her lap and looked hopefully at the doctor. "He's only four years old, and last week he was running around laughing. What is it, Doctor Ross? What's the matter with Little Sam?" She waited for Robert to speak.

Robert looked at the youngster, his head lolling against his mother's shoulder, legs hanging loosely.

"Let's have a look on the examination table. Can you set him down there please, Mrs. Walkerson?"

The little boy whimpered as Mrs. Walkerson placed him on the table, but his body was limp and hot, and when Robert checked his reflexes, there was hardly any response.

The frightened woman was silent as the doctor examined her son, but her expression beseeched Robert to reassure her.

"Little Sam needs to go to the hospital right away. My nurse will come in and take a blood sample immediately to be sure we know what is causing this, but I am afraid it is infantile paralysis. We will make him as comfortable as possible, and you need to know that many, many times this muscle weakness and pain is temporary, and with care it will pass. He may recover completely. Our job now is to try to stop the disease from worsening."

Silent tears ran down Mrs. Walkerson's cheeks as she listened to the diagnosis. She knew what it meant, and her agonized worry about her son was evidence of that fearful knowledge.

Robert arranged for the child to be admitted to the newly established isolation ward in the hospital and silently prayed to what he hoped was a merciful God that the paralysis would be temporary and would not affect the boy's inner organs, especially his brain and spinal cord. He also prayed that no other children would be affected.

But this was not to be. Many children became ill as the polio epidemic of 1927 swept across North America. Several children in Drumheller, including Little Sam, died when the paralysis reached the muscles of their chests so that they could not breathe, but many more who recovered from the initial illness were left with permanently twisted legs or an arm that dangled uselessly.

Robert and the other doctors had no idea what caused the disease to reach epidemic levels in Alberta and the other prairie provinces or why it seemed to be at its worst in the summers. Most medical men believed that poor sanitation was an underlying cause; others thought it was waterborne; many believed that overcrowded cities were the cause. There did seem to be evidence that newly arrived immigrant children were less susceptible to the illness, but no one knew why.

For now, Robert and all the doctors and nurses in Drumheller did their best. One late evening, he paced the living room in frustration and anger at the medical communities' inability to combat this horrible illness.

He turned to Jennie, where she sat quietly watching him, but all of her reading of medical journals offered little help as there was simply no more information available.

Robert was almost shouting in his anger. "Why do they get sick? If we knew what caused this, we could do something about it. Why does it strike healthy, well-nourished children? What about this convalescent serum in Manitoba? Does it do any good? Perhaps I should phone the Minister of Health in Manitoba. Perhaps he knows something that could help?"

"Robert, please sit down. You know that if there was anything, I would have told you. You are doing all you can."

"It is not enough, Jennie. Don't you see? It is not enough. They're dying or paralyzed for life."

"But you and the others have done something. You have established an isolation ward in the hospital to keep the disease from spreading. Many patients are recovering..."

"Yes, but they do that on their own, and I don't know why!" Robert was again up and pacing.

"Robert, the church groups have arranged for extra help in the hospitals, even though it puts them at risk, and we are taking care of families. I pray every night for the afflicted children."

"This time, Jennie, I don't think your God is merciful. Too many children are dying, and I am helpless."

Robert left the room and stormed up the stairs to his bed, leaving his wife in shock at what she considered close to blasphemy. "He is distraught and didn't mean to say that." She murmured a prayer for her husband. "He is so tired."

Despite the Herculean efforts of the doctors and nurses, children continued to die or were left crippled that summer as the worst of the epidemic ran its course. Finally, it was over, and, as summer changed to fall, the medical people slowly relaxed their vigilant watch, but no one knew when another fearsome wave of this dreaded disease would sweep across the land.

***

The house seemed very quiet and peaceful through the fall days of 1927. Douglas was now enrolled in Arts and Science at the university in Edmonton, and Gordon spent his days either at the bank or studying in his room. Robert and Jennie were relieved that he had chosen to live at home. This was a good period, and he was making a concerted effort to follow his father's instructions both with his diet and insulin and his concentration on his studies. His health and attitude towards his diabetes were inextricably linked, and when he rebelled at the necessary regimen, he and everyone around him suffered the consequences.

The use of the Reo was a powerful incentive to behave, but he also thoroughly enjoyed the accountancy courses he was taking.

And it seemed as Gordon's health went, so went Jennie's. Though she tired very easily and had to sleep for several hours each afternoon, when she was well, she spent a lot of her time helping Gordon with his course. The remainder of her time was allocated to a growing role in the management of church business.

Robert's practice and his active involvement in community affairs continued to grow. He was always on the go, from hospital to office to meetings to office again. He and Jennie now had little time together, meeting for the noontime meal and again in the evenings when he returned from work, but the long conversations they had once shared were a thing of the past. Life was simply too busy, and their interests too separate.

Drumheller had grown rapidly, and while initially the population had been largely male, the miners and merchants had soon sent for their wives and children. By the late 1920s, young families made up the larger part of Robert's medical practice.

One such family suffering from what Robert was quite sure was red measles lived on a low hill overlooking a brush-filled ravine on the edge of town. When the mother had called the office to say that two of her children were ill and described their symptoms — a red angry rash, headache and fever — Robert had quickly advised his nurse what to say to the mother.

"Don't bring your children into the office. Doctor Ross will call at your house later today following afternoon office hours. He says that you and the children are to stay home, and none of the children are to go beyond your yard if they go outdoors. Keep the ones who are sick indoors and quiet, and keep their room darkened."

It was Robert's aim if at all possible to keep the measles, if that was indeed the cause of the illness, confined to this family. He had his doubts that this would be possible but thought he would try; he knew that most people did not realize that there could be serious complications from measles. He also knew that rubeolla was highly infectious, and the whole family would probably succumb, but with luck and care, it might be contained in this one house.

"Thank you for coming, Doctor Ross. The twins are in their room, but I let the others outside to play in the yard. It is such a nice day. Billy is beginning to sneeze and cough, though. Do you think he will get sick, too?"

"I'm quite sure all the children will get sick if this is what I think it is. I'll examine the twins now."

The twins had all the signs, including small red spots inside their mouths, and they complained of fierce itching and scratched at the rash on their faces and necks.

"Did you and your husband have measles as children? If so, you will probably escape this time."

"Yes, I think so, but I don't remember being sick. I do remember my mother's friends bringing their children over to the house so that we would all get it at once."

"That is probably not a good idea, Mrs. Blakely. Red measles will usually run its course without any problems, but we do know that there are sometimes further complications for adults and for children who are not as well nourished and healthy as these rascals of yours. So plenty of rest, lots of fluids, and, this is important, no aspirin. Have you a soothing lotion in the house? I'll give you a note to take to the drugstore. You do not need a prescription; it's just for a calming lotion to ease the itching."

"How long will it last, Doctor Ross?"

"About two weeks per child, Mrs. Whitley. And no school. Remember, we are trying to limit the spread."

Weeks passed, and several more families were affected, but there was no epidemic this time, and, to the relief of all, no complications or loss of life. All the medical men knew that they had been spared the worst manifestations of this disease and longed for a vaccine that would prevent it entirely.

Another childhood disease that they dealt with on a regular basis was German measles, similar to red measles in its initial symptoms but a much milder disease that lasted only about three days. Most people did not even know they had it, which meant that others could be unknowingly infected with dire consequences. Robert's recent research had shown him that German measles could be a hidden killer in that it posed a significant health risk to pregnant women, who very often miscarried, delivered far too early, or gave birth to infants with a variety of birth defects, including profound deafness. If a woman was infected with rubella, especially in the first three months of her pregnancy, the doctors were always anxious. It was very difficult to convince families of the danger as they did not connect the miscarriages or birth defects with what they saw as a mild illness.

An epidemic of German measles almost always resulted in at least one such tragedy, and as an obstetrician and a father, Robert hoped that would never happen in the Drumheller Valley.

Chapter 25
Dr. George and Economic Disaster

Robert nodded pleasantly to Reverend Leitch when they happened to meet in front of the Knox United Church. The two men often met in the minister's office in the church where they enjoyed philosophical and theological discussions. Today, however, Robert was on his way to make a house call.

"I look forward to you and your good wife joining us for dinner this Saturday evening. Mrs. Ross has no doubt informed you that we will be joined by Mr. and Mrs. McVeigh and my brother George."

Reverend Leitch smiled in return. "Yes, Robert, it will be a pleasure. My wife and I look forward to an evening of excellent food and lively conversation. The McVeighs are good people, and Doctor George always has something interesting to add to our conversations."

With that, the two men parted, both smiling at the prospect of Robert's older brother contributing to the "lively conversation," and chuckling quietly to themselves.

George was known affectionately by Robert as a "rapscallion," and Robert recollected his discussion with Jennie when the dinner party had been planned and he had insisted on George's presence. "He is my brother, Jennie; they are family, and we must entertain them whenever possible."

"Of course, Robert, but please remember that there will be no alcohol served in this house. Reverend Leitch and his wife will be our guests, as will the McVeighs. Mrs. McVeigh and I enjoy one another's company at church meetings, and I know how much you enjoy your conversations with Reverend Leitch. He is a good man."

Nodding, Robert silently made plans to get over to Rumsey for a visit with George within the week. He and his brother found it relaxing to meet in George's small office. Robert, a teetotaller, would have tea while George sipped on a glass of whiskey as they caught up on family and medical matters. Both men were sharp observers of the foibles of humanity and shared a broad sense of humour. Robert also admired George's cavalier attitude to life in general.

In the event, the dinner party went smoothly as Dr. George, who also had great respect for Reverend Leitch and had been raised to act honourably when ladies were present, behaved with admirable decorum.

George had served as an army doctor during the First World War. Like so many others who were caught in the horror of the Great War, he returned to Canada suffering from shell shock. Unable to settle back into his old life in eastern Canada, he followed in the footsteps of his younger brother to Alberta.

George Ross was a year older than Robert and had also been employed by the Hudson's Bay Company as a young man, not as a trader or a clerk but as a sled dog driver. He had loved the sled dogs his family and the nearby Ojibwe had kept when he was a boy in northern Ontario, and as he grew up discovered that he had a talent for training the dogs. This suited him much better than any indoor life. He had even travelled to England as a dog driver when the HBC had supported the Shackleton Expedition, but his fondness for alcohol meant he was not taken on the mission. Also, rumour had it that he had also shown a somewhat casual attitude to some HBC accounts when he was taken on as clerk at one of the posts. This meant he could not remain with the company that valued sobriety and trustworthiness above all. So George instead obtained his medical degree from Bellevue and followed his younger brother's footsteps to Alberta.

Dr. George first practiced in Rumsey, about thirty miles from Drumheller, arriving there in 1918 just as the 'flu epidemic swept across Canada. He was very well liked in the area, and all his patients were gratified that he was willing to do what was called "barter doctoring," whereby goods from scrawny chickens to vegetables were traded for his services.

Robert was a great friend to his younger brother and understood how the experiences of the war had affected George. The two doctors often met to talk over national and world affairs and medical matters. They also shared a strong sense of family, and both missed their brothers and sister in eastern Canada.

After George purchased a motorcar, he often drove to Drumheller and would sometimes drop in, unannounced, at the Ross home. Unbeknownst to Jennie, he always let Robert know he was coming so that he would be sure to be home when George arrived. He knew very well that his "rough diamond" manners and boisterous humour were not appreciated by his brother's wife, who also disapproved greatly of George's drinking. It was also illegal during Prohibition, but alcohol was available through prescription, and Jennie firmly believed George prescribed for himself too often.

In 1928, George and his family moved to Big Valley, some distance south of Drumheller, so the visits became less frequent, but he was still liable to appear and was always made welcome by Robert.

***

Only a very few lights shone from the windows of early risers, and the street was cold and dark when Robert left the house this morning in 1928 and walked to the office in the predawn chill. He had left the Reo behind as he needed the time spent walking alone to think of what he had to do in light of the collapse of the grain market.

The news had come to him from one of his business friends the previous afternoon, and his thoughts had gone around like rats in a cage ever since. He simply could not tell his wife. Jennie, innocent of the immediate repercussions for the family but always worried about finances, had commented last evening on the sudden drop in wheat prices.

"Robert, this will be so hard for the farmers and the town. How will they manage, do you think?"

"I don't know, Jennie. No one foresaw this. We all thought the grain prices would continue to rise."

"Shouldn't the wheat pools have ensured that wheat prices were stable?"

"Apparently not, my dear. They gambled and lost. But we don't know enough yet."

Jennie's thoughts went immediately to her own family's welfare. "Robert, how will your farm patients pay their medical bills? What of our expenses? And Gordon and Douglas have university fees?" She waited for Robert's reply, anxiously twisting her hands. "Do we have enough savings?"

Robert leaned forward in his chair and took her small, cold hands in his own. "Jennie, this news just came. I don't know yet how bad it will be, but I'm sure we'll be just fine."

However, Robert was not at all sure all would be well, and after a sleepless night, he left his bed at four o'clock in the morning to walk alone through the dark streets.

He raged at his own stupidity and what the devastating news was now costing him. As had many of his friends, he had enjoyed the steady profits his investments in wheat futures had brought him and had continued to reinvest his profits, sure that his money was safe. He had chosen to ignore the rumours he and the others in his group had heard about the reckless marketing strategy of the combined prairie wheat pools, choosing to believe that the pools' decision to carry fifty million bushels of wheat from last year's crops into 1928's sales would only mean more profit for the farmers and himself as an investor. However, these bushels had no price protection, and the gamble on higher prices failed. This resulted in financial ruin for the pools and loss of their savings for those, including Robert, who, gambling that prices would go up, not down, had invested in wheat futures. Every farming nation in the world had bumper crops this year, and the price fell dramatically.

"What am I going to do? Thank Heaven I still have some savings; that money will all go to pay off the debt I owe to the traders. I am left with nothing but regular income for Gordon and Douglas's university education. Jennie must not learn of this; her heart is already weakened with the rheumatism. It would make her ill with worry, and she would be furious at this loss of the family's savings. It will also mean that she cannot go to the West Coast during the coldest months until I have somehow recouped my losses. How am I going to explain that?"

Robert continued to agonize about his sons' future. "What can I sell? Fool, no one has any money. All my friends have also been caught out. Thank the Lord, I still have a job, but I'll have to talk to Jennie, and without letting her know that this financial catastrophe has hit closer to home than she realizes, find a believable reason to economize...thank goodness she is no longer doing my accounts. Perhaps I can take on more work...maybe a bank loan to tide me over until this financial situation improves."

But the economy did not improve. The men who had met so optimistically in the café for coffee and conversation over the past years sat in gloomy silence. Wheat made up seventy percent of the prairie grain crop and sixty percent of that was exported. That export market ground to a brutal halt as Europe had placed an embargo on North American wheat. The other major economic driver in the valley also suffered dramatically as the price of coal dropped. From a record high of over nine dollars per ton in the early 1920s, the price plummeted to less than two dollars in 1929.

The mine owners at the table groaned in despair. "I've cut every job I can and cut back on wages to try to keep the mine going...there is little money for more mechanization, but I have to look at that, too. And of course, mechanization means fewer jobs. The unions are gaining strength; the politicians do nothing to help. We have to deal with the bloody Communists. Can it get any worse?"

The bank manager offered his glum opinion. "The Americans are getting even more protectionist, cutting their own throats, I think, but certainly not helping our exports. My God, what I'd give for a political party with guts. This WLM King seems useless. What do we know about this man Herbert Hoover who is running for election as president in the States?"

Robert, usually the most optimistic and cheerful of men, listened to his friends' bleak comments, quietly reflecting on the desperate situation in the town and the surrounding areas.

Am Rosain, who, along with Sid Hopkins, owned the town's meat market, said anxiously, "It doesn't promise to improve, does it? You all realize that our livelihoods depend on the farmers and the miners earning enough money to pay our bills and purchase our goods?"

"Of course, man, of course we know that; no one will escape this." Bill Crowly of the telephone office expressed his frustration and despair.

"People are going to starve if the farmers don't produce food. And taxes will still have to be paid, the 'temporary' income tax of the war years is still with us and looks likely to stay, and we all have expenses and debts!" Bert Toshach contributed angrily.

An uncomfortable silence followed this statement as most of the men around the table had, to a greater or lesser extent, been caught short by the collapse of the wheat market and had their own debts to pay. What no one could predict was that the situation, already bad, would get much, much worse over the following decade.

On October 29, 1929, the Stock Market on Wall Street crashed, and the whole world was thrown into the terrible decade of the Great Depression. After years of booming growth, desperate times had arrived. Along with this huge economic downturn, the "dirty thirties" were still to come to the prairies provinces. Drought, searing winds, and plagues of locusts would finally destroy what meagre crops remained.

Chapter 26
The "Persons" Case

The valley was again in the grip of winter. The window panes were glazed with ice, and a shrill wind had clawed at the house all morning. But in defiance of the weather, the postman had delivered the morning's mail, and to Jennie's joy, a letter from Nell had arrived. The familiar handwriting tempted Jennie to open it immediately. But it was almost time for luncheon, so she placed the envelope reluctantly on the tray in the hall, knowing that later she would have time to read it and linger over the news from her beloved cousin in Victoria.

For now, she continued her preparations for the meal and the church business meeting to follow. She wanted everything to be just right when the ladies of her church group arrived. There were so few occasions now to set a pretty table.

Jennie was confident that the meal would be perfect. She and Martha had put up jars of fruits and vegetables from her garden this past fall, and shining sealers lined the shelves of the cool room in the basement, sufficient for the winter and more. Milk was delivered daily, and farmers often paid their medical bills in eggs and butter and chickens so they had an ample supply for soups and stews and jellied chicken. It did seem that in the last years there was more and more barter of this nature.

Jennie was puzzled by Robert's continuing focus on scrimping as she knew he still received money from his contract work. They had no extra money but were still able to live quite comfortably. Sighing, she put her worries aside and returned to her plans. A savoury chicken stew accompanied by cheese and Martha's fresh biscuits would make a fine lunch, and then coffee or tea would be served in the front room where the business meeting would be held.

"Mrs. Ross," Martha's voice startled Jennie out of her reverie, "the ladies have arrived."

After a last glance at the table, Jennie went immediately to the front hall to greet her friends. Her next-door neighbour, Mrs. Ewing, led the group, and Myrtle Toshach and the rest of the women were close behind. After removing their warm outer clothes, the women gathered around the table and bowed their heads as Jennie said Grace. They settled to eat and to talk about topics ranging from families and the recent bitterly cold weather to the latest news from Ottawa of the decisions regarding the rights of women to be considered "persons."

"Whatever does that mean for us, do you think?"

"I have always considered myself a person. No one in England needs to tell me that," said one of the women.

"Yes, but remember, we were not considered persons in the eyes of the law. Although we have finally been given the right to vote, we could not take political office or sit in the Senate."

"Rubbish," one of the older women snapped. "Do you want to sit in the Senate?"

"No, but I want the right to sit there."

"Nonsense. Women already have too much to do. Who will look after the homes and the children?" The church secretary was firm in her opinion.

"But," the young wife of one of the new doctors spoke up, "even if you don't want to, this means that you could. It is much like being able to vote. Even if you choose not to, you can. And if women don't speak up, the world will continue to be run as men like it."

"But our husbands will always tell us how to vote anyway," was the inevitable reply.

"Of course, but it is a secret ballot. They don't have to know how we voted unless we are foolish enough tell them," another of the younger women interjected shyly, unsure of how her contribution would be received.

All the women smiled at her comment as Jennie and the women left the table and moved the discussion to the business meeting in the front room.

There was great anxiety among the women about the deepening economic crisis and its effect on the town's business. The difficult times being experienced by the farmers and miners were discussed and the repercussions on the merchants and their families' incomes. No one had any answers, but all were most willing to discuss what the church groups could do to help.

"We need to find more ways to help those less fortunate than ourselves, especially as the times get harder, and it seems likely they will. Robert says this downturn is going to last, and I know that Mr. Toshach agrees, does he not, Myrtle? Do we have any ideas?"

The other women all nodded, and suggestions were offered. "Perhaps we could hold our church suppers twice a month, instead of just once, to ensure that more families come and get baskets of food out to those whom we know are in the greatest need."

"Of course, we could do that. Those of us who are fortunate enough to have a garden will have much we can share."

"And any winter coats or other warm clothing we can spare could be collected and distributed."

"How would we do that?"

"Well, we could make arrangements with the Salvation Army. They have an excellent distribution system and would welcome our help."

"What a good idea. What else can we do? It will be a long hard winter for many."

The women did not need to be reminded and began to consider how else they could help. Several hours were spent exchanging ideas and making plans.

Jennie presented the church financial report for discussion, and then, after a few final moments spent in prayer, the women left for their homes. All thought this winter would be difficult for everyone, but none of them could foresee just how badly the recent October stock market crash would affect their small town for the next decade.

Satisfied with the business of the afternoon, Jennie glanced with longing at the letter from Nell but knew she was too weary to read it before she had her afternoon rest. There would be time for it later. She would sleep then have her tea and wrap herself snugly in the warm afghan on the big chair in the front room or sit by the warmth of the stove in the kitchen. Her bones ached so badly in this cold weather.

Gordon was rarely home in the evenings, spending most of his time with his friends or at the home of Elsie Gabriel. Much to the delight of his mother, and with the approval of Robert, Gordon had asked Elsie for her hand in marriage shortly after receiving his accounting degree.

"Elsie is perfect for him," Jennie drowsed beneath her warm quilts. The housekeeper had placed hot water bottles in the bed so that it would be warm when Jennie lay down for her afternoon rest. "She will look after him, I know. He is so fortunate to have found such a kind, sensible woman. And they'll live close by," was Jennie's contented thought as she drifted into sleep.

The early dark of the winter evening was dispelled by the glow of the lamp over the round kitchen table when Jennie arose and came downstairs for her tea. She had decided to sit in the kitchen to enjoy the warmth from the stove and now finally had peace to read her letter from far off British Columbia.

The family news from Nell was comforting. Her husband, TJ, had died eight years ago, but the rest of the family were all well, though Horace, Nell's oldest son, was suffering again with earache after a bad cold. Jennie could easily picture the large house near Beacon Hill Park as she had last seen it, full of books and young people.

"Let me see," she thought, "how old would Nell's youngest, Harold, be now? My goodness, he will be twenty-seven. Horace is thirty-two. They have all grown up."

Jennie knew that Nell had not practiced medicine since leaving Sudbury in 1907 but had been a strong advocate for women's rights and very busy with her work for the Women's Franchise, travelling around British Columbia. Sure enough, following the news of the family, Nell wrote jubilantly of the passage of the Persons Bill that officially recognized that women were persons in their own right.

> *This is such a victory for us, Jennie. As women, we have contributed so much to this country, both in our homes and now in the workforce. To think that, until now, we could not hold office as we were not even considered to be "eligible persons"...thank goodness for the Judicial Committee of the British Privy council and its realization that excluding women from all public office, especially the Senate, was a barbaric idea. We are making progress.*

Jennie smiled, realizing that many of the issues of which Nell wrote had been echoed in the comments of the women at her own small lunch today. How she missed Nell and her own family in Ontario and how she longed to have the strength to do more. And how did Robert really feel about the question of rights for women? He would often smile indulgently when she spoke of Nell's efforts in this area. Although he had great admiration for Nell's work as a doctor and thought it was a waste of a fine physician when she was unable to practice in Victoria, he somehow didn't seem to link the issue of women's rights to the ban on women doctors.

He had even remarked that women having the vote was all very well, but many women did not want to vote or did not understand the larger issues. To Jennie's tart rejoinder that many men did not understand the issues either, he only smiled benevolently and said, "As for political life, my dear, who would look after the homes and children?" He obviously believed that not too much would come from these changes.

Jennie picked up her pen to write a reply to Nell, telling her that she shared her joy in the passage of the Persons Bill, and of the reaction of her own small women's group.

We are all well here. Robert is very busy with work, leaving early and coming home very late, though more and more patients are without money to pay. He travels a great deal in his role as treasurer of the Alberta Medical Association but should be home within a few days. Douglas will also be home for Christmas, but I fear that he will spend most of his time with the Stevenson family. He is quite taken with the daughter, Elizabeth, and is good friends with her three brothers. Elizabeth is planning to become a teacher and will go to Calgary to Normal School for her studies then hopes to get a teaching position. Gordon is doing well as an accountant and is feeling quite strong at this time. He is very good about taking his insulin, though I fear sometimes his friends lead him astray with their parties. He is to be married next year to Elsie Gabriel, a fine young woman who will make him an excellent wife. Both Robert and I are happy with his choice. Please write again soon...I long for your letters and miss you all.

Lovingly,

Jennie

Jennie put her pen down and sat for a long time, enjoying the warmth of the kitchen as her thoughts turned to her absent husband. He was away so often, and with the boys gone, she felt she was alone too much of an evening. "I don't like that too well. Though one would think that by now I would be resigned to his absences," she told herself, sternly.

Rising a bit stiffly from the table, she slipped her letter into an envelope and placed a stamp on it ready for the next morning's post, noticing in passing that the stamp was bilingual. "Robert would like that, with his French," she murmured and then began to make a list of things to be done the next day. Elsie and her mother were coming for dinner, so Gordon would be home.

DRUMHELLER 1930-1939

Chapter 27
Destroyed by the Great Depression

On a beautiful spring morning in 1930, Gordon McLeod Ross married Elsie Edna Freda Gabriel in a quiet ceremony at the Knox United Church. The sun streamed in through the stained-glass windows, and warm light danced over the bouquets of flowers that the ladies of the church had placed along the aisle and in front of the altar where the young couple stood to say their vows.

Both Robert and Jennie were pleased with the match as they knew that Elsie was a happy, well-liked, and very kind young woman. Jennie in particular believed Elsie would be a steadying influence on her elder son and would look after him in his frequent periods of illness and depression.

On a break from his last year of pre-med courses at the University of Alberta, Douglas was best man and smiled proudly at his brother and his new sister-in-law. He, too, was fond of Elsie.

After the ceremony, the guests gathered at Robert and Jennie's home for refreshments before the bride and groom left for their honeymoon. Douglas spoke quietly to his father, "Dad, it is good to see Gordon and Elsie looking so happy. Are they moving to Calgary right away?"

"Yes, Gordon is doing very well there as an accountant with a small prosperous firm. Elsie will be an excellent wife. She makes friends easily everywhere, and she is so kind."

"I like her very much, too. I only hope she can cope with Gordon's periods of unkindness. I'm sorry, Dad, but we both know how miserable he can be when he is feeling ill. I know, I know. I won't say anything to Mother about my concern, but dammit, Gordon has used his diabetes as an excuse for his behaviour for too many years."

"Don't swear, Douglas. Your brother has been ill for a long time."

"Dad, you know others who have diabetes. You have patients who manage very well. They don't use it as a reason to be miserable to others, and Gordon's drinking only makes it worse. I see how distressed Mother is."

"That's enough, Douglas, and surely this is hardly the time to discuss it. Now, how long are you able to stay this time? Will we be able to have a good visit?"

Douglas looked at his father in exasperation. They had grown very close over the past three years as Robert travelled to Edmonton on AMA business, but it was evident that Gordon's lifestyle and behaviour were still topics that would not be discussed. Douglas could see that his father was also deeply troubled about other matters and was unwilling to talk about them, either. And Robert was right; Gordon's wedding was not the place for this discussion.

"Let's find some time to talk, Dad. I'm here for a few more days, which I intend to spend relaxing and visiting with my friends. Then I'm back to Edmonton. I have a summer job there, which will help a bit with my expenses for McGill in the fall."

A frown passed quickly over Robert's face, but he shook his head when Douglas questioned him.

"No, it's nothing, Son. I'm fine and so is your mother. Her rheumatism has been bad this year, but she makes sure to rest often, and the warm weather helps. Now, let's join the happy couple and wish them well before they leave on the train for their honeymoon," he said. Then he smiled and added, "No, I don't know where they are going."

Robert touched Douglas fondly on the arm, and they walked over to the front door to join Jennie who stood with Gordon and Elsie. The happy couple were surrounded by their friends as they prepared to depart. Elsie looked very pretty in a blue suit with a tiny matching hat and dotted veil.

"Good luck to you both. Bon voyage," Robert shook Gordon's hand and smiled fondly at his new daughter-in-law.

"God bless you both," Jennie murmured as she kissed their cheeks.

As always, Robert kept his misgivings to himself. He believed Elsie would make a good wife for Gordon, but whether Gordon would appreciate his new wife's strength and generosity of spirit was another question.

His thoughts turned again to his finances. Robert had managed to pay off his debt to the wheat brokers, but that had used most of his savings. Bit by bit, he was managing to once again build up his funds but was still concerned that there would not be enough money for university for Douglas in the fall. Although he had said nothing to Jennie, he knew she was aware of how careful he had become and how he watched every penny. He was grateful that her horror of ostentation meant that the wedding was very small but grieved that he could not have managed a larger wedding present for the young couple.

September was rapidly approaching, and the economic climate on the prairies and worldwide was steadily worsening. The stock market crash of 1929 had destroyed so many families, and their hopes and dreams were literally dust. Although his family was secure, there was no extra money. Somehow, if he was careful, he would find a way to manage the costs of his younger son's medical education.

***

"Good morning, Doctor Ross. May I take your coat and hat? Looks like we'll have a good trip to Edmonton today. Visiting young Mr. Douglas are you? Please give him my best regards."

Robert took his usual seat in the passenger section of the morning train to Edmonton as the porter continued to chat while making sure the doctor was comfortable.

"Morning, William," Robert smiled and thanked the porter for his help. "Yes, I'll see Douglas during this trip. I'd enjoy some tea in about an hour, and please bring my lunch at noon as usual, thank you."

For the last three years, Robert had been travelling throughout Alberta as required by his duties on the Executive of the Alberta Medical Association, so William's was a familiar face. Robert always enjoyed his travels to various cities in Alberta, seeing the growth of small towns and the cities of Calgary and Edmonton. The paper on chronic appendicitis presented by Dr. GH Murphy at the September 1929 convention in Lethbridge had been most interesting. Robert dealt with that condition frequently and knew that one of the reasons appendicitis became a chronic condition was that the farmers and their families often ignored the pain because they could not afford the necessary surgery. And, of course, Robert had enjoyed revisiting the Galt Hospital and seeing the changes that had occurred since he had worked there in 1910.

The trip to Edmonton was always his favourite as he could fulfill his duties as president as well as visit with Douglas. Robert also liked Alberta's capital city on the North Saskatchewan River and all it had to offer. He was sorry that Jennie did not feel well enough to accompany him this time because Edmonton was also one of her favourite cities.

When Jennie came along, she was content to spend hours in the campus library while Robert went about his AMA business, and when the weather was clement, she particularly enjoyed the time they spent strolling on the beautiful university grounds.

The daylong train trip also gave Robert time to read and think. This year was particularly worrisome as Alberta, indeed all of Canada and the world, was in the depths of the Great Depression. Although it was generally accepted that the stock market crash triggered the Great Depression, many in Alberta believed that it had instead been brought about by the enormous 1928 wheat price slump. As a result of the record grain crops in Europe, the overseas market, upon which North American farmers depended for the bulk of their income, was no more. They could no longer sell their wheat globally. The income for farmers, the backbone of the prairie economy, fell to less than a quarter of what it had been before 1928. To make matters worse, prairie farmers had stored three years of bumper crops, driving the prices for their wheat down even further.

Robert himself had been caught short in the wheat market crash, but he had managed to pay his bills and support his sons at university through his regular income.

He knew that his wife suspected he had lost a great deal of money, and she was coldly withdrawn and furious, but she never questioned him and silently made do when required. Robert also knew that Jennie was very aware that his regular income protected them from the worst of it. They both knew that for many others, the Depression meant financial and personal ruin.

Robert saw his patients in great distress. These were proud independent men who, in 1932, had been forced to accept financial relief in order to feed their families. They were humiliated that their wives had to take any jobs they could find to augment the dwindling family income, with little children left alone on farms to fend for themselves as their mothers and fathers sought work elsewhere.

The effects of desperate worry and poor nutrition were taking their toll on all ages. Young men were forced off the family farms as the little monetary relief that was offered was automatically cut back when children turned sixteen, and struggling parents could no longer afford to feed them. Wandering the roadsides hoping to find a little work or shelter, this displaced generation sometimes starved to death or froze in the ditches.

Robert's dark thoughts were interrupted by William.

"Here's your tea, sir, can I get you anything else?"

"No, thank you, William. May I ask if you have a family?"

"Yes, sir. Thank you for asking. My wife lives in Vancouver."

"And you are able to manage with what you earn on the railroad?"

"Just about, sir. I am grateful to have this job. But I'm ashamed to say my wife also has to work. She does laundry for rich folks in Vancouver. I see the poor souls who haven't got any work at all. They keep looking and looking for work, and I wonder if it will ever get better," he paused for a moment then continued, "Sorry, sir, I don't mean to complain. May I get you anything else?"

"Nothing, thank you, William. Just one more question, if I may? Do you think the work camps are of any help?"

"I wouldn't know, sir. Will that be all?"

The porter was obviously uncomfortable with the discussion, so Robert nodded his thanks and quietly determined to leave a much larger tip than usual.

He then tried to return his mind to the work he had brought with him. There was some possibly good news. A powerful antibacterial medicine called penicillin had been discovered by a Dr. Alexander Fleming and was being used in trials. No one knew yet quite how it worked, but it seemed to have great promise for treating infections. Robert read the article that Jennie had marked for him in the June issue of *British Journal of Experimental Pathology* and wondered if anything would come of this hopeful discovery.

RB Bennett was the new Prime Minister of Canada, and although Robert had very little faith in eastern politicians who had done so little for the people of the West during this terrible time, he read with interest that Bennett seemed to be pushing for sovereignty for Canada. Robert considered his own feelings as a member of the British Empire and realized that while he would always be loyal to the monarchy, he believed as a proud Canadian that it was past time for Canada to stand on her own and looked forward to the passing of the Statute of Westminster.

And thinking of Britain, he wondered if Jennie would be interested in a trip to England. Her health was always precarious, but maybe she would be well enough. They seemed to spend so little time together now, so perhaps once Douglas was enrolled in McGill, they could travel east and then on to Britain. A journey on an ocean liner would be quite something, and his position as a CPR doctor meant he would have little difficulty finding a berth on one of the new Empress Liners. It would be good to go on a longer journey. He remembered their last trip together in late winter of the previous year. They had travelled to Banff, a beautiful resort town in the Canadian Rockies, about four hours by train from Drumheller.

They had enjoyed a visit of several days with Robert's younger brother Arthur Howey Ross, of international hockey fame, and the group who had accompanied him from Boston. Arthur's wife, Muriel, a kind and loving woman, had created an instant bond with Jennie. Along with their other friends from the East Coast, they had all enjoyed their excursions to the Banff Hot Springs and the surrounding area. It had been a happy time.

Watching the flat prairie landscape become more rolling as the train entered the region closer to Edmonton, with more hills and trees and lush river valleys, Robert's thoughts inevitably turned again to the Depression. There had to be a solution, but certainly the politicians did not seem to have any answers, and life was growing harder and more desperate for the farmers. Another dry year would finish those who had struggled to keep going.

"Your lunch, sir."

"Thank you, William."

The hours slipped by. Robert reviewed his notes in preparation for the upcoming discussions regarding the sponsorship by the AMA of the Canadian Medical Education program at the University of Alberta and the beginnings of the Canadian Cancer Society, both very important topics.

George Hoadley was the Minister of Health and was certainly pressing for government involvement in health insurance. Robert mused on this topic as it related to the subsidies doctors in the southeast of Alberta received to treat families in the area known as the "Dry Belt," who were now sorely affected by the Depression. Robert himself had a contract with some of the mining companies to treat the miners and for years had also been a CPR doctor providing medical services to the railroad workers. These two contracts had made all the difference to his income when the Depression hit. But what of the families of the farmers and miners?

His thoughts were interrupted by the conductor's voice. "Edmonton, next stop. Final stop for this trip. Please collect all your hand baggage before disembarking."

William's friendly face appeared, and the porter offered to help Robert with his coat and hat. "Have a good visit, Doctor Ross. Perhaps I'll be your porter on the return trip."

Robert thanked William for his help throughout the trip and agreed that they would likely meet again on the return journey three days hence.

Robert was pleased to see Douglas waiting for him at the Edmonton Station of the Canadian National Railway, an imposing brick-and-marble building not far from downtown.

"Good evening, Douglas. Thank you for coming to meet me. You are well?"

"Just fine, Dad. Here, I'll get your baggage from the cart. Thanks, William, good to see you again. All your family well? My regards to your wife." He turned to his father and smiled. "Dad, I have a hired car waiting for us as you requested. Your usual hotel?"

"Yes, the MacDonald always provides good service. It is a treat to see you again, Son. After I freshen up, will you have time to have a late supper with me? I don't want to take you away from your studies for too long."

Douglas grinned, "I've been looking forward to your visit for a while, sir. My studies can manage without me for this evening."

"Good, we'll meet in the dining room here at about seven. We have a number of things to discuss, including those studies of yours."

The two men enjoyed a quiet meal in the hotel restaurant, and their conversation turned to Drumheller.

"Douglas, the townspeople are struggling but seem to be managing a little better than the farmers. I am afraid that anyone with a bit of money is doing better than those whose income is tied to the land, but we all depend on the farmers for our livelihood. And people who have barely enough to eat and feed their families certainly have no money for anything else. They cannot even sell their farm equipment as there are no buyers. I had a sad and frightening case the other day of a man driven mad by despair. Let me tell you the story."

Douglas nodded and settled back in his chair, well used to his father's tales.

"As you know, Son, the terrible financial hardships of the 'dirty thirties' have hit all businesses hard. An economic downturn of this magnitude spares no one, and in this particular case, the loss of his income and status in the town hit one businessman, let's call him Mr. X, very hard. You'll know who I'm talking about when you hear the story.

"Well, it hit him so hard that his sanity was affected, and he began to imagine that everyone in the town was mocking him. His pride was badly bruised when his financial woes resulted in the loss of his business and thus, to his mind, his social standing in the town. He, of course, did not consider that he was in the same sorry state as thousands of others. He also began to imagine that his wife had abandoned him and was seeing other men when he was not home. For some unknown reason, he fixed on me as a culprit in all of this and determined to get his revenge.

"About eleven o'clock one evening, as I was retiring after a long and busy day at work, I received a telephone call from a fellow I knew asking me to go and see this friend. I'd never met the man but had heard of him as one of those whose business was suffering badly. As usual, I asked my informant what seemed to be the trouble with Mr. X. He replied that he didn't know but understood that he was suffering from some sort of brain trouble and was in a bad way.

"Later, I realized that I should have given this brain trouble comment more thought, but I asked him where his friend lived and said that I would go and see the man.

"He told me that I would find his house easily. It was one of the few three-story residences in town."

At this, Douglas smiled, knowing exactly whose house his father was describing.

"Anyway," Robert continued, following the good directions, I soon pulled up in front of the house.

I was puzzled, because all the lights were on in every room. That was odd. But I thought that maybe they were having a party. I figured the man couldn't be that ill if that was the case. I went through the front gate and up to the house but was further puzzled by the complete absence of noise. Dead silence greeted me as I walked up half a dozen steps to the front door. I was about to put my hand on the doorknob when the door opened without me touching it. It swung silently inward, and I walked into the front hall, which also had all the lights blazing.

"There was no one to meet me. The place was utterly silent. I stood for a moment and then spun around as I heard the door close behind me. There stood Mr. X, naked except for a short woollen undershirt, locking the door behind me. I was startled to say the least.

"In his right hand, he held a revolver that he raised and pointed at me, shouting that at last he had me right where he had wanted to have me for a long time. He accused me of coming to see his wife for months when he was not around but declared that I would never come to his house again, as he was going to finish me off."

At this, Douglas murmured in alarm, which brought a smile to his father's face.

Robert went on. "I saw at once that I was dealing with a man whose 'brain trouble' was insanity, and I realized that I was in grave danger. Mr. X was shaking with rage, and his pistol was cocked and ready to fire. My only hope was to stall, and I decided to try to talk the man out of his angry state.

"I told him that he was probably right when he said that someone has been coming to see his wife in his absences. I said that I had heard that she was a very beautiful woman but that I had never seen her. I reassured him that I was a doctor and that I had come to see him because someone had telephoned me and said he was sick and needed a doctor's attentions. I asked him if he remembered me and reminded him that I had purchased a motorcar from him three months earlier. I said that it was the first car that I had ever owned, and I liked it very much.

"Surprised by this reaction from me, Mr. X asked me if I wanted to buy another car. He told me that he had a great number of them because no one was buying them anymore.

"Well, thinking fast, I told him that I would very much like to buy another motorcar, or more than one, from him, seeing this as an opportunity to distract the man from his murderous intent.

"Did I mention he was half naked, Douglas? Thankfully, he was delighted with my offer and invited me into the dining room, telling me that he would sell me all the cars I wanted. And cheap, too!"

Douglas laughed out loud at the picture his father's words were painting. "Then what?"

"Well, it wasn't over by a long shot, so to speak, but much relieved, I went into the dining room with the gun still pointed at my back and sat in the chair the man indicated that I was to take. Still with one eye on me and the gun held steadily in his hand, Mr. X opened a cupboard and took out a stack of papers. I glanced around the room to see if there was a door leading to the outside, but there was none. It was probably just as well because if I had made any effort to escape, the man would surely have shot me. I knew my best chance continued to be to face the distraught businessman and try to talk him out of using his gun."

At this point, Douglas indicated to the hovering waiter that they would both like more coffee. Robert continued the story.

"Remember that Mr. X now sat across from me at the table, with his bare bottom on a hard wooden chair. The papers on the table between us consisted of order forms for cars from his defunct dealership. As soon as he made out one form, he would pass it to me for my signature. Every little while, this madman would stop writing, raise his revolver, and point it at me and ask me what I was doing there.

"Each time he did this, I repeated calmly that I was there to buy cars from him. I also asked him each time to please put down his gun, telling him that it was loaded and if it went off he would kill his best customer.

"This gun pointing and threatening was repeated every few minutes, and each time I reminded him that he didn't want to kill one of his best customers.

"This went on all night, during which time I'm sure I had ordered trainloads of cars. Once I tried to grab the gun while the he was writing, but Mr. X was too quick for me. By now, Douglas, I had determined that if I did get possession of the gun, Mr. X would not live long. I had had enough of this bargaining for my life.

"Once again, hoping the man was tiring and becoming distracted, I tried to get the gun. Again, Mr. X was too quick for me and kept his hand firmly on the weapon. The third time, I grabbed for the gun, the madman looked at me, smiled coldly and told me that it would not be long now, as he had sold me almost all his cars, and when they were all gone, he was going to kill me for visiting his wife."

Douglas, who had been listening to the story with a smile on his face, asked, "How the hell did you get out of there, Dad?"

Robert laughed and continued. "I could see the front door from where I was sitting, and when daylight finally broke at about six o'clock, I saw, through the window beside it, two mounted police officers standing in the road by the front gate. Someone, perhaps my informant of the night before, had called them and alerted them that Doctor Ross had gone into the house but had never come out and was being held at gunpoint by a madman. I realized that I had to get Mr. X to the door, but he was still holding the gun.

"I told him that he had some callers that morning. I said that I could see two men standing in front of his door and suggested that they were probably there to see his wife.

"As I had hoped, he rose to the bait. He stormed to the front door, pulled it open, and charged out onto the front porch brandishing his gun at the two officers. They rushed up the steps and lunged at this maniac, knocking his feet from underneath him. He fell backward, his pistol went off, and the bullet buried itself in the wall."

By this time, Douglas was weak with laughter but encouraged his father to finish the story.

"He begged them to let him up and insisted that his gun was not loaded, sobbing, 'I give up.'

"The police did let him up, and he raised his arms over his head, saying that it was Ponoka for him.

"Of course, he was still half naked at this point, so the officers took him back inside to dress under guard. He was then led away to jail, and thence to Ponoka, for admittance to the Provincial Asylum. I signed the necessary papers to have him committed, and three weeks after his admittance there, Mr. X died a broken man and another casualty of the despair of the Depression years."

Sobered by the sad ending to what had been a humorous, if frightening, tale, Douglas said, "My God, Dad. You could have been killed. That poor man."

"Yes, it is very sad, but there is more to the story, Son. Shortly after news of his death reached Drumheller, his widow telephoned me and asked me what my bill was for the call on her husband. I told her that I didn't know what to charge her, Douglas. I would not have taken ten thousand dollars to go into that death trap had I known in advance what I was facing. In the event, she sent me a cheque for fifty dollars."

The two men sat in silence for a few moments, Douglas shaking his head at his father's narrow escape and both considering their helplessness in the face of the terrible hardships the Great Depression had brought to this once prosperous land.

"That's a heartwrenching story, Dad. I can see the dark humour in it, though. I'm sorry to end the evening, but I do have classes in the morning, and I know you have AMA meetings. Let's meet again for dinner tomorrow evening."

Chapter 28
England, State Medicine, and Cleveland

"A most enjoyable three days." Robert boarded the morning train to Drumheller, his satisfied thoughts on his time in Edmonton. "The AMA is doing good work for the medical men and the people of Alberta. I'm proud to have been president of an association that is determined to put patients first. And Douglas is getting along very well with his studies. He works hard, but his quirky sense of humour is refreshing. It's important to have some fun, too. I'll miss him when he goes to Montreal. But an excellent visit. Now to plan the next trip: England."

Robert was pleased to see William's smiling face when he found his seat. "Good morning, Doctor Ross," William took Robert's coat and hat. "A successful trip, I hope?"

"Very much so, William. Thank you. I'm happy to see you again. All is well?"

"Yes, sir, thank you."

Robert settled into the comfortable seat and placed his valise beside him but chose not to begin his paperwork immediately.

"I'm planning a much longer trip next time, William. I have to go to England on business so will travel across the country by CPR to Halifax and then board ship to go across the Atlantic."

"My goodness, sir, that is a long trip. I don't work on the cross-country routes, so I won't see you. I hope you have an excellent journey. I'll bring your tea shortly."

As the porter moved along the aisle, Robert considered his travel plans and smiled inwardly at his "business" in England. How he wished that Jennie would change her mind and accompany him. He thought about the discussion they had had when he first broached the idea of a trip over the Atlantic Ocean to the British Isles.

Jennie had smiled at her husband as he had paced around the room, as he often did when he was excited.

"We will go to London, Jennie. We will travel across Canada to Halifax then on the new CPR liner, The Empress of Britain. My privileges as a CPR doctor will smooth the way, and of course, I will not be expected to pay full fare, so we can afford it. It will be a wonderful trip. We have not travelled together on a long journey for quite some time. We will be gone at least two months."

Robert paused to catch his breath then went on, "It will be a marvellous holiday. I want to go to Edinburgh to find out what is required for me to apply for a fellowship with the Royal College of Physicians and Surgeons, and there is a guitar in Manchester that I plan to purchase. I will make arrangements at the hospital and the office, and we can visit Douglas at McGill on our return..."

Robert, realizing that Jennie did not seem to share his excitement, paused and looked at his wife's solemn face.

"Jennie, what's wrong?"

"Of course, you must go, Robert. You have often spoken of your desire to visit England. But I cannot go."

"What? What are you saying?" Perplexed by her words, thinking that this time she would surely travel with him and they would have some time together away from their work and the demands on their time in Drumheller, Robert could hardly believe that she would not be thrilled to journey overseas. "Are you saying that you will not come with me? Jennie, we may never again have such an opportunity. And London, we would visit London and go to Buckingham Palace. Jen!"

"Robert, you know that such a long trip would simply be too exhausting for me. And besides, Elsie and Gordon's baby, our first grandchild, will be born during that time. I must be here for them and that event."

Stunned by her words, Robert sat down heavily in his chair, closed his eyes, and struggled with how to respond.

"Elsie is very healthy, it has been a completely normal pregnancy, she has an excellent doctor, and her mother is here; there is nothing you can do."

Jennie sat silently with her hands folded in her lap. Exasperated at the idea that his wife would not go on this great adventure with him, Robert stood again and paced around the room. "I do wish you would accompany me, Jennie. It would be a wonderful experience for both of us to travel to England."

"I cannot leave, Robert. Now, we need to discuss your travel plans and your wardrobe. You will, of course, need several new suits."

And so shortly after his return from Edmonton, complete with new suits, Robert set off alone for Halifax and then on to England.

He made many friends on the beautiful new ship and during his travels by train around England and Scotland. Robert was a keen observer of life and found the gently manicured landscape of England very beautiful, and the Scottish Highlands reminded him of the Canadian Rockies.

London was exhilarating. Robert smiled at the pomp and ceremony of Buckingham Palace, so different from prairie informality, and was very proud of his king and queen. He found Queen Mary particularly impressive; her dignified, gracious demeanour reminded him of his mother, Maggie.

He attended the theatre and had a good time at several social events and on tours of London where he met another Thomas Robert Ross from Australia. The two "colonials" had a fine time together, laughing at some of the protocols and ceremonies. The two men parted fast friends when Robert left London and boarded one of the fast trains to Manchester. There, he completed his business in England when he purchased his dream guitar, an 1846 Louis Panormo.

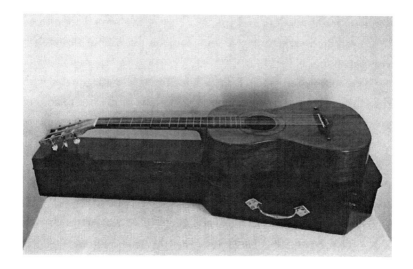

The Panormo Guitar, 1932

"Now," he thought, "I can go home. It has been a wonderful trip," he reflected, his happiness tinged with regret. "I wish Jennie had come. She would have loved it all, I know."

***

"Tonight's dinner party promises to be interesting," Robert murmured to his reflection in the pier glass mirror in the corner of his bedroom. His usual suit coat and vest had been exchanged for a soft velvet dinner jacket, and he found his image quite satisfying as he straightened his tie.

Two young doctors and their wives who were interested in moving to Drumheller were guests this evening. Robert knew that after the usual niceties had been observed, the conversation would turn to the growing discussion about prepaid voluntary medical care, or as it was being called, "state" medicine.

"Robert, our guests will be arriving soon." Jennie came into the room to be sure he was ready. Her gown was a soft and simple long-sleeved burgundy crepe de chine, with a high collar and slim skirt, which she wore over high-buttoned boots.

"I am ready, my dear, and you look elegant as always. I am pleased to see you are wearing the gold and diamond pin at your throat. It is very becoming."

"Perhaps it is too much, Robert, but I thought it was suitable with this dress. We must go down now; I wish to be in the front room to greet our guests. Martha has everything ready. And, Robert, please remember, no appendectomy conversations during the meal."

Robert chuckled. "Of course not, Jennie. We will speak only of pleasant things. I would not want to see Martha's good cooking go to waste."

Their company was welcomed and offered glasses of Martha's excellent chilled grape juice before they went in to the dining room for dinner. The conversation flowed easily. Robert regaled the group with a few of his Hudson's Bay stories, and Jennie's knowledge of current affairs and medical news balanced Robert's tales. Her most exciting medical news was the discovery of a drug called sulpha. There was no official information available yet, but the rumours told of a powerful anti-infection medicine developed in the Bayer Laboratories in Germany that would stop infection when sprinkled on a wound.

For several minutes, the doctors sat in silence imagining the miracle this would be if these rumours proved true.

"Mrs. Ross, that is amazing. How did you learn this?"

"We receive medical journals regularly, and Doctor Ross's colleagues in the East are a constant source of new information. And of course all the doctors in the office here are keeping up-to-date."

Robert smiled proudly and remarked that Jennie had always been a trusted source of information.

Inevitably, though, as coffee and tea were offered and the couples moved into the front room following dessert, the conversation turned to the idea of province-wide health insurance.

Local voluntary health insurance programs were not new. Mine owners had contracts with certain doctors to provide medical care for injured miners. Robert himself was also a CPR doctor, which meant he was on contract to provide medical care to railway workers.

At the provincial level, the United Farmers Association had passed several motions over the previous two years requesting that the government conduct an inquiry into state-supported medicine. The Dry Belt doctors of southern Alberta already received a bonus to encourage them to remain in the area when their patients, hard hit by drought and the depression, could not pay for medical care.

Jennie, to Robert's surprise, initiated the evening's discussion by referring to the debates held in Cardston, a small town in the Dry Belt. She acted as devil's advocate by drawing their attention to an editorial written by W.O. Wright, in *The Cardston News*, of 1932. She said, "Wright urged, '*solving the conundrum which exists today in the medical profession*,' and he briefly outlined what he saw as major problems. He further asked, '*what is our Public Health system for, if not to prevent disease and enable doctors to practice preventative medicine? In many cases, the current contracts covered men only, not their wives and families. Prepaid medical care would be more inclusive. Finally, doctors would get their bills paid.*'"

Jennie then presented a counter argument to Wright's words, asking the others, "Do you not think that such care, with the state paying the bills, would take away a man's independence and limit doctors' incomes? Someone else would decide how much each of you would be paid and could limit your income no matter how hard you worked."

Jennie finished speaking, and Robert waited for a response from the young men. Again, to his astonishment, it was one of the wives who spoke politely but firmly.

"Mrs. Ross, I understand what you are saying about limiting a doctor's independence, but I, too, have been reading about the United Farm Workers Association Women's group. And what they are saying is true. The present contracts are for men...miners, railway workers, and farm labourers."

She continued her argument, "My husband is interested in the specialty of obstetrics, and he has not yet been paid for many of the babies he has delivered. It is not that the families don't want to pay; there is just no money. And many poor women and their families have no income at all, so they get very sick before going to the doctor. This costs them more in the long run, but they still have no way of paying. We understand that there is just no money, but my husband and I have to live, too. I don't believe people would abuse a state system," she paused then went on, "and I do believe in preventative care."

Her face flushed as she realized she had perhaps spoken with too much enthusiasm for a dinner guest.

"It may be that my wife is too passionate about the subject, Mrs. Ross, but she has a kind heart," Dr. Black spoke somewhat apologetically.

"Your wife is right to speak her mind," Jennie replied. "It is a topic deserving of our passion."

Mrs. Black, relieved at Jennie's response, gestured to her friend, the other young doctor's wife, who then said quietly, "I, too, have been following the Cardston debates, and the actions being taken now at the provincial level. There are many good points being made in favour of state-subsidized medicine."

Her husband also smiled apologetically at his wife's fervour, but it was evident that he was proud of her grasp of the facts.

Robert listened carefully, and while honestly stating that his household would not have survived the dark years since 1928 without his income from contracts, he carefully expressed some of the views of those who opposed state medicine, making sure that everyone understood that the opinions expressed were not necessarily his, nor those of the AMA. "First, there would no doubt be an increase in taxation, and we already pay enough. It could take away some of the independence of doctors; perhaps standards would drop. People want to choose their own doctors. Would that change? What happens when doctors or patients move? Would there be refunds to be paid? Money is already tight and liable to get tighter, and finally, think of the humiliation to those classed as indigent."

The spirited discussion continued and gradually became more general and anecdotal, and no real conclusions were reached. It was, however, clear to everyone that change was coming.

As the guests left, Jennie's exhaustion was apparent, but she smiled contentedly. It would not be the last time the topic was discussed, and she had enjoyed speaking her mind and the lively exchange of views.

"Nell would have been proud," she thought, "especially of the women and the way their husbands supported them."

***

Late autumn of 1933 and the early months of 1934 had seen a continuing epidemic of both red and German measles spread across North America. Although many of the cases were mild, some children and adults became very ill. Complications from red measles often resulted in weakened hearts for survivors. For Robert, as an obstetrician, the resulting miscarriages and tragedy of birth defects caused by German measles made it a long and sad spring.

He sat sombrely over his tea one evening, discussing the day with his wife. "Two of my patients suffered miscarriages today, Jennie. I know that the miscarriages are nature's way of sloughing off a foetus that would not survive, but my dear, it is so sad."

Jennie, who continued to read all the medical articles that Robert received, commiserated with him but also reminded her grieving husband that a child carried to full term after the mother had been infected with German measles was often born with birth defects. "This is God's way of sparing mothers the tragedy of such births."

"You are no doubt correct, but that is small comfort to these bereft women today."

"God will comfort them, Robert. He has taken their little ones to Himself. I will visit these poor women tomorrow with Mrs. Ewing."

"Thank you, my dear, you will be most welcome, especially if you are able to take a basket of food. There is little enough for their other children, and the women will be too weak to do much for a few days."

"Of course, Robert. There is always soup and bread available from the church kitchens."

"Good, that will help. Thank goodness that our granddaughter was spared this infection. Remind me, though, when are Gordon and Elsie and little Shelagh coming to visit?"

"They will arrive this weekend, Robert. I hope they will be able to stay for a few days, but Gordon is very busy."

While the family sat over lunch on Saturday, Gordon made a surprising announcement. "It really is time that Shelagh met her great-grandmother and my aunt Sybil, so Elsie and I are taking our daughter to Cleveland this summer. Are you well enough to travel, Mother? Dad, how about you; can you get away for a visit? It's been a few years since you saw Grandmother McKenzie, and she is getting very old."

Jennie was taken completely aback by Gordon's words. She knew that she did not want to travel to Cleveland, in part because her health had been so poor the past winter but also because she had absolutely no desire to spend time with her mother-in-law. But she was hurt that Gordon had planned this trip without her knowledge, and she was very sure that Robert would go, with or without her.

Gordon went on, disregarding his mother's consternation. "Dad, you still have CPR privileges, don't you? Could we take advantage of family rates, especially if you come with us?"

Robert, equally surprised, asked, "Why are you going now, Gordon? What about your job in Calgary? Can you get away so easily? It is a long time to be away from your position."

"I have been offered a job in Montana. It has better pay and would be good experience for me. I thought a trip to Cleveland now would be a welcome break before we move to the States."

All this talk of moving was news to Jennie, and her heart sank further at the idea of Gordon and her granddaughter being such a distance away.

"But you haven't yet decided to take this position, have you?" she asked.

"Not yet, Mother." Gordon replied, "I needed to talk to Dad first."

Elsie, who had been unusually quiet, now spoke softly to Jennie as Gordon and Robert began to discuss the possible move. "I know that you are worried about Gordon's weight gain. He is all right, Mother Ross. He still takes the daily insulin but sometimes gets very moody. I think this change might be good for him." She paused then spoke tentatively, "May I ask if you could look after Shelagh while we move to Montana, if Gordon does take this new job? I don't know how I could manage to look after her and care for Gordon while we moved into a new home. Just until we get settled, of course."

Jennie, who was very fond of the little girl, agreed. "Of course, our new housekeeper is very good with children; we will manage nicely."

Robert had overheard this last conversation and knew that Jennie would indeed be pleased to have Shelagh with them for a time, but he also knew that his wife tired very easily and an active toddler could quickly disrupt a household.

"We'll hire a young woman as a nursemaid if Shelagh is staying with us. But all this is uncertain. First things first: When do you plan to take up this position?"

"I plan to go to Montana after we return from Cleveland. Elsie and Shelagh will stay with Elsie's mother here in Drumheller while I see if the job suits me."

During this conversation, Jennie had come to another decision. "Meanwhile, I wish to accompany you to Cleveland. I am feeling quite strong just now, and it is time I went on a journey."

Robert was delighted that Jennie had decided to make the trip but, thinking about it, realized that she would be eager to spend time with Gordon and Shelagh. The long ride on the train would offer an excellent opportunity to visit.

"Good, my dear, very good. We all need to get away for a bit. If we make arrangements to go now, it will be full summer when we arrive back home. And you are correct, Gordon, I do need to see my Mother again. She is eighty-three, and although she has always been healthy, it's probably not wise to delay a visit."

Robert also planned to take the train from Cleveland to Montreal to see how Douglas was getting on with his internship. He wanted to talk to his younger son about the work of Dr. Wilder Penfield who was in the process of establishing a Neurological Centre at McGill. Penfield, with whom Douglas had studied, was already famous for his discoveries of how the brain worked, an area, Robert was the first to admit, he knew very little about.

"But," he thought. "I'll say nothing of a side trip to Jennie right now. I know she would not want to come with me to Montreal, but she could spend that time with Gordon and Shelagh and visit with Sybil in Cleveland."

It was quite likely that other members of his family would be in Cleveland as Sybil's house was a favourite location for them all to gather. He would let the eastern Rosses know he was coming. Perhaps Art and Muriel would be there.

It had been a morning of surprises, but it certainly helped to take his mind off the measles.

Chapter 29
Speaking for the Ojibwe

Robert loved to tell stories of his early years growing up as the son of a Hudson's Bay trader in the wild North woods of Ontario and Quebec where his best friends were the children of the Ojibwe Indian tribes. He also enjoyed recounting tales of his adventures as a Bay Man, living and working with the Ojibwe for fourteen years before his marriage and subsequent arrival in Alberta. He had great respect for the philosophies and spiritual beliefs of his Indian friends and spoke often of their culture and strong family lives.

Robert was a founding member of the Drumheller Rotary Club, an active participant in the organization's community activities, and a welcome raconteur at their regular meetings. So, when in the fall of 1934, an opportunity arose to speak to the club members and their wives at a dinner meeting, he jumped at the chance. His good friend, W. R. "Bob" Johnston, a local druggist, had mentioned to Robert that he was responsible for the programme for the next club dinner. Bob wondered if Robert would be interested in being the speaker.

"Gladly, Bob. This is my chance to explain, without offending anyone, that the Indians are not the ignorant savages they are made out to be. I will be happy to speak to the club and will call my presentation 'The White Man as Seen through the Eyes of the Indian.'"

"How will you do that, Robert? People here will be angry if you tell them they are wrong in their beliefs."

Robert, who had a very broad sense of humour and loved to play jokes on people, smiled and said, "Leave it to me. I will not offend anyone, but I think I know my friends well enough to believe that they will listen to another point of view. Are you willing to play a part in this?"

Bob was dubious but willing, so the men planned for the coming meeting, a few weeks away.

Late afternoon of the meeting day, Robert secretly transported his Ojibwe garb to his office. This consisted of deerskin trousers and beaded jacket, along with a brightly coloured cap and headdress of feathers over a wig of flowing black hair. There, he changed and made up his face with ochre paint, including a dab of ochre-stained cotton in the deep dimple on his chin. He then covered this regalia with a long black coat and headscarf and made his way along the darkened streets to the nearby hall. Dinner was in progress when he arrived.

Bob Johnston introduced him as an honoured guest, Chief Morning Cloud, head of the Ojibwe of Ontario. He told the group that he would translate the chief's words into English.

An astonished and attentive audience hung on every word as the Chief spoke to them in Ojibwe. His speech, which included a brief history of the Ojibwe people and a discourse on Ojibwe culture, customs and spiritual beliefs, stressed that they were a people of kindness and strong family values.

He also included the story of a white man, a graduate of McGill University who had taken an Indian wife and chosen to live contently with the band.

At one point in his presentation, the chief teased the solemn Rotarians with talk of fire water, braves, and scalping but insisted that he came "to pledge goodwill and friendship" as he asked them to look at the White Man through Indian eyes. He compared the relationship of White Man and Indian to the Biblical story of an older brother who sold his birthright for a mess of pottage. Chief Morning Cloud said, "The Indian people have sold our birthright to the White Man, who have obtained our broad lands, our majestic mountains, our great lakes, and immense rivers with their thunderous waterfalls. We cannot say the White Man has been generous, but he has tried to be fair."

He talked of the White Man having a large brain but a small weak heart and how afraid he is to go hungry so does not share what he has. On the other hand, the Indian has a large heart and shares his wealth because he knows everyone will share with him.

The chief then had the audience somewhat embarrassed when he said the White Man was afraid of his woman, teasing the men in the group about having only one wife.

Gales of laughter accompanied his remarks about the number of wives the men in the group had, and his pointed question to the post-master, who shouted in broad Scots to the chief that, "I have only one wife, you auld bugger, you."

Inwardly delighted with the response, the chief talked of his three wives and many children and solemnly advised all the men to fill their homes with "the gladness of young lives." In the hush that followed this announcement, the chief then spoke of the folly of competing religions and stated that the Indian's belief is that, "the Great Spirit is as big as his universe and cannot be contained in walls built by human hands. He worships his God in his great out-of-doors. He hears His voice in the thunder and the storm and the stillness of night. He sees His face in the sunlit clouds and feels His gentle caress in the sunshine and the rain."

For a long moment, there was silence, and then the chief, who had held his audience enthralled for over two hours, sat down to thunderous applause.

Chief Morning Cloud quietly left, ostensibly to catch his train out of town. In reality, he was driven home to change out of his deerskins.

Jennie, who normally would have been in bed at this hour, was waiting up for him. She looked at him in astonishment when he entered the house in full regalia.

"Robert, whatever are you doing dressed like that? I thought you were at the Rotary dinner. Why are you dressed as an Indian chief? Your foolishness is so embarrassing sometimes."

Robert's good humour drained away as he faced his wife's questions and disapproval, and he suddenly thought of how she would feel if she ever heard his comments about wives and filling the home with many children. But he was determined to enjoy the warm afterglow of his successful performance so simply stated, "Jennie, I will tell you all about it tomorrow. But now I have to change and get back to the office. Good night."

"Well, that will be quite a conversation," he thought as he hurried back to meet with Bob Johnston at the office, "especially when I tell her I have agreed to give the speech again for the Rotary ladies. But so far no one knows it was me, so perhaps all will be well. I'll just have to swear my secretary and the other men to silence. It is a better joke if no one else knows anyway. Maybe I should have told Jennie in advance of my plans, but she has never shown any interest in the Rotary Club meetings. And I think I achieved my goal of opening some minds to the truth about my Indian friends."

He laughed out loud as he hurried along the darkened streets. "I enjoyed every minute of it tonight."

Robert was still smiling when he arrived at his office where he and Bob were met by Dr. Robertson, a dentist who shared the upper floor of the building. To Robert's surprise, Dr. Robertson grinned at them and congratulated Robert. "That was a priceless hoax and splendidly executed by you and Mr. Johnston. But how ever did the two of you manage it? I know that Mr. Johnston does not speak Ojibwe, but he translated perfectly."

Robert looked at his secretary who stammered sheepishly that she had inadvertently given the game away, "I did not know it was confidential, and I asked how your speech went at Rotary, Doctor Ross. I am sorry."

"No harm done as long as it goes no further," Robert told her then sat in his big chair and chuckled contentedly. Bob explained that the secretary had typed the English version for him to read as Robert, in his role as chief, spoke in Ojibwe.

For several hours, the men laughed together as they went over the evening. Robert firmly swore all of them to silence.

Needless to say, the whole town was talking about the mysterious Indian chief and his speech for weeks to come, but to Robert's great relief, Jennie, who did not belong to the Rotary Women's Club and prided herself on not listening to town gossip, did not put the pieces together. At least, Robert hoped she had not as nothing further was ever mentioned.

Chapter 30
Spousal Abuse

Most afternoons in Robert's office were spent dealing with the ordinary illnesses and concerns of any small town, from sore throats to sprains and pregnancies to pneumonia. But this summer afternoon in 1935 was going to be quite different and would end in a tragedy that severely tested Robert's support for the work of the mounted police.

When, at his usual hour of two o'clock, Robert arrived at work, the receptionist admitted a middle-aged couple and their adult daughter into his office. The Bauers, who lived on a farm several hours drive from Drumheller, were of German descent and had been in Canada for many years. Their daughter, born in Alberta, was a beautiful, fair young woman of medium height with clear skin, dark blue eyes, and a mass of curly auburn hair.

Her mother told the doctor that Stephanie had been married about a year ago to a young man from Medicine Hat, a CPR employee.

"I remember the wedding being reported in one of our local newspapers," commented Robert. "It was a swell affair and a great event in the family papers. Don't I recall that the happy couple went to live in Beiseker?"

At this, Mr. Bauer snorted in angry disbelief, "Happy couple? Bah!"

"How can I assist you?" Robert asked them.

Mrs. Bauer spoke to her daughter, "Stephanie, we agreed. You must tell the doctor your story."

Stephanie hung her head and remained silent.

"Perhaps," Robert encouraged the mother, "you could tell me the story, Mrs. Bauer."

"My daughter has been subjected to terrible abuse by her husband. Please let the doctor examine you, Stephanie."

Mr. Bauer left the room for a few moments to give his daughter some privacy. Upon examining the young woman's arms, chest, hips, and legs, Robert found that there was hardly a spot on her body that was not terribly discoloured with fading bruises from the blows she had received.

"Tell me how this happened, Stephanie."

But Stephanie still would not speak, hanging her head in shame.

So Mrs. Bauer continued, "After being in bed with my daughter for a short time," she said, "her husband would go into a sort of mad frenzy and would beat Stephanie, after which he would drag her by the hair out of bed and onto the porch and leave her there. When she was recovered enough to move, she would slip quietly back into the house and lie down on the couch until daybreak. When her husband arose, she would get his morning meal ready and fill his dinner pail.

"Following a breakfast eaten in silence, he would take his dinner pail and leave for the day only to have this terrible abuse repeated upon his return in the evening."

The woman had spoken clearly, but her anguish was obvious.

Unhappily, Robert had seen this behaviour before so knew better than to ask why Stephanie had not left her husband.

"What else?" He gently questioned the young woman.

At this, Stephanie began to speak so quietly that Robert could barely hear her, and the rest of the story tumbled out. "He told me that if I left him he would follow me and shoot me and kill my parents as well. So I stayed with him, but I began to hide some food outside in the shed. Some weeks ago, instead of going back into the house after he threw me on the porch, I knew I had to get away. My only choice was to go home to my parents.

"I had no means of transportation and was too afraid that my husband would discover my plan if I telephoned my father to ask for help. It took me two weeks to get home. I walked from Beiseker to my parents' farm by night, always afraid my husband would find me. I travelled just along the edge of the roadways and only when it was dark. Once my food ran out, I ate berries and whatever else I could find, drinking water from ponds."

Relieved to be telling her story at last, Stephanie continued in a halting voice, "I hid in ditches or in haystacks during the day, creeping occasionally to the doors of farmhouses where I knew the women would keep my secret and give me something to eat. Although these kind farm wives fed me, they could not hide me for fear of the disapproval of their own husbands and because they said it was not for them to come between a husband and his wife."

This last was said with no trace of bitterness, only gratitude to those who had given her food. For two weeks and nearly ninety miles, she had pursued this gruelling journey.

"When I finally got to my parents and learned that my husband had not been there, I was so thankful."

Mr. Bauer had returned to the room to hear the story and now spoke to Robert, "We were surprised and horrified when Stephanie arrived at our home this morning. As soon as she told her mother what had happened, we brought her to see you. What is your advice, Doctor? I do not feel safe about keeping my daughter at our house, for her sake or my wife's. And does my daughter need medical care?"

"As far as I can tell, Stephanie has no broken bones. She managed to walk home, so internal injuries are unlikely, and her bruises, although extensive, are beginning to heal. However, you must go to the police immediately and tell them her story. Show them her bruises. Tell them I believe you all need police protection right now. You are dealing with a dangerous lunatic who has beaten your daughter over and over again and threatened to kill both you and your wife. The police must apprehend him before he beats Stephanie to death or kills someone else."

"Yes, of course, we must go to the police. Thank you, Doctor Ross. We will go there as soon as we leave here."

Robert then asked, "Do you have a gun in the house?"

"Yes. I do."

"Good. Keep your gun loaded, and keep it handy by you at all times. If that crazy man appears, shoot him on sight."

Mr. Bauer hesitated and said, "I do keep a revolver in the house. I know how to fire it, but I have never had cause to use it."

Robert met his eyes and said gravely, "Remember, this man has beaten your daughter and has threatened to kill you and your wife. Your only defence is to shoot him first."

"I will, Doctor. I will have my gun ready, and I will shoot him if the police do not capture him first."

The family left, and Robert phoned the Mounties to tell them to expect the Bauers and stressed that they needed police protection immediately. The constable thanked Robert and said he would report their story to his superior.

The next afternoon, Robert received a phone call from the matron at the hospital saying that Mrs. Bauer had been shot in the abdomen and was in serious condition. Her husband and daughter were bringing the injured woman to the hospital as fast as their automobile would travel.

Disturbed, and somewhat puzzled, by this news, Robert drove to the hospital, wondering what could have happened.

Mrs. Bauer was carried into the operating room upon arrival, but there was no doubt her wound was fatal. All Robert and the nurses could do was administer opiates to lessen the agony of her death.

After she died, Robert sat with her grieving husband. "What happened? Was this an accident, or did that madman do this? I thought the police were going to protect you."

Ashen-faced, Mr. Bauer struggled to recount the story. "When we left your office, Doctor, we went right to the station and reported the man's actions as you had advised. We told them the story exactly as we told it to you." Mr. Bauer shut his eyes for a moment and then continued. "They told us to go home and forget about it. That there was nothing they could do. That they could not interfere between a man and his wife."

Hardly able to contain his anger at the police, Robert gritted his teeth and asked as gently as he could, "Why did you not shoot the man as I had advised?"

"He arrived at our farm early this morning, banged on the door, and loudly demanded to see his wife. I had taken your advice and had my gun loaded and ready. I held it in my hand, cocked the trigger, and pointed it at the closed door."

Silent tears coursed down Mr. Bauer's face, and his voice shuddered as he went on.

"I told my wife to go to the door and open it. To tell the man Stephanie was inside and then move quickly out of the way. This she did, and as the crazy man stepped into my house, I raised my gun and took aim. But I couldn't shoot him! My finger froze on the trigger, and I just couldn't pull it. Oh Mein Gott, I couldn't pull that trigger."

For long moments, there was silence, and then Mr. Bauer continued in a monotone. "He shot my wife and then ran off. I have just learned from my neighbours that when Stephanie and I left the house to rush her mother to the hospital, the madman burned down my barn and killed my horses and cattle. He set the chicken coop on fire and burned two hundred hens and chicks. After that, he shot himself through the head. They say he is dead."

There was nothing more that could be said. Robert ensured that the neighbours were prepared to look after Mr. Bauer and Stephanie. As soon as the devastated pair left the hospital, he contacted the mounted police to express his anger and frustration at their apparent dismissal of the Bauers' story and the resulting tragedy. "I sent those poor people to you," he stormed. "They trusted me, and they trusted you. And you did nothing. Nothing! Don't tell me about the law. If you had sent someone back to their home with them, you might have prevented this senseless death."

Robert was even more infuriated when, several days later, he heard that the police had appeared at the Bauers' farm to express their interest in the safety and well-being of the family. The sum total of their actions, however, was to advise the young widow to have her blood tested for syphilis. Too little, too late.

His anger smouldering, Robert began to give serious thought to using the agency of the press to expose the manner in which the police had disregarded both his urgent warning and pleas of the family. However, he hesitated to take the story to the newspaper. He knew that William Aberhart, then Premier of Alberta, was trying to get rid of the mounted police and substitute a provincial police force in its stead.

In his conversations with Jennie, they had gone over the tragic results of the inaction of the Mounties. Still distressed and angry at the needless loss of life and his inability to do anything about it, Robert remarked, "I believe an exposé of the negligence of the police in failing to give that family the protection they urgently needed is the right thing to do. The Mounties ignored both my warning and the pleas of the family. But taking this sad tale to the papers won't bring the poor woman back, and I greatly fear Aberhardt, whose motives I simply don't trust, would use the story to further his own agenda."

Jennie agreed. "You are correct, Robert. Going to the press will not bring Mrs. Bauer back nor would it mend this family, and it would be a powerful argument for Aberhardt. Remember, for the most part, you have a good relationship with the mounted police here, and they usually do listen to you."

"Yes, I know, my dear. You're right. And we don't know that Aberhardt's provincial police force would be any better than what we have right now."

"Robert, it is the law that needs to be changed so that husbands cannot beat their wives in this way and go unpunished."

Robert sat for a few moments, knowing his wife was correct but still struggling to determine his best course of action. Finally, tired beyond words, he made his decision.

"Of course, Jennie, of course," he sighed. "I am too weary to even think about the politics of it all right now, but I won't go to the press with this story. I will keep my silence."

Chapter 31
A Wedding and an Undertaker

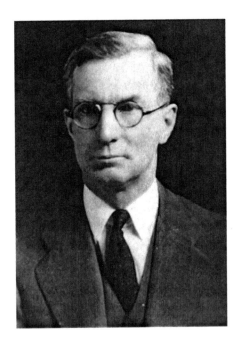

Robert, Drumheller, Alberta, 1935

A much happier event was to occur in late summer of that same year, although the morning of August 6, 1935, got off to a slightly shaky start.

"Robert, where is Douglas? He knows the ceremony begins at eight-thirty. Reverend Shortt has another wedding in Calgary this morning and must leave just after this ceremony." Standing at the front of the church, watching their guests arrive, Jennie's voice was tight with anxiety, and she turned to apologize again to the minister. "I'm sure Douglas will be here momentarily. I do apologize for his tardiness as I know you are pressed for time. So thoughtless of him to be late for his own wedding and inconvenience others."

"Jennie, Reverend Shortt," Robert spoke quietly, "Douglas was in surgery all night. There was a terrible accident at the mines. A cutting machine fell on several men. He was in the operating room until six o'clock this morning, but I know he arrived home an hour ago. He will be here on time." Robert glanced at the gold watch he wore on a chain across his vest. "It is just gone eight o'clock. He will be here."

Jennie's face was tight with worry, and she turned back to the minister and Gordon, who had a half smile on his face. His wife, Elsie, was Elizabeth's matron of honour, and Gordon was best man, although he was aware that this was against Elizabeth's wishes. He disliked her for her quick mind and sharp comments, and he knew she returned his dislike. She believed that as his mother's favourite, Gordon had subtly encouraged Jennie's criticism of Douglas. There was evident tension in the little group that waited at the front of the Knox United Church on this warm August morning.

"Elizabeth and her father are waiting outside for Douglas's arrival." Apparently enjoying his brother's predicament, Gordon spoke again, "I do hope my brother gets here. It would be a shame if he missed his own wedding. It is almost eight-thirty, and Reverend Shortt must leave by nine-thirty."

Robert took a deep breath and said firmly to his older son, "We know that, Gordon."

Much to Robert's delight, the small group of guests included Douglas's cousin, Colin, from Montreal. They all chatted happily, and the music from the organ played gently in the background.

The side door opened. The groom had arrived.

"Good morning, Mother, Dad. Good morning, Reverend Shortt. Sorry for the delay. It was unavoidable, I assure you." Douglas was pale with exhaustion, and his black curls were in disarray as he walked briskly to take his place with his older brother at the front of the church. He smiled at the minister and at their guests, with a special nod to Colin with whom he had stayed in Montreal. The family, especially Jennie, had hoped one of the Victoria cousins could attend, but Horace had already been to Drumheller that year, so he could not make the trip over the mountains again so soon.

Robert and Jennie moved to their seats in the front row, and the organist began to play Mendelssohn's triumphant "Wedding March."

Douglas turned to grin, not at all solemnly, at his bride as she entered the church on her father's arm, a smile of the purest joy on her beautiful face. She was preceded by her matron of honour, Elsie, and three-year-old Shelagh, who carried a tiny basket of flowers. Elizabeth, dressed in a simple white gown, moved gracefully down the aisle toward her husband-to-be. Her father placed her hands in Douglas's, and then Morris Stevenson joined Elizabeth's three brothers and their mother, Charlotte, who were already seated.

Robert's watch softly chimed eight-thirty, and he sighed in relief and slipped it back into his vest pocket. His younger son was marrying the girl he had loved for nearly a decade, and Robert knew it was a perfect match. He, too, loved Elizabeth and was quite sure the young couple would follow their dreams. A feeling of great contentment swept over him, and he turned and smiled at his wife. "It is all right, Jennie, both our sons are married, and it is all right."

***

The warm days of fall were only a memory, and November's freezing winds brought tiny hard pellets of sleet that tapped angrily on the windows of her bedroom. Bedridden for the last few days, Jennie's rheumatism was always bad when the cold came, her joints ached, and even the soft weight of the blankets was painful.

This morning, the new housekeeper brought her tea and helped her move to a slightly more comfortable position. Jennie asked her to run a hot bath, hoping the warmth of the water would ease the pain enough for her to dress in time for lunch with Robert. It was difficult, but with Ethel's assistance, she managed and was sitting at the dining room table when Robert came home from the hospital.

"Ah, you are able to be up today. I am so glad. This has been the worst spell you have had for some time. Is the aspirin helping at all?"

"Yes, thank you, Robert, I am feeling better, and I detest lying in bed. There is much to be done. We have another dinner planned to raise funds for the church. The hall basement is leaking, and repairs are necessary as that is where Sunday school classes are held. It seems there is always something."

"Jennie, please try not to overtire yourself. You know that the pain is always worse when you are fatigued, and this winter promises to be long and bitterly cold. I am sorry our finances are such that you will not be able to visit Nell and your cousins on the coast this year. We did enjoy the visit from Horace in the spring when he came here for his surgery. Have you heard any word of his health since he returned to Victoria?"

"Horace is fine now, quite recovered from his abdominal surgery, though his ear still bothers him. Don't fuss about me, Robert. I know very well how to manage this disease. I have had it since I was a young girl. I will do my best to keep warm and rest each day, but I cannot lie abed forever just because the weather here is so cold."

Robert knew that there was no more he could say so instead asked if she was pleased with Ethel's work.

"She is doing very well. She is an excellent plain cook, as you can tell from your lunch, able to make delicious meals from very little, and is a most caring, Christian woman. I am pleased. Perhaps now that Douglas has graduated and we seem to have a little more money, we could once again have some friends here for dinner? I know Ethel would cook an excellent meal for us. She is used to preparing meals for a large family, and we could hire a maid to help her serve that evening. Goodness knows, there are so many looking for work right now."

Robert looked sharply at his wife, considering her comment about Douglas and the drain on the family finances but wisely chose to let it go. "Yes, a dinner party would be a good idea, my dear. And speaking of Douglas, I had a letter from them today. He is enjoying his locum in Shawinigan Falls, and Beth says that her French is improving daily.

But Douglas has had no success in finding a position in Quebec or Ontario. He tells me that most of his graduating classmates are also having similar difficulties; there are just no jobs. Older doctors are hanging on as they cannot afford to retire during these hard times, and there is not enough money available to risk starting a new practice. The promised economic recovery is a long time coming even with the efforts of Roosevelt's New Deal in the United States."

Jennie was not surprised that Douglas had written to his father rather than to her, although she had received a polite note from Elizabeth, telling of their daily news and the happiness Douglas took in his medical practice in Shawinigan Falls. Jennie was pleased to know that they were well, but she knew that the locum would end in February when the absent doctor returned.

"Do you think they will have to come back to Drumheller, Robert? There is very little money here now, and another doctor would perhaps be one too many."

Robert was angry at her question but spoke quietly as always. "Jennie, Douglas is our son, he is an excellent doctor, and he and his wife would be welcome in our home, anytime. I know he hopes to find work elsewhere, perhaps on the West Coast, but if not, this is, and always will be, his home."

There was silence for a few moments, and then Jennie turned the conversation to Gordon's daughter, Shelagh, who was very much her grandmother's pet.

"Elsie and Gordon are bringing Shelagh for a visit this Christmas. It will be good to see them again. I am glad he did not take the position in Montana. He continues to do very well in Calgary."

Robert, who took great joy in his granddaughter, smiled and agreed that it would be good to see them at Christmas, although he knew that the excitement would be a strain on Jennie's health. He did not mention that Douglas had asked if he and Beth could return to Drumheller in February to stay with them if he was unable to join a practice in eastern Canada. He also did not mention that Beth was expecting a baby in April. Time enough for that.

"The house is very quiet, Jennie. It will be good to have Gordon and Elsie and Shelagh here for a while. I miss them; I miss them all."

Robert headed up the stairs to have a brief nap before he went to the office at two o'clock. He found his own back was beginning to bother him after a long morning of surgery, "Well," he mused, "I am sixty-five after all. I must expect a few aches and pains, especially in this cold weather. And," his thoughts turned to a young patient as he drifted off to sleep, "I need to decide what to do about little Tommy Jackson's earaches...I have an idea...I think George will help."

**

Back at the office, Robert telephoned George, who confirmed with his brother that there were two unidentified and unclaimed bodies waiting for burial in one of the towns where George practiced. Accordingly, the next evening, masked, gowned, and accompanied by a similarly attired graduate nurse, as well as Mr. Saunders, the owner of the funeral home, Robert moved quickly and quietly through the parlour's cool room, where the two bodies, which had been packed in snow to keep them cold, now lay on trestle tables.

On their arrival at the funeral parlour in the small town, about a two-hour drive from Drumheller, they had been handed a message from George. *"Tied up tonight with a patient. Do wish I could have been with you on this adventure."* George's note continued, *"I am sorry to miss this opportunity to work with you, Robert, especially in a somewhat secretive mission. But I wish you well. I am sure your real surgery will be a success. Mr. Saunders is most willing to help."*

Robert was disappointed to read that his brother would not be able to assist him in his plans to use the unclaimed bodies to review and practice the tricky procedures involved in a procedure called a myringotomy. He planned to operate on the middle ears of both cadavers in preparation for performing the same operation on his living patient, Tommy Jackson. He was particularly pleased that it was a body of a young man, as it would allow him to practice in the smaller surgical space an ear of that age presented.

Robert had seen Tommy in his office too frequently of late, and the youngster had been complaining of severe earaches for some time. Despite the best efforts of the doctor and the excellent care of his mother, who had trained as a nurse and was now accompanying Dr. Ross to his practice session, Tommy was showing no improvement and suffering increasing pain. Robert, though fully apprised of the work of Dr. Blake and Ashley Cooper, had not performed such a delicate operation for some time. He was nevertheless determined to do the necessary procedure, realizing that Tommy's ear infection had worsened, and pressure on the eardrum was becoming more and more severe. The only way to stop the infection was to operate and insert a tiny tube into the eardrum to allow the fluid to drain and equalize the pressure between the outer and middle chambers of the affected ear. If he did not operate, the infection could spread to the mastoid bone surrounding the ear canals, and the child would lose his hearing and quite possibly his life.

Tommy would be in a hospital bed waiting for surgery the next morning, but before going ahead, Robert had decided to avail himself of the two unclaimed cadavers in the funeral home to practice the precise surgery required. Although deeply saddened by the fact that one of them was a boy in his teens, he was comforted by the knowledge that the young man's death would at least help a living child in some way.

"I assure you, Mr. Saunders, the bodies will be restored to their original condition before burial."

"Nobody has claimed them, Doctor Ross. We've tried, but all our efforts to identify the young man who was found starved to death in a ditch by the side of the road have failed. And the other one, well, looks like he was in some kind of accident. But the police can't find anything about him."

"Hmm," murmured Robert, "what a dreadful shame. But this young man is the perfect choice to help Tommy, so his death is not a total waste."

Robert had brought with him all he would need, including his otoscope, which he had acquired from Queen's University. It was a recent version of Dr. Clarence Blake's invention of 1884 and had excellent magnifying lenses. This was not his only new tool. He had also brought with him the latest innovation from Eveready, a flashlight with a prefocused bulb. This was a vast improvement over the 1906 version, which flashed intermittently. In addition to this equipment, Robert had also had with him several fine metal tubes. He would insert one into each ear drum during his practice surgeries this evening.

In a living patient, this tube would allow drainage of the infected fluid from the middle ear and would remain in place while the ear healed. It would also greatly relieve the pain as the pressure between the middle ear and the eustachian tube leading to the back of the throat was balanced.

Carefully, with as much respect as he would have shown this lost young man if he were alive, Robert asked the undertaker to clamp the dead boy's head firmly. With the nurse's assistance, he proceeded to wash the whole side of the head thoroughly. The nurse then swabbed the area with antiseptic and cleaned the outer ear and ear canal.

Mr. Saunders, fascinated by what was happening, aimed the flashlight at the dead boy's head as the doctor prepared to operate.

"Hold the light so that the beam shines into the ear canal." Robert ordered Mr. Saunders. "And do not move."

"Now," he spoke to his nurse, "clean the eardrum, be very cautious, but get it clean, and swab it with antiseptic." Tommy's mother, realizing that the same procedure would take place with her son the next morning, steadied her hands and proceeded as Dr. Ross had requested.

Then, with great delicacy, Robert made a small incision in the thoroughly clean eardrum and inserted the tube just as he would the next morning for Tommy.

"We may have to use a siphon tomorrow to be sure the fluid begins to drain, but this is not required now," he said as he trimmed the tube to size and left it in place with the exterior end just visible in the outer ear.

"I am satisfied that this procedure will work," stated Robert as he removed the tube and then said, "We are now going to repeat this procedure on the other ear and then again on both ears of the other cadaver." And so they did.

"Thank you for your cooperation, Mr. Saunders. As you can see, we have been most respectful of your charges, and your willingness to permit this and your help has meant that a young living boy will be spared a lot of pain."

"You are most welcome, Doctor Ross. I am beholden to Doctor George for his care of my family."

Dr. Ross reassured his nurse that all would be well when he operated on Tommy. "Your son is strong and well nourished, and if we can get the fluid draining properly, and I am confident that we will, his own healthy body will do the rest."

By eight o'clock the following morning, Robert and the boy's mother had returned to their homes in Drumheller. After taking time for a quick breakfast, Robert drove to the hospital, fully prepared for the surgery he was about to perform. Tommy's mother, who had been sworn to silence about the previous night's work, knew she had to wait in the room outside the operating theatre as relatives were not permitted by the hospital to take part in an operation on family members. She was completely content that the doctor was prepared, and she had confidence in the skill of the surgical nurses attending the surgery. She knew that Tommy would be all right. And although she would say nothing about the nighttime practice session, no one had told her that she could not sing the praises of her doctor, which she did on every possible occasion as the weeks passed, pointing proudly to her happy son.

Chapter 32
Prairie Madness

Douglas and Beth returned to Drumheller in February of 1936. They lived with Robert and Jennie while Douglas worked in his father's practice. This arrangement was to last until the younger doctor found a house to rent and employment elsewhere.

Their first child, Robert Douglas, named after grandfather and father, had been born in April, a healthy, happy baby boy who was the centre of attention. Jennie was fond of the newborn but found the pressure of sharing her home and the attendant turmoil of a baby difficult. Robert was certainly aware of the rising tension between his strong-willed wife and his equally strong-willed daughter-in-law, especially as the drought and the hardships of the Depression dragged on and the heat of the summer continued unabated.

His mind on the unvoiced discord in his home, Robert was on his way back to work. As he walked through the tree-lined streets, he hardly noticed the town drowsing in the scorching temperatures of a dusty summer afternoon. Even shady front porches were deserted as people sought relief in their cool homes.

Nearing the office, he turned his mind to a problem he had to solve that afternoon. A patient was due to arrive in about an hour, a young mother, and he was very concerned about her and the request her father and brother had made when they booked the appointment for her.

Lucy Brady was about thirty, and Robert had delivered her of four babies in the last five years. He also looked after her other two children. She had six in all, the oldest a boy of ten.

Robert had been worried about Mrs. Brady. She had seemed very depressed and lacking in her usual energy in recent months. However, she had never complained of feeling ill when she brought any of her children in for the doctor to tend to their various ailments.

She was a proud woman and very softly had told Doctor Ross that she would bring him some eggs as soon as possible, as she had no money now. And with good reason, as he well knew. She and her husband had homesteaded in a fertile valley several miles from the town. After the initial brutal struggle to till the land and plant their fields, they had done quite well. But the loss of any market for their crops followed by years of scorching drought had destroyed their livelihood.

There was no money from the land, their animals were dying for lack of water, and along with thousands of other men, her husband had left the area in search of work, seeking some income in the work camps or cities to the east. The young mother had buried her pride and moved with her children into her parents' home, but they, too, were struggling.

Her mother had tried her best to help her daughter's family, but within a year had succumbed to pneumonia and died. This left Lucy's father and her younger brother struggling to wrest a meagre living from the land. They carried water from a distant, muddy creek for the family to drink and tried to grow vegetables and raise a few chickens and a cow.

It was Lucy's father who had set the appointment with Dr. Ross for today, telling the receptionist that Lucy was ill and broken in spirit and had just given up. Her father and brother wanted to commit her to an asylum and send the children away, each one to live with a different relative or friend in order to get them something to eat. The father had said that he could not cope any longer and maintained that Lucy was unable to work on the farm or care for her children. According to his story, she simply sat in a corner and ignored the pleas for food from her children.

Robert knew what the law said he could do in cases such as this. According to the Mental Health Act of 1927, if a doctor's certificate was obtained, and a justice of the peace agreed, a woman could be committed to an insane asylum such as the one in Ponoka.

The moral and ethical considerations were not so clear, and Robert struggled, as did every doctor, with the consequences of whatever decision he made. He knew Lucy Brady. He knew that she had broken under the terrible strain of seeing their farm destroyed, of trying to care for her mother until her death, of looking after everyone without her husband's support, of trying to feed her children while watching starvation creep up on her family. He knew she had borne too many children too close together, that her absent husband might never return, and that her father resented having to feed her and the children when he could barely feed himself and his son. Robert suspected that Lucy's father also blamed her for her mother's death. He knew her father's land, like all the prairie farms, would soon be stripped bare by the incessant wind and drought and dust storms. And Robert knew that these thoughts tormented the young mother.

If Robert decided to commit Lucy to an asylum for the mentally ill, he knew that she would receive food and care, but she would never see her children again. He also knew that what little was left of her dignity and her mind would soon be gone.

"And what of her children?" he thought as he paced along the dusty street. "Willing neighbours and relatives have little enough for themselves, and one more mouth to feed would break many of them."

He continued to turn the problem over in his mind. "Her father and brother might be able to scratch enough sustenance from their land to feed themselves, but the children, the youngest of whom is just a year old, would not be welcomed in homes where the same bleak conditions obtained. The older children might be worked to death or placed in orphanages." Robert knew that this had happened in several similar situations in the valley.

"But if I don't sign the certificate, what then?" He understood that the father and brother would search for another doctor — one more willing to comply — that the children would have their mother but only until they all starved or she was committed by another physician. She would soon be truly insane without food for her family or some care for herself.

Robert knew that Lucy was not insane. She was not violent and posed no threat to society. Exhausted? Yes. Depressed? Yes. Ill and broken of spirit and body, she needed rest and food and help. She was only one of the thousands whose families were trying to find a similar answer to a seemingly insoluble problem.

Robert had encountered this agonizing dilemma before, and unless the rains came, the economic situation improved, or the government in Ottawa provided more relief, he and other members of the medical profession would have to deal with it again and again.

By the time he reached his office and waited for Lucy Brady and her father and brother to arrive, he had reached a decision. They entered his office and sat down, Lucy sitting silently between the two men.

"We can't look after her, Doctor Ross. We can't feed ourselves, never mind her six children. She can't work, can't do nothing. Her mind is gone; she needs to go to the asylum."

Lucy sat, slumped against the chair back, her hands nervously pleating the coarse fabric of her dusty skirt, her eyes blankly staring at the floor.

Robert spoke to her, "Mrs. Brady...Lucy, you know me, Doctor Ross. You brought the baby to see me only a month ago for an earache. Tell me, why are you here?" Robert leaned toward her and took one of her twitching hands, gently holding it until it was still. Slowly she raised her eyes to his, and for a few moments her gaze was focused on his face.

"No, no, not my babies. Don't take my babies." It was no more than an agonized whisper. "Not my babies. My babies are gone. Please, Doctor, please."

"She don't know what she's saying, Doctor. The children are back at the farm."

Robert looked sharply at the men and made a decision. "We'll go back to the farm together and see your babies, Lucy."

At this, Lucy's father and brother looked nervously at the doctor, and then the younger man spoke hastily. "Doctor, we sent the children to the neighbours a few days ago. Lucy wasn't looking after them, and we couldn't. They're not at the farm anymore. They were hungry, and so are we…" his voice trailed away.

On his walk to the office, Robert had thought of a temporary solution if he decided that Lucy was indeed sane. He had quietly supported the Ursuline Sisters in their convent with regular donations from his own kitchen and pocket as they did great good in the town. Although he was Presbyterian and a staunch supporter of the Knox United Church, he did not believe religious dogma should ever stand in the way of helping those in need. Indeed, he and Douglas provided free medical care to the Sisters on the rare occasions when they sought help.

Annoyed that the children had already been taken from their mother, Robert turned to Lucy's father and made his decision known. "Your daughter is going to stay in the convent for two weeks and get her strength back. You will go and fetch the children immediately. Bring them here to me. I will ensure that caring families take them in. They will be fed and clean and safe for the two weeks. After that, we will see how Lucy is faring, and at that time, I will make my final decision on this matter. Meanwhile, you must do whatever is necessary to get her husband back home. You have no right to do this to his wife without his permission."

Robert knew it was only a short reprieve, but perhaps it would allow sufficient time for this one young woman to recover and care for her family again.

"Would this Depression never end?"

Chapter 33
Norman Bethune

It would seem not, as the "dirty thirties" continued with all the horror and pain of the Depression grinding down the communities of the prairies and indeed the whole of Canada. An unprecedented decade of drought savaged the Great Plains of North America. Even as the price of wheat tumbled from $1.23 a bushel in 1929 to $0.27 a bushel in 1932, the once fertile fields dried up, and what crops there were burned in the sun. It was 1937 before there was some faint hope that the global economy was in the beginnings of a recovery, but across the prairie provinces, financial woes and drought continued unabated.

Wars in Europe seemed very far away and unimportant to those facing starvation in Alberta, but some people understood the looming threat. Newspapers were full of stories of the civil war in Spain, thought by many to be a war against fascism and a precursor to a larger European conflict. Rumours of the Nazi's growing power in Germany filled the airwaves.

Canada had her own hero of the Spanish conflict in the person of Dr. Norman Bethune. He had set up a mobile blood bank close to the front lines in support of those rebelling against Franco. At one point, Dr. Bethune and his field team were giving up to one hundred blood transfusions a day.

Robert, Jennie, Douglas, and Beth often spoke of the events in Europe. The men particularly admired the work of Bethune, who had been a lecturer at the Royal Victoria Hospital in Montreal when the younger Doctor Ross was at McGill University. Douglas had attended several lectures and had been very impressed by Bethune's innovative approach to tuberculosis and thoracic surgery.

When Norman Bethune returned to Canada to a hero's welcome in 1937 and announced that he would crisscross the country on a fundraising tour for the victims of fascist oppression, it was inevitable that Robert would invite him to stay at his home in Drumheller. He and Jennie had room for guests now, as Douglas and Beth had found a home nearby.

Dr. Bethune was due to arrive at the Drumheller station on the noon train on a freezing day in January. Robert, well bundled up in his warm winter overcoat, got to the train in good time to meet him. However, when Robert arrived at the station, he was told that their guest had mistakenly left the train at Rosebud, a small stop several miles down the line. Concerned that Bethune would be waiting in the cold, Robert drove as rapidly as possible along the icy roads, only to discover the famous doctor shivering in the winter wind. Bethune had not thought to bring a heavy coat, so Robert promptly shed his own treasured beaver coat from his HBC days and handed it to Bethune. Grateful, but too chilled to speak, the doctor wrapped himself in the warmth as Robert said, "This coat is a gift to you. Keep it. You will need it on your journeys across the prairies. Get in the car, and we will go to my home. My wife is waiting for your arrival."

Jennie was not opposed to Bethune as a person. She believed that he was a good man, whose work for the poor and oppressed was commendable. But she struggled with his support for the establishment of socialized medicine in Canada and especially his membership in the Communist party. Her own Methodist beliefs reflected the avowed goals of the Communist party to change the world for the better. However, Wesley's teachings were firmly rooted in the words of the Bible, and the Communist party rejected religion, which upset her dreadfully.

Her quandary was resolved when her husband and her younger son made it clear that the medical advances Bethune had made, especially in thoracic surgery, far outweighed their own discomfort with Bethune's political beliefs. Beth's father, Morris Stevenson, was a coal miner who had been reviled by strikers for his refusal to support what he believed to be an illegal strike, so for her, Bethune's Communist dogma was anathema. However, Beth had deep respect for her husband's decision to rise above politics and support Dr. Bethune's advances in medicine.

Norman Bethune was a brilliant and charismatic man, and conversation over the dinner table during his visit sparkled. Each family member argued their points persuasively, fully supporting Bethune's medical skill while challenging his political stance. Just as alarming to them was his belief that Europe would soon be embroiled in another war.

"The Spanish Civil War is merely a rehearsal for a much larger conflict to come," he contended, "and it will come soon, with Germany at the centre."

"Surely not," Beth protested. "The rest of Europe and Britain trounced them so soundly. They would not allow it to happen again."

"Germany and its people have resented the terms of the Treaty of Versailles for twenty long years. The monetary penalties alone beggared the country, and this depression has increased the misery a thousandfold," Douglas replied thoughtfully. "Right or wrong, they blame all of us for Clemenceau's revenge. I am also uneasy."

Bethune nodded in agreement, "As you all know, Adolf Hitler has used the rest of Europe's concern about the rise of communism as a shield behind which he has built up the German Army. What you may not realize is how weak Britain and France are in respect to Germany's territorial advances. Germany has taken over the Rhineland, and, Hitler's promises be damned, Austria is next. I apologize for my strong language, ladies, but it is an extremely likely scenario. He will not be stopped, mark my words."

Robert noted solemnly that there had been news of German pacts with Italy and Japan. "It is frightening, but surely Britain and France will have to stop him now. And what of the Americans?"

Bethune groaned in frustration. "The Americans wouldn't even support the League of Nations, although it was Wilson's idea. Even Roosevelt can't break through their isolationist stance, and most people choose to believe that geography and distance will protect them from a European conflict. And, of course, the League has no real power."

Jennie spoke up. "The politics of appeasement have always been disastrous. But time is slipping away, and Doctor Bethune, you and your party have a train to catch. If I remember correctly, you are due in Edmonton tomorrow."

"Of course, Mrs. Ross. Thank you for the reminder and for your wonderful hospitality." He turned to Robert with a smile. "Doctor Ross, I will be forever grateful to you for your gift of a warm coat and your generous donation to the cause. My future plans include a trip to China to assist the poor people in the terrible wars being waged there. I will wear this coat on my travels. Watch for me in newsreels from the northern areas of that great country."

He shook Douglas's hand and said, "Douglas, it has been a pleasure seeing you again and meeting your beautiful wife and little son. Now, I must go."

Bethune left to catch the 11 o'clock train to his next destination. Douglas and Beth and baby Robert returned to their home just down the street, leaving Robert and Jennie to sit by the fire and review the evening.

"A most interesting houseguest Robert, but I am glad the visit is over. I am exhausted. I feel as though we have all been walking on eggs for the last two days."

"Jennie, sometimes it is important to do this sort of thing. You were a wonderful hostess despite your firm beliefs. Thank you."

Jennie smiled at the compliment and spoke, "I am truly sorry Gordon could not have been here. His opinions would have been valuable. Douglas, I'm afraid, suffers somewhat from hero worship as far as Doctor Bethune is concerned. And Elizabeth will always support her husband's views."

"Jennie, you are not being fair. Beth has a mind of her own."

As always, Jennie simply ignored remarks that challenged her convictions. "Do you know if Doctor Bethune was able to raise any money here in Drumheller? Even the miners who support his beliefs have little enough as it is, and I'm quite sure the local merchants would have no time for a Communist."

Chapter 34
Looking Better

Communism was the last thing on Robert's mind as he and Douglas sat in the office late one afternoon discussing an upcoming strabismus surgery scheduled for two mornings hence. Robert had realized the need for this operation upon the discovery that one of his appendectomy patients also had a condition known as "walleye."

Although the operation to correct strabismus was rarely performed outside of a university hospital setting, Robert could not abide any suffering when he believed it could be alleviated through his own efforts. He was also supremely confident in his surgical skills and experience. Since he had been joined a year earlier by his son, a gifted surgeon in his own right, Robert felt that together they could successfully perform any operation necessary. Along with his up-to-date medical knowledge, Douglas also brought with him from McGill the very latest in medical equipment, and he enjoyed the same confidence as his father.

Some months ago, Robert had examined a young woman who had come to see him complaining of severe pain in her abdomen, and he was quite sure that an appendectomy was required within the next twenty-four hours. Her abdomen was very tender, and as he palpated it, her mother, who accompanied her, inquired tentatively, "Ellen doesn't fuss much, but she says her stomach is really sore, and it feels like something is pulling her insides. Could it be something she ate?"

Ellen said nothing but sat gripping her stomach with her head turned sideways and her eyes downcast. When Robert was examining her, she grimaced in pain but kept her eyes shut throughout the examination.

"The severe pain you are experiencing is not indigestion, Ellen; it is acute appendicitis, and we must operate by tomorrow at the latest." Seeing Mrs. Johnson's alarm and hesitation, Robert stressed, "Mrs. Johnson, without this operation, your daughter will assuredly die a painful death."

"Oh, please, Doctor Ross, you must do the operation. Somehow, we will find the money to pay you."

Robert stepped out of the examining room to make the necessary arrangements with the matron at the hospital to have Ellen admitted immediately and prepared for surgery. However, he had noticed that throughout the examination Ellen had kept her head turned away, looking at him only rarely and always from the side, her eyes downcast or even closed. Determined to find out why, he returned to the waiting pair and spoke directly to Ellen.

"Please look at me, Ellen. I need to tell you about the operation." He was taken aback when she reluctantly raised her eyes to his, and he saw that she suffered from such a severe strabismus, or walleye, that her left eye was facing almost impossibly to the left while her right eye was straight and focused on him.

"Why did you not tell me about this condition?" He looked at her mother, as Ellen again gazed at the floor in obvious embarrassment.

Mrs. Johnson hastily answered the doctor. "She was born that way, Doctor Ross. It's God's will, and we accept it. Otherwise, she's perfectly healthy and a good worker. She always does her chores without complaint."

Robert was a strong supporter of his church and a believer in the Creator, but his faith was based on a much kinder Supreme Being, so he spoke firmly to Mrs. Johnson." Nonsense, God would never punish someone who has done nothing wrong. It is a medical condition that I have seen before and operated on with good success."

Robert did not feel it was necessary to mention that his strabismus surgery had been on cadavers during his student days at Queen's. It was not important that Mrs. Johnson knew that. The important thing was that he had done the operation and was sure he could do it again, especially with Douglas's assistance.

"I cannot say I will be able to improve her ability to see properly at this stage of her life, it is likely too late for that, but I can certainly straighten her eyes so that she will appear normal. It will improve her appearance and she will feel much better about herself. Poor creature, I can imagine the remarks made about her."

The young woman whimpered both in fear and in hope as she looked from under her half-closed eyes at her mother.

Robert continued, "I'll operate on her eye when she has recovered from the surgery to remove her appendix; about six weeks from now should be sufficient time."

"Will it cost more, Doctor? We don't have much money. I know she has to have the stomach operation, but the eye....I don't know, perhaps it is God's will."

"No, Mrs. Johnson, it will not cost more. I'll do the eye surgery for nothing. I don't believe God would be so cruel. Perhaps He brought Ellen here today so that her eye could be straightened. She is a strong and healthy young woman who may be able to marry after her eye is fixed. You may have grandchildren yet. But you must decide right now."

Robert was concerned that after Ellen had recovered her strength and was back to work on the farm, her parents would again ignore the problem with her eye, so he insisted on a commitment now.

"The appendix surgery cannot wait, but I also want you to agree to the eye surgery. It is very important to Ellen's future."

A long moment of silence followed then a nod. "I will pray for the Lord to guide your hands tomorrow, Doctor, and Ellen will have the eye surgery when she is recovered from having her appendix out."

Six weeks after the successful appendectomy, Ellen was admitted for her eye surgery. Robert had requested a specific nurse whom he knew would be up to the challenge, and he would also be assisted by his son. Douglas was more than willing and, like his father, relished the challenge.

The two doctors had already spent some time reviewing various options. They knew that Ellen, as an adult, was not a candidate for optical management through the use of special glasses, and her family could not bear that expense. They also considered a process whereby the strabismus would be corrected through a gradual stretching and tightening of the horizontal muscles of the eye. This procedure, called the O'Conner Cinch procedure, had been developed in 1916, and Douglas was quite familiar with it. However, it could mean several returns to the doctor's office, and both Robert and Douglas knew that was not feasible for the Johnson family. They settled on a simpler surgical procedure.

Robert chuckled, "We will have need of your shiny new instruments, Douglas, especially those clamps that you showed me. They will do a wonderful job of holding the eye open throughout the operation. We will also make good use of your very fine retractors and the tiny speculum and scalpels when we operate on Ellen's eye."

Douglas replied enthusiastically, "I haven't done one of those since I left McGill. I'm looking forward to it, Dad"

"Good, I'm pleased to hear it, Douglas, because I have decided that you will do the surgery and I will assist you. I've noticed a very slight tremor in my left hand, which normally doesn't bother me at all, but for this surgery your steady young hands might be the best idea."

At Douglas's instant frown of concern, his father replied, "No, it's nothing at all to worry about, but that is my decision. Please get the new anaesthesiologist you spoke of when last we met. This surgery will need a cool head and a smart hand for the anaesthetic."

Just after eight o'clock in the morning, six weeks after her appendix was removed, the young woman, nervous but hopeful, was asleep on the operating table with her mother again praying for God's guidance for the surgeons.

Once Ellen's head was held firmly in a padded clamp device that was used for patients who required surgery for head wounds, the two doctors commenced their work. Measurements of Ellen's eyes had shown that the wide angle misalignment was almost completely a horizontal deviation, and the vertical muscles holding the eye would not need to be altered. The nurse swabbed the eye area with a dilute solution of iodine, and then the eyelids were held securely open with one of Douglas's new clamps. Using his very fine instruments, the young doctor located and loosened the muscles holding the eye to the left and tightened those that pulled the eye into its central front-facing position. This caused the pupil of the left eye to assume a more normal alignment. Douglas used the very finest of silk for the stitches required in the muscles. Robert assisted him throughout the operation.

"There, we have done all we can, thank you, Douglas." Robert smiled, "She will not regain depth perception, of course, though perhaps her mother's prayers will have some effect. But if she cannot see better, she will certainly look better." Robert chuckled again. He dearly loved word play. "Thank you, Son. I've always wanted to do this surgery on a living patient."

The surgical nurse looked a little startled at this statement but took over, and the area was lightly covered with a stiffened buckram disk placed to keep the dressing away from the eye. Although the bandaging was not necessary for healing, it was absolutely necessary to keep the eye clean, and this extra protection would help with that. Robert knew the nurses would follow his instructions to the letter.

"She must not touch her face when she awakens or even move her head very much. And of course, the room must be kept very dim. As long as we can avoid infection, she will heal quickly. I will check on her later today, and tomorrow we will have a look and see how she is doing. Thank you, Nurse."

The next day, the covering was removed. The nurses carefully bathed the area and removed the crusty residue, allowing the doctors to assess the results of their surgery. True to Robert's prediction of a speedy recovery, the young and healthy woman was already beginning to heal.

"Good afternoon, Mrs. Johnson, this young lady is getting better quickly. How are you today, Ellen?"

"There is some pain in my eye, Doctor, but it is not too bad. It hurts mostly around the outside of my eye, like I have a bruise there. Now that the nurses have cleaned my eye, it is no longer stuck shut, but it still feels very swollen. When will the swelling be gone so that I can open my eye completely?"

"Another few days, Ellen, we cannot rush this part."

"Mother says I must be patient and wait while God does His work."

"Mmmmph," Robert smiled, thinking about the fine work Douglas had done but said no more and nodded to Mrs. Johnson who spoke to him as he was leaving the room.

"My daughter needs to get home soon, Doctor Ross. We need her on the farm. How much longer do you think it will be?"

At this, Robert paused and spoke quite sternly, "I will not discharge her until the eye has healed, and you must understand that she can only do light chores in the house for some time. She must not lift anything heavy or do any hard work until the appendix surgery has completely healed as well as the eye. We will talk again in a week's time."

Mrs. Johnson was anxious about her daughter, but she was also a practical farm wife, and on the farm, every member of the family had to work hard if the family was to survive. Robert, however, was adamant. He had no intention of seeing the fine work he and Douglas had done ruined by sending Ellen home too soon. He would extend her hospital stay as long as was necessary.

The two doctors checked the eye again in a few days. Robert chortled with delight at his own response to the challenge posed by Ellen's strabismus and was overjoyed to have worked so well alongside his son. While he was not a particularly introspective person, he nevertheless savoured this moment of happiness, then shook his head at his maundering, and returned to thoughts of the successful surgery and, on a more practical basis, to his own pleasure as a surgeon in using those fine new instruments and learning new techniques from his son.

Robert had a sense of all things being right in his world now, as though he had reached a goal he hadn't known he was seeking. "A good collaboration," he thought, contentedly, "Youthful skills and new knowledge matched with my expertise and experience."

The next day, he saw Ellen. She had been supplied with a hand mirror by the nurses and was thrilled with her straight eye and was eager to go home. Robert again counselled patience. He reassured her, "One or two more days, Ellen. Your eye is now straight. Although it is still a bit red, that will go away with time, and you will look just like everybody else. You will be able to look straight at people, and they will look straight at you."

With these reassurances, and a few words with the nurse, Robert left the hospital room to attend to his other patients. There were always other patients waiting, other challenges to be met.

Chapter 35
Sadness, a Snow Baby, and World War II

It was a month since the baby had died. The grief Elizabeth felt was a constant ache throughout her body, but she loved her father-in-law and so had agreed when he had asked to visit her and his namesake, young Robert. She held her little boy on her lap, knowing that his determined happy presence was her lifeline as she mourned the death of her baby girl.

Elizabeth Ann had lived for only eight days. Born with an incompletely developed intestinal system, it was evident from her birth that despite all the care she received, she would not live. Douglas and his wife comforted one another, but he had to return to work and buried his grief in being busy. He was at the hospital now, so Robert took this opportunity to visit his beloved daughter-in-law.

They sat quietly, little Robert toddling happily back and forth between the two of them while they talked of Beth's pain at the loss. Robert knew there was little medical information he could add to what Douglas had already said, but he was very concerned about Beth so was determined to help her talk about her fears.

Her dark hair, usually a mass of shiny curls, lay limp around her pale face, and she gazed at Robert with dull, reddened eyes. "Douglas tells me that we will have more healthy children," she whispered. "I have to believe that, Dad, but I am so frightened. I don't even want to think about it now, I know I should not worry, but I can't help my thoughts.

They are like rats in a cage, going around and around with no escape. What if we have another child who has the same problems and dies? I can't bear the idea; I just can't." Beth thought she had no more tears to cry, but as she spoke, she again felt the moisture on her cheeks.

"Mommy?" Young Robert climbed back into her lap and gazed anxiously at his mother, touching her face.

"Shhh, Robert, it's all right; it's all right. Mommy's all right."

"Come to Granddad, Robert. See, I have a treat for you." Robert hugged the toddler and pulled a little wooden toy from his waist-coat pocket.

His voice was quiet and reassuring, "You will have more healthy children, Beth, and soon, I hope. Of course, you are frightened, but remember, Elizabeth Ann's death was no one's fault. The condition is very rare. I have delivered close to a thousand healthy babies, and I know. It is so hard for you now, so very hard, but both Douglas and I know that the next baby will be strong and healthy. I can predict that with no doubts. Look at your healthy young son, and you will see the wisdom of our words."

Beth smiled gratefully at her father-in-law. "Now," he continued, "I cannot predict a girl next time, but for that we can hope. Though, looking at this fine fellow, another little one like him would be wonderful, too." Beth cuddled her son, who clutched his new toy firmly and then nodded off to sleep in his mother's arms.

That Christmas, Douglas and Beth were pleased to tell Robert and Jennie that Beth was again pregnant, and the baby would be born in July of the coming year, 1939. Elizabeth hugged Robert as she told him their happy news. She knew that he was mourning the death of his own mother, Grandmother McKenzie.

Robert had travelled alone to Cleveland for the funeral as Jennie had not been well. His mother had been a central focus of Robert's life, and although she had lived far away, he had always depended on her letters to sustain him.

"I am so glad we visited her in thirty-five" he said to Beth, "when she was still healthy and able to enjoy seeing us. I wish I had been able to go back to Cleveland last year. But, she was eighty-eight when she died, and she lived a long and interesting life."

The conversation turned to the news from Europe, which was bleak. Germany had annexed Austria; then, convinced that the major European powers would not oppose him, Hitler's troops had occupied the Sudetenland in Czechoslovakia. Germany had risen from the ashes of Versailles and was once again a major military power in Europe.

Robert spoke sadly, "Bethune was correct; it means another war, Douglas. And Canada will be drawn in again. We are loyal subjects of King George."

Walking home through the snowy evening with young Robert asleep on his shoulder, Douglas spoke of their good news and how pleased his father was about the new baby coming. "He has been very sad about his mother, Beth; this helped."

"He is so kind, Doug, but what of this war? We knew it was coming, but I suppose we just hoped it would not."

"Will your brothers volunteer, do you think?" Douglas asked.

"Probably," Beth sighed, "they are young enough to think it will be an adventure. But their jobs in the mines support the family now. You know my father has not been well this year. He is still very tired after that bout of pneumonia last spring, and the problems in the mines continue. Are you on call tonight?"

"No, but I have an early surgery tomorrow morning then a busy day at the office. We are seeing a lot of miserable 'flu cases. In this cold and for those who do not eat well or get enough rest, influenza is often a precursor to pneumonia. Be sure your dad takes good care of himself."

"Oh, my mother will make sure of that," Beth laughed. "But is there nothing else that can be done to treat pneumonia?" She tucked Robert into his crib and readied herself for bed, still worrying about her father.

Her husband thought for a moment then replied, "Well, we know that some pneumonia is caused by bacteria, more than one organism, especially streptococcus. We can identify the bacteria using the Gram stain in the lab, and we are beginning to see some good results with sulpha drugs against strep. The problem still arises from the dosage.

Sulpha is a very powerful drug, almost miraculous, but how much is too much, especially with infants and the elderly? We are seeing some worrisome side effects, especially stomach problems. And there is some pneumonia that does not respond at all to drugs. We need more research…"

Doug realized that Beth had fallen asleep, so still musing on the possible harm this "wonder drug" could do, he crawled beneath the quilts, hoping to go to sleep as quickly as his wife had. There was a worrisome case he needed to discuss with his father after surgery tomorrow.

***

Robert abruptly stood up from his noon meal and announced, "I'm off to a birth in the Hand Hills region. It is about a four-hour drive to get to their farm, and this is the young woman's first child, so I want to be there. The baby was due a week ago, and I heard from the midwife this morning that the mother-to-be seems very uncomfortable. That baby should have arrived days ago, and I'm somewhat concerned."

He had fretted throughout lunch and, having made his decision to go, was now impatient to be on his way. "I must leave right away. I should be back in a day or two, but Doctor McGregor knows where I am going, and Douglas will take my patients if any problems arise."

Jennie quietly instructed the housekeeper to put together a large package of food, a covered pail of distilled water, and a vacuum flask of hot tea for Robert. He had a valise of clothes already packed for occasions such as this, but she reminded him that blizzards were not uncommon in late winter.

"Yes, of course, my dear," he replied impatiently, "You know I am a careful driver."

Jennie knew no such thing; rather she knew that Robert was a dreadful driver, completely ignoring other vehicles and any rules of the road that might apply. Still, she also knew Robert had relied on his own resources all his life and was always prepared for the worst, with his old buffalo robe, warm blankets, winter boots, snowshoes, and a shovel in the boot of the motor car. The Plymouth was a heavy vehicle, good in the snow, and it had given him solid service on his calls to outlying farms this past few winters. If necessary, it would provide adequate shelter for several days should there be a storm.

The winter snow lay brittle and frozen across the fields, but the gravelled road was fairly clear, the sky was a bright crystal blue, and there was no wind, although it was bitterly cold.

As he drove, Robert's thoughts moved from concern for the overdue baby to musings about the dark rumours of war spreading across the land. In Germany, Hitler had taken over Austria and then had promised to go no further.

"Britain and France are continuing their policy of appeasement. That's a mistake. Adolph Hitler will not be stopped." Robert muttered gloomily to himself then, remembering what had occurred in the Great War of 1914 to 1918, began a mental checklist. "We must be prepared at the office. And the hospital. If there is war, medical supplies will once again be in short supply, especially analgesics, bandages, and sulpha. I must talk to the other doctors in the clinic and the matron at the hospital."

His worries naturally turned to his family. "If Canada joins Britain, what of Douglas? Gordon is thirty-five now and a diabetic; he will surely be considered medically unfit. But Douglas? The army will need doctors, especially surgeons. He is thirty-one now, not likely to be called up in the first wave, if we have conscription. But Drumheller will also need doctors. I know Douglas will try to enlist. And Beth is expecting this summer. After the loss of Elizabeth Ann last year, they are hoping so much for a healthy little sister for Robert Douglas. Will Douglas have to go? I hope not." His anxious thoughts went round and round as he continued his long drive across the prairie.

Seeing the little weathered farmhouse just ahead, he shook himself out of his dark rumination of war and pulled the Plymouth into a space by the tiny porch of the two-room shack. By now, the sky had darkened to the deep indigo blue of late afternoon, so he was glad of the light and warmth of the kitchen and the welcome from the nervous young farmer, Will Voortz, and the midwife, Mrs. Whitley.

Robert immediately walked into the small bedroom and examined the mother-to-be, who seemed fine except for a slightly elevated temperature. Her eyes were darkly circled, and her face was pale against the pillow. "Is the baby all right, Doctor? It was supposed to be born a week ago, and it's not moving as much as before. I am so afraid."

Robert smiled at her and said, "First babies always arrive when they choose, and this one has chosen to come a little later than expected. But, here, listen with my stethoscope, and you will hear a strong heartbeat. We won't start worrying for a while yet."

It was some time since Robert had induced labour outside of the hospital, and he mentally reviewed the procedures and the instruments he would need and began his "just in case" preparations. He decided that if his patient had not gone into labour by the following morning, and the weather held fine, his first choice would be to transport her to the hospital, but he had all he needed if the procedure had to take place in the farmhouse.

Robert conferred with the midwife who knew the young woman well and who confirmed for him that it had been an uneventful pregnancy. Mrs. Voorst was strong and healthy. They both felt another twelve hours could safely pass before they would need to consider moving her to the hospital.

Reassured by the doctor's presence, the mother-to-be relaxed and slipped into a peaceful sleep.

"Let me get you something to eat, Doctor. The neighbours have been generous with covered dishes, and I have become quite good at warming things up," smiled the young father-to-be, "No, no, Mrs. Whitley," he continued, as the midwife began to rise from the table to help him. "I'll do it. You and the doctor sit now."

The three of them had just finished their meal when Mrs. Voorst called from the bedroom, and within a few hours, she was delivered of a healthy, seven-pound boy. The midwife took care of the afterbirth chores and, once new mother and son were content, settled herself to sleep on a straw pallet by their bed.

Robert and Will congratulated themselves on a successful evening then rolled up in buffalo robes and blankets and fell asleep on the floor of the warm kitchen.

Shortly before five o'clock in the morning, the men were awakened by a sudden drop in temperature and the thump of a gust of wind slamming into the side of the little house. They jumped up and in the predawn dark pulled on heavy jackets. The farmer opened the door just enough to see that a good foot of snow now covered the ground, and thick swirling flakes were piling up against the farmhouse and the outbuildings.

Struggling into his boots, Will shouted over the noise of the wind, "I must get to the barn while I can still see the way, Doctor. I must see to my animals."

"I'll come with you, Will." Robert, too, had pulled on his boots and heavy outerwear. The men cracked open the door again, slipped out, and stood for a moment in the slight shelter of the porch before Will grabbed a large spool of rope hanging on the outer wall. One end was firmly attached to the railing; the other would be fastened to the barn when they reached it, thus ensuring safe handholds to and from the house during the blizzard.

Will forged ahead, breaking trail through the rapidly deepening snow, with Robert behind him, muttering that he should have brought his snowshoes into the house.

When the rope had been securely tied to the barn, the men slipped inside, and Will panted his thanks to the doctor.

"I really appreciate your help, Doc, but who knows how long this blizzard will last or how much snow we will get? You won't be going anywhere for a while in that motorcar. Can you ride a horse?" By now, Robert's Plymouth was buried in the snow.

"Can I ride a horse?" Robert chuckled. Although his back was stiff after spending the night on the cold floor, he was thoroughly enjoying the adventure. "Absolutely, of course I can ride, but I'll stay with you here 'til the storm passes. You're going to need help getting the animals in and getting hay out to those who are in the fields. I'll enjoy being a farmhand for a few days, and Mrs. Whitely is here to look after your wife and new son."

The men looked at each other and laughed out loud. The Depression had nearly destroyed Will's farm, war would likely be declared, they were cut off from everything by a blizzard, but the new baby was healthy and strong, kind neighbours had left them food, the barn was redolent of the warm beasts, and there was hay to feed them.

"My son will be named Thomas William if you don't mind, Doc."

"Mind? I'm honoured. Now, let's get these beasts fed and their stalls mucked out. I see you have lots of hay. Any grain to make mash?"

Will grinned and set to work. He had a son, and the doctor was working as his farmhand. Life was good.

As it happened, the blizzard raged for ten more days, and all communication with the outside world was cut off. For Robert, it was a happy time; he enjoyed the hard physical work, although his aching joints reminded him that he wasn't as young as he once was. Along with the family and the midwife, he ate his way hungrily through all the covered dishes the neighbour ladies had brought in anticipation of the baby's birth. It was a pleasure for him to be there to watch young Thomas William thrive.

Robert, who had no sense of time when he embarked on an adventure, was completely sanguine about his absence from Drumheller. "My wife is used to my absences and knows not to worry about me." He reassured the young couple. "I spent my youth, often completely alone, in the North woods of Ontario and Quebec, summer and winter. This absence is nothing. There are lots of doctors to take care of my patients back in town. This is a holiday for me."

DRUMHELLER 1940-1950

Chapter 36
Innovations and Accidents

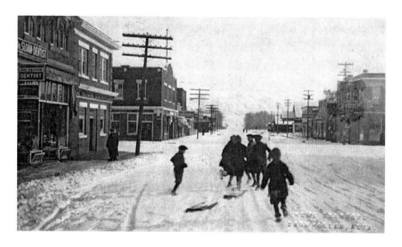

Winter in Drumheller, Alberta, 1940's

Drumheller averaged four mining deaths a year, and almost every death meant a widow and young family without a breadwinner. The neighbours did their best, and churches were helpful, but all the kindness in the world could not replace a husband and father, so the forgetfulness that came from "patent" medicines, such as those containing laudanum, was welcomed, even when it resulted in addiction.

And although an average of four deaths a year might not seem so many, frequent dreadful accidents that resulted in painful, often life-changing injuries were commonplace and formed a large part of Robert's practice.

When the temperatures dipped every winter, the demand for coal increased, and miners who had struggled to make enough money during the summer months gladly worked as many shifts as possible when demand was high.

The weeks leading up to Christmas were the deadliest for mining injuries as men risked their lives pushing further and further into the underground seams to extract as much coal as possible. In winter of 1925, at least a dozen miners were killed and fifty more seriously injured.

Robert and the other doctors in Drumheller were always dealing with mining injuries. For a general practitioner, this meant doing one's best to stabilize the injured man, cleaning wounds and alleviating pain as much as possible. Frequently, these injuries involved broken bones, and usually these fractures were simply immobilized in a cast and left to heal, often with resulting deformities.

For an expert surgeon such as Robert, with his years of experience treating injured miners in Coleman and Lethbridge, dealing with more severe injuries meant putting his skill and experience into the battle to save broken and crushed bones and mangled and torn muscles. While he was of course familiar with traction and splinting, his determination to stay current with the latest orthopaedic techniques had also led him to explore the use of intramedullary rods. One late evening in 1940, exhausted by many hours of surgery on badly injured miners, he described the day to Jennie.

"I had an audience of younger doctors today. They are eager to learn that bones must be properly set, not just patched up on the outside and splinted. Of course, first aid training ensured that the injured had been washed at the mines and the wounds had been cleansed thoroughly before the men had been brought into the hospital. That initial treatment at the mine meant that the risk of infection had been reduced."

Jennie nodded at this, pleased to hear that Robert's hard work and time spent teaching first aid had been well spent.

Her husband continued, "You know, my dear, we have such an excellent staff of doctors and nurses. The Drumheller Hospital should be known as one of the top centres in Alberta for dealing with mining injuries."

His pride in the hospital was evident as he continued to describe the day. "My plan as always was to try to rebuild limbs to be as long and straight as possible, so the operations took much longer than just patching and splinting would have. Several of the younger miners had relatively simple fractures, but I made sure that the ends of the bones did not overlap before splinting. Thankfully, the hospital had received a supply of the new intramedullary rods."

Jennie had done the research on this new orthopaedic technique and was delighted to hear that Robert had put them to use. "Those are the ones that can be inserted into the leg where the break is severe and bone has been crushed and must be removed, are they not, Robert?" She asked, with interest.

"Yes, Jennie. The very ones. Just as the article you found described, the rods are now holding the broken bones in place so that new bone can grow to fill the break. I also had to lengthen and re-attach the tendons and ligaments. It was complicated, but the young heal quickly as long as we can fight infection." He paused to sip his tea then shook his head sadly.

"One older man had a terrible back injury. I operated on him, but I do not yet know if that surgery will result in a complete recovery for him .The spine was crushed in several places. However, we did what we could, removing shattered bits of bone and fusing some of the vertebrae. It should heal well. It appeared that the spinal cord itself was intact, but I just don't know...I just don't know."

Robert paused, his face grim as he contemplated paralysis for the man. "Right now, I can do no more. His back will be stiff, but providing the damage is not too severe, he may be able to walk again. Whether he will be able to go back into the mines is another story." Robert's voice faltered, and he slumped into his chair, his second cup of tea untouched. "Another family bereft of an income."

Jennie, who had not interrupted while her husband described the spinal surgery, sighed and spoke quietly, "Robert, it is now in God's hands. You will have more surgery tomorrow so you must sleep. Go to bed. I will see that any calls tonight go to another doctor."

Robert nodded then, utterly weary, climbed the stairs to his bed, thinking sadly of the homes where no father would return, and the bleak Christmas that awaited those families.

***

Robert and Douglas paused for a few moments of rest on a bench in the doctors' change room in the hospital, both weary after the morning's surgeries. Inevitably, following discussion of the operations, the conversation turned to the war.

Canada had officially entered the war on the tenth of September the previous year, and although conscription had not been declared, eager volunteers headed to the nearest recruiting office. For many men, enlisting was not only patriotic, but it also offered a way out of the joblessness and desperate times of the Depression.

Douglas was among those who had gone into Calgary to join the army, but now, slumped in despair beside his father, the younger doctor spoke, teeth clenched in anger. "They wouldn't take me, Dad. Said I was too old, for God's sake! Damn it, I'm only thirty-two, and I'm a doctor, a surgeon. And I was completely fit at the physical, except they say I'm colour blind. Even if I was, it has never affected my skills as a surgeon. It makes me so angry! All these young men going to serve this country, and here I am, hale and healthy and I can't go!"

Robert recognized the conflict Douglas was experiencing at the rejection, but privately his feelings were those of relief. However, he was wise enough to say nothing. Logical, reasonable reminders about how the War Office had determined which doctors could leave and which ones must stay, that Drumheller still needed doctors, and how Douglas would be serving his country here would not be welcome now. He merely nodded sympathetically as he listened to his son's frustration and rage. He also thought of Beth, hiding her fears, and of the two little ones who didn't need to lose their father.

His sad rumination then turned to all the wives and children who would be fatherless after this war. And he sent a silent prayer to the Great Creator to let it end soon. He remembered the length and terrible toll of World War I and was not particularly optimistic that this one would be a short conflict.

Over the next years, conversation about the war and those who had gone overseas and, worse still, would not be returning to Drumheller was a constant in everyone's life. Brothers and sisters left to join up or work in the factories established as a major aspect of Canada's contribution to the war. Doleful newscasts on the radio, rationing of gasoline, the absence of certain foods and supplies in the stores, but most of all fear for those who had left to fight overshadowed everything in the small prairie town.

But life went on, and in 1940 another grandson brought needed joy to the family when Thomas Arthur, Elsie and Gordon's son, was born, and in 1941 Beth and Douglas had another child, Colin Morris, both healthy, sturdy little boys.

Gordon joined the war effort in 1941 when he accepted a position as an accountant with the Allied Purchasing Commission in Montreal, and he and Elsie planned to take their new son with them to live in eastern Canada. Their daughter Shelagh, now nine, was in school so rather than disrupt her education, Gordon and Elsie asked that she be allowed to live with Robert and Jennie.

Gordon had already gone to Montreal on his own, but Elsie remained in Drumheller with the baby until he was old enough to travel. Robert, concerned that looking after an active nine-year-old would be too much for Jennie, who was now sixty-six, insisted that she must have more help. Accordingly, a young farm woman was hired to look after Shelagh as well as assist the housekeeper.

Elsie was to take baby Tommy to Montreal to join her husband but asked if the infant could also be a member of Robert and Jennie's household when he was a bit older. The toddler would then live with his grandparents until the war was over.

"This would really be too much for you, Jennie." Much as he loved his grandchildren, Robert was uneasy when it was suggested that in a year Tommy would join them as well. "Even with the nursemaid, two young children will put quite a strain on the household."

"I will have lots of help, Robert. Gordon and Elsie travel so much with Gordon's work. It will be best to keep the children here. It would only be for a short time, just until the war is over. Elsie would be here often."

"Jennie, it is best for children to be with their own parents, but it is your decision. What about Elsie's mother and sister? Couldn't they help?"

"They have moved to Manitoba. When the time comes, we will manage. Others are much worse off than we are, and Mrs. Hall and the new nursemaid are both excellent with children."

Jennie's mind was made up about taking Tommy as well as Shelagh. Robert knew that she would do anything Gordon asked and that she found the house lonely. She and Mrs. Hall also enjoyed the presence of the children and their nursemaid. "I feel that this is a way that I can contribute to the war effort, as it allows Gordon to travel freely which is an important part of his job." Jennie said no more, and Robert knew her decision was final.

"Just be sure you don't become overtired, or you will become ill yourself. Now, I plan to travel to Montreal with Elsie and baby Tommy when she goes to join Gordon. I will visit with our son and my brothers' families while I am there." He looked at his wife hopefully. "Although it will not be an easy trip as the trains will be full of troops and businessmen, it would be a change for you. Will you not come with me to see Gordon? The visit will be short, but it would be good to get away. Shelagh is happy at school with her friends, and she will be fine with our housekeeper and the new nursemaid."

Jennie considered the matter. It was difficult for her not to go and see Gordon, but she simply did not have the strength for such a long trip, and she and her church groups had much to do with the war effort. "Not this time, Robert. You will give them my love and my blessing."

Her husband, who had not really expected her to come, rose to his feet, the matter settled, and gathered his coat and gloves. "Rotary tonight. I'll be late home as I have a call to make after the meeting."

The trip to Montreal with Elsie and the baby was uneventful, though Robert was quietly amused by how very social his daughter-in-law was, visiting cheerfully with other families and making new friends every day. She also had harmless, flirtatious conversations with the young soldiers who admired the vivacious young mother and her baby boy.

"They are going to war, Father Ross, everything is very proper; we're just having a laugh."

Robert agreed with Elsie. "It doesn't hurt to smile."

He enjoyed the time in Montreal; he was very proud of his son's contribution to the war effort but expressed his concern at the lack of routine and skipped meals, "This is not good, Elsie. Now that you are here, you must see that Gordon eats regular healthy meals."

"Father Ross, I cannot make him eat. His schedule is too change-able. I never know when he will be home, and I am busy with the baby and often out visiting myself. Gordon usually gets something to eat in the cafeteria at his office so there is no point in my preparing meals. He takes his insulin; he is fine. And he gets very angry when I fuss over him."

Robert attended Rotary meetings whenever he found a branch of the organization. He planned to attend one in Montreal with his brothers Simon and Colin. Colin lived in Montreal, and Simon had come to join them for a few days from Philadelphia where he practised as a doctor of osteopathy. All three brothers were delighted to hear that Dr. Dafoe, the medical man who had become the most famous obstetrician in Canada when he delivered the Dionne quintuplets, would be the speaker.

Robert had a good visit with his brothers but was concerned about Simon's appearance. "Simon does not look well," Robert thought uneasily. "He is very busy, too busy, perhaps. But there is nothing I can do for him."

His thoughts turned to Jennie. "Sometimes Alberta seems very far away. I will miss my family here in eastern Canada. But I need to go home."

While the journey from Drumheller to Montreal had been uneventful, the return trip on The Dominion passenger train was certainly not. Robert was sitting happily chatting to several army medics who were on leave and travelling home to Saskatchewan, when, just outside of the small Ontario town of Tripoli, their train met another coming from the opposite direction on the same line. The head-on crash threw them all out of their seats, injuring many passengers and crew and killing the engineer on Robert's train.

Robert, along with a trained nurse and the army medics provided first aid and saw the injured safely to a nearby hospital. After the railway inspectors and local police had gathered descriptions of the accident, those who had not been hurt were housed in local accommodation until they could be put on the next available train heading west.

"Thank goodness Jennie was not with me," Robert thought, as he settled in for the remainder of the journey, and then, "What a story this will make for the next Rotary meeting."

Chapter 37
An Operation, Uncle George, and a Party

As he sat down in his office chair, Robert checked his appointment book. "Only one patient this afternoon, good."

He was gradually limiting his practice now, moving more into a consultative role and taking only surgeries that really interested him. He found the arthritis in his spine to be very painful after several hours bent over an operating table, and the slight tremor in his hands was becoming bothersome for delicate work.

He was puzzled by the name in his appointment book. It seemed familiar somehow, but he could not place it. "Please send in Mr. LaChance, Agnes."

A well-dressed and fine-looking man in his middle years came into the office for a consultation. After listening to his complaint, Robert picked up the man's card to make some notes about his case and when he read his name and address, his curiosity was piqued again.

"Say, there was an old man by that name, LaChance, whom I operated on about ten years ago. Did you ever hear of him? I think he was from your part of the country."

"Yes," the man smiled, "he is my father."

"Your father? Surely, by this time he will have passed away." Robert replied.

"No, he is very much alive and well up into his nineties," Mr. LaChance continued. "We never saw such a change as came over him after your operation."

"What kind of change?"

"Well, before that operation, he was a great homebody. Never went out at night. Seldom went to the hotel and then only for one drink of beer and, after that, home for the night and to bed early. He was always up before daylight, out to the barn, did all the chores, and fed the cattle."

Robert smiled, having a good idea where the story was going.

"Since the operation, all this has changed. Now he sleeps until nearly noon. Gets up in time for dinner, goes to the hotel after eating, and stays there until the beer parlour closes. He then visits the neighbourhood, catting around until one or two o'clock in the morning. Then he comes home and sleeps all forenoon, gets up at noon, and proceeds to do the whole thing over again"

Robert's chuckle changed to a roar of laughter at the son's next statement. "We have often said at home, we wished you had killed the old bugger."

Robert laughed heartily at the story and after sending his patient on his way, picked up his case files from ten years previous and reviewed his notes. He remembered that on the morning the old man was admitted, surgery had just been completed and the doctors were on their way down the main stairs when Robert had been intercepted by Matron.

Drawn back in time, Robert could hear Matron's voice as she said, "I think you should see a patient who has just been brought in to the hospital, Doctor Ross. He is in room fourteen and appears to be very ill."

"Do we know anything about him?"

"No, he seems to be from the country; he is all alone. I think you should see him at once."

Without another word, Robert turned and headed to room fourteen. He saw a man who looked to be well along in his seventies, in a comatose condition.

"How did he arrive, Nurse?"

"I don't know, Doctor Ross. He just appeared at the front door, and some of the nurses going off shift saw him on their way out and brought him in. All we know is that his name is LaChance, he's unconscious, and he has a raging fever."

Judging from his ragged clothing, Robert assumed the man was a worn-out farmhand who had been brought to the hospital to end his days. He had probably been working for a mere pittance, so by leaving him at the hospital, the farm family, who no doubt had little enough themselves, ensured that there would be no trouble to them.

"Thank you, Nurse, I'll examine him now."

Robert examined the man and discovered a badly infected and misshapen foot, with signs of blood poisoning beginning to streak up his lower leg. Clearly, the fellow had had some sort of accident and had not been treated. This, in combination with his advanced age, general poor health, and malnutrition had resulted in a complete collapse. Although it looked very bad, Robert felt that using a combination of drainage and sulpha, he could get the infection under control and the swelling reduced. Then he would be able to use the X-ray machine to see exactly what the problem was. He suspected that the foot had been crushed and had not been set properly, likely because the poor fellow did not have the money to pay a doctor. The patient was not sufficiently conscious to tell anyone how long he had been suffering.

"We'll have to use drainage to be sure this infection is cleared up. Thank God for sulpha drugs. That is the only way we are going to save his leg. He must also be rested and ready before we can operate. Perhaps once his fever breaks and he regains consciousness, he will tell us what happened to his foot. Keep a close eye on him; call me if there is any change. Thank you, Nurse."

When Robert saw the patient the next morning, he was much improved, although still not coherent. His fever was gone, the infection was responding well to the sulpha, and he was sleeping peacefully.

On the third day in hospital, the swelling had reduced enough for X-rays to be taken, and Robert's suspicions that the foot had been crushed were confirmed. Happily, he also determined that the damage to the foot was not as bad as he had initially feared and that it could be mended. Surgery would give the man back the use of his foot.

For the first time, the silent old man spoke, "Are you going to operate on my foot, Doctor?"

"Yes, I am. But it will take several more days to get you strong enough for surgery. How did this happen? What can you tell me about yourself?"

"Got nothing to say, Doc. Just want this better."

Nobody came to see him, and he said no more, so Robert decided he was a homeless old man without friends or relatives in the country.

When his patient appeared to have regained a reasonably healthy condition, Robert operated. The foot healed well, and seven days later the old man was sitting up in bed quite happily.

"It is time for you to get up and walk. You need to practise getting around with that cast on your foot, and you will have to use these crutches for the next six weeks. In the meantime, we will see about finding a place for you to live," Robert announced.

There was no answer from the old man, but as Robert walked out of the room, he detected a small smile on the patient's face.

After he had been up and walking, the old man asked, "When can I go home?"

"You can go home anytime, if you have a home to go to and someone to look after you until that cast comes off."

"Fine, I'll take the train this evening if you will sign me out. How much did the operation cost?"

"The usual price is $150.00, but if you cannot pay that much, I'll cut it down to what you can afford."

The patient replied, "Give me a blank cheque, and I will pay you the full amount"

As Robert accepted the cheque, made out to a bank in a neighbouring town, the old man said. "You will find that the cheque is okay, and I am glad to pay you the full charge for a very satisfactory operation. You have given me a new lease on life, and I intend to make the most of it."

Robert discharged him, the bank honoured the cheque, and the old man was not heard of again until his son walked into Robert's office ten years later.

Still smiling at his memories of the story, Robert's thoughts returned to the present day as he gathered up his notes and placed them in the file. "I'll have to write that story someday, but for now, I'm tired and I'm going home."

His plan was to hold office hours only three days a week by the end of the year, though he would act as a locum when required and would certainly see his obstetrical patients through to full term. He was now delivering babies of the babies he had brought into the world when he first came to Drumheller. It was definitely time to slow down and spend more time with friends and family, especially his grandchildren.

He laughed out loud again as he put on his coat and hat and prepared to leave the office to go home for his tea. It had been an eventful couple of weeks.

He had had a visit from his brother George the previous week, and he was still smiling about it.

George had driven from Big Valley to Drumheller in freezing weather with the top down on his new Packard convertible. It was a beautiful bright March afternoon, but there was still lots of snow on the ground and ice in the river down the hill from Robert's home. Standing at the front window, Robert had been watching his oldest grandson and his friends sledding down the icy slope in front of the house when he saw George, well wrapped up in coat and muffler, arrive and park his car at the top of the hill.

The boys had paused to admire the automobile and six-year-old Robert had waved cheerfully, calling, "Hello, Uncle George," as the doctor exited his car with a flourish, slamming the door behind him.

"Hello, Robert, hello boys, good day for sliding," George had called out as he strode up the walk to the house.

The boys had watched the beautiful car in silence for a moment, and then one of them said in a quiet voice, "It's moving. The car is moving!" Stunned by this development, the wide-eyed youngsters had watched in awe as the Packard had very slowly gathered speed and begun to descend the slippery road.

Then, after shouting, "Hey! Hey! Uncle George, Granddad!" at the top of his lungs, young Robert and his friends had pelted down the hill beside the car, astonished at this wonderful event happening in front of their eyes. They had run alongside all the way to the river's edge at the bottom of the hill where the stately car had slid nose first into the icy water.

By this time, of course, George and Robert had rushed out of the house and had slipped and slid down the icy hill in fruitless pursuit. The boys had looked at the men and looked at the car, and then all of them had collapsed in helpless laughter.

"Oh, dear, oh dear, Jennie will be furious," George had gasped for breath. "I have embarrassed her again."

"You have a rare talent for it, George," Robert had replied as they began the trudge up the hill, "but, my word, that was a sight worth seeing." He had slapped his brother on the back. "I know a man with a team who can pull it out of the river for you, but you'll have to stay the night until we can arrange for transportation home for you. Why on earth did you have the top down?"

"Oh, just for fun. I know how my antics annoy my good sister-in-law, but I really didn't intend this to happen. Must have not set the brake properly. I've been warned about that."

The men had stopped walking and had burst into laughter again thinking of the reaction of George's long suffering wife to this latest news.

By this time, a small crowd had gathered as the boys, sledding forgotten, had raced off to share the news with their families, before returning in hopes of seeing the team of horses arrive to drag the car out of the water.

"Dad will really enjoy this story," young Robert had declared gleefully, grinning, "I'll tell him when he gets home from work. He loves Uncle George stories."

***

The story of the runaway Packard was to be repeated to uproarious applause at an impromptu party held in Douglas and Beth's home later that year. Robert had tried to coax his wife into attending.

"Douglas and Beth and several of the nurses and doctors and their wives are having a get-together this evening. And we're invited, Jennie. It will be good for us to get out and enjoy good food and good conversation. The party is really for the wives of those doctors who are away in Europe. They need cheering up. I think we should go."

"Robert, don't be silly. The young people don't want us there. I really don't feel up to the noise, and all they'll talk about is the war."

"Oh, my dear, I think we will be very welcome. And the war talk is more positive this year. The Big Three are getting together to discuss what will happen after the war is over. Surely it will end soon. We need a party."

"Robert, you go along. I'd rather stay home. I'll invite Mrs. Ewing over for company, and I have a great deal of work to do for the church." Jennie was now on the board of directors of the Knox United Church and, in addition to her other church duties, was in truth sometimes overloaded with paperwork.

Sighing, Robert went back to the office. He had a few hours of his own paperwork that needed attention, but he intended to go to the party later on by himself. He enjoyed a bit of fun, and Doug and Beth's house was the heart of what social life there was for the medical office and hospital staff in Drumheller. He looked forward to a pleasant evening there. Everybody brought whatever could be spared to share, and the party was in full swing when Robert arrived at the big old house overlooking the park. The young couple had rented it while their new home was being built.

The lively conversation jumped from difficult cases to new babies, from music to politics, from new cars to the question of Poland still unresolved at the Tehran Conference.

"Do you think Mackenzie King will impose conscription? Quebec is dead set against it."

"No, it will tear our country apart. Besides, there have been just as many volunteers from Quebec as from English Canada. They just don't want to be forced to join."

"Well, maybe they should be forced to enlist. We sure can't have conscription just for English Canada. And it's coming. We have to have a big push to finish this bloody war. Sorry, ladies."

"Listen, I'm really excited about this new medicine, streptomycin. *The Journal of Medicine* says it will cure TB; for God's sake, that would be wonderful."

"What about side effects? Remember how we all jumped on sulpha drugs?"

"Yes, and I also remember how well they worked! This is supposed to be better. Even better than penicillin, if you can believe that."

"I wish we could get all the penicillin we needed. The war effort has severely limited our supplies, and it made such a difference for our pneumonia patients."

"Good thinking to stock up on analgesics before the war, TR." Robert smiled at the nickname the doctors and hospital staff had given him when Douglas had joined the Medical Practice in 1937. "Wonderful food, Beth, how are the children? Did you enjoy young Robert's story about Uncle George?"

Beth smiled, "The children are all well, Dad. Your grandson thoroughly enjoyed his storytelling role, and we all need a funny story these days." She paused and then asked sadly. "Did you hear that all the

Hansen girls' husbands have gone overseas? Can you imagine how that family feels about conscription?"

"It will come unless this war ends very soon."

The group was quiet for a few moments, lost in contemplation of those who were not present.

"What do you think about these terrible stories we have been hearing about those horrid concentration camps and the poor Jews?"

"It is beyond awful if they are true. That German madman is attempting to exterminate a whole race of people."

"Gas chambers? My God, it can't possibly be as bad as they say. And our Canadian government is refusing to take in any Jews who have escaped and have asked to immigrate here. What are we fighting for anyway?"

"The Americans are accepting them, though they have a quota and other restrictions. Makes me feel small."

On that sad and frightening note, the men and women began to gather up their belongings.

"Doug, before we leave, will you play the piano for us? Maybe something we could all sing along with? How about *Tipperary*?"

Douglas had already played several popular songs, including *On the Road to Mandalay*, which was a great favourite of everyone, but happily returned to the piano and began to play the famous World War I song. Everyone joined in, and as they said their goodbyes and left the house, most were humming or singing the lyrics that ended with, "*It's a long way to Tipperary, but my heart's right here.*"

***

It was 1943, and Robert's reflection in the pier glass mirror showed a gentleman whose hair was now grey and whose back was somewhat stooped with arthritis, but, all in all, at seventy-three, he was content with his appearance. His body was not so lean as in earlier days; however, his new vested suit had been well cut, and as he dressed, he looked forward to the dinner with his old friends Reverend Moss and his wife.

It was a clear, cold January evening following a windless day of brilliant sunshine. A coal-burning fireplace warmed the room, and the round oak table was set with damask and silver. Mrs. Moss murmured her appreciation of the pretty scene as they sat down to dinner.

The United Church minister and his wife were particularly welcome guests. For the last three years, Robert had enjoyed his frequent weekday conversations with the minister, on the rare occasions when the two men were able to steal a few moments from their busy days. They had tea in the small church office and discussed philosophical and spiritual questions as well as local and world affairs. Jennie often commented to Robert about how impressed she was with Reverend Moss's interpretations of scripture. She felt Drumheller was fortunate to have such a fine man, and she hoped his tenure at the Knox United would be a long one.

Their housekeeper-cook, Mrs. Hall, also a member of the Reverend Moss's congregation, was pleased to prepare a special meal for them, using the family's ration coupons and fruits and vegetables put up last summer from the garden.

The minister, as did Robert, firmly believed that one should not separate spiritual and emotional well-being from bodily health, so was keenly interested in the advances being made at the provincial and federal levels in the area of state-supported medicine for all his parishioners.

"I hear that the Dominion government is considering support for a program similar to the Alberta Health proposal. Have you heard any news, Robert?"

The doctor smiled, "No more than you, Reverend. I am always impressed by your knowledge. You must realize that Federal funding is absolutely required if we are to move any closer to a universal healthcare system."

Jennie broke off her conversation about church business with Mrs. Moss to ask, "Is this the same proposal supported by the Canadian

Medical Association? Robert, you are a member. Surely you know whether the proposal would gain support in Ottawa?"

Mrs. Moss quietly added her own question. "Would that mean that every Canadian would be assisted in obtaining medical care and hospitalization and not just those who could afford the payments?"

Reverend Moss added, "Obviously, my good wife is concerned about those of our parishioners who have no means, even with the pittance they receive for food from the government now."

"You know that no doctor would ever turn away a woman or child in need," Robert replied.

"I do believe that, but sometimes there are those who do not know that and are fearful or are just too proud. The stigma of the Depression and having to beg for help still throws a long shadow over the lives of many."

"Indigent is such a demeaning term for human beings," Mrs. Moss's soft voice was sad. "We must all help."

"We in the medical field have been working towards this full coverage for quite some time now, and this latest report looks promising. Unfortunately, the war effort overwhelms everything else, but when it is over, and it looks to be soon, I am confident that things will change. The governments of the provinces will be able to turn their efforts to building more hospitals and funding a more comprehensive health plan."

"I am pleased to hear that," the Reverend's eyes twinkled, "but meanwhile, we who are in the business of saving souls will continue, funding or not, to provide comprehensive coverage."

Robert, who appreciated the minister's dry wit, chuckled and nodded to Jennie. "Shall we move to the front room for coffee or tea, my dear? Please thank Mrs. Hall for the delicious repast. Mrs. Moss, how is your family? I apologize for not asking sooner."

The conversation turned to places and friends they had in common before the Mosses bundled up to take their leave and walk home beneath the starlit sky.

As they made their way carefully down the front steps, Mrs. Moss paused and turned to Robert and Jennie, smiling as she said, "A lovely evening, thank you, Jennie and Doctor Ross. Please give our thanks to Mrs. Hall."

Reverend Moss added, "We are encouraged by the promising news about healthcare. Our duty is clear: We must all continue our endeavours on the home front." He smiled at his good friends, "I look forward to seeing you both on Sunday. I have prepared a sermon of hope for all of us in this terrible time. Good night."

Chapter 38
The RCMP and Surgery

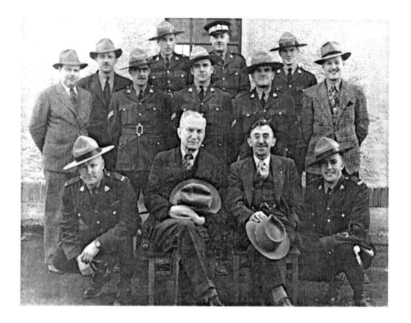

Robert, the R.C.M.P, Surveillance & Investigation Unit, and
Mine Rescue Representative, Drumheller, Alberta, 1940's

Some months later, Robert received a request from the staff sergeant
of the local RCMP detachment to meet with him and discuss some
concerns the Federal government had expressed regarding the possibility of Communist agitators in the mines. Robert understood
that his own involvement with the miners through his first aid and
mine rescue work as well as his contractual position as a mine doctor
meant that he had excellent knowledge of what was happening in the
mining community. However, he also had an excellent reputation as

a trustworthy person of great personal integrity and did not want to damage that in any way.

He agreed to the meeting, to be held in his office, but made it clear that he had no time for any spying on the men or the unions.

"I share your concerns about Communist agitators and want to avoid any problems in the mines, but I have to chuckle at the 'cloak and dagger' aspects of this consultation. This is a small town, and everyone knows who you are and why you are here."

The local RCMP Sergeant looked at the plainclothes men from Ottawa and smiled but said nothing.

Robert continued, "We've had strikes and agitators here for years. These miners are, for the most part, good hardworking men who only want to raise their families and do their jobs safely for a decent wage. They have little time for rabble-rousers and commies, though of course the idea of Russia as a workers' paradise has swayed some of them. I doubt that many of them follow the news of the Tehran Conference and realize how bloody-minded Stalin is becoming."

Several of the RCMP Surveillance and Investigation men who had been seconded to the Drumheller detachment looked at one another, and it was evident that they thought the doctor did not understand how serious Ottawa believed the situation to be in the valley.

Robert noticed their skeptical glances and spoke again. "How much do you know about the background to the current situation here in the mines?"

They readily admitted to knowing very little about the history behind the present-day unrest.

Robert nodded and went on, "Well, at the risk of this sounding like a lecture, I think it might help if I gave you some history of Drumheller and the mines. If you have time to hear it, that is?"

The staff sergeant, familiar with Robert's encyclopedic knowledge of all things Drumheller, welcomed this and indicated that Robert was to continue.

A story was a story, and Robert happily settled in to tell this one. "The unions have been a strong force in the valley for years, beginning with the United Mine Workers of America in the early 1900s. The formation of the O.B.U., or One Big Union, in 1919, believed to be the brainchild of radical Communists over forty years ago, resulted in conflict. In 1927, the two unions clashed again when they competed for the support of the miners. There was also a strike to try to improve working conditions. Many of the miners believed then that the Canadian Union had been infiltrated by Communists. This belief led to some violent altercations between opposing groups with frequent attempts to intimidate, and they used physical violence from stones and clubs to guns to make their points. In all of these disputes, the police forces, from the Northwest Mounted Police to the RCMP, conducted themselves bravely and honourably."

The sergeant nodded his agreement with Robert's words as the doctor went on. "It's important to know this history if one is to understand the current situation.

"At this time, the UMWA is the sole union in the valley, and things are reasonably peaceful, but I know that rumours of Communist support continue. However, there has been more anger recently as the distrust and suspicion of the growing power of the USSR has increased. You must remember that many of the men who have gone to war from here are miners' sons, and they are fighting for Britain, not Russia."

Robert paused then said firmly. "Here is my advice: You need to get to know these miners, and the best way to do that is to meet them in a useful role, so I'll introduce you to the leaders of the mine rescue team and some of their members. I presume, as members of the RCMP, that you all have current First Aid Certificates?"

The men all nodded.

"Good, because that is a prerequisite to mine rescue, and you might be called upon to help."

The uniformed members of the local detachment all knew Robert well. They were also familiar with the miners and recognized the good sense of the "stitch and patch and send home" medicine that the doctors practised. Police were not interested in the usual payday brawls that occurred every other Saturday night, unless serious injuries involving guns and intent to kill were the case. Fortunately, this was a rare occurrence.

The sergeant spoke. "Meeting the men from the mine rescue teams is an excellent idea, and there will be no secret attempts to infiltrate. Doctor Ross, could you also introduce these men to the mine owners and to the shop stewards of the union?" Robert nodded his assent.

The sergeant made several points clear to all present. "We have spent half a century building goodwill for the police here, and I think we have earned the respect of the majority of the miners. Of course, there have been incidents when the police have had to establish order, especially during the strike of 1927 to which Doctor Ross referred, but in every case, the force has prevailed justly. Remember also that most of the miners want to avoid trouble and do their jobs. We'll take your advice, Doctor, and appreciate your help. I know some of our members already take part in the mine rescue courses, so that will also help."

Robert looked at the plainclothes men in the group. The Surveillance and Investigation men were here to determine whether or not Communist supported agitators in the mines were being paid by the Soviets to disrupt Canada's wartime production. How would they take to his advice?

"This way, you will get to know these men and the hardships of their lives without subterfuge. You will learn about conditions in the mines, and you will soon hear if there are instigators and how the men feel about them. As I said, everybody in town already knows why you are here."

The four Surveillance and Investigation men looked at one another but knew that they had no choice but to comply, as they had been seconded and were under the supervision of the staff sergeant and must obey his orders. "Of course, Doctor Ross. We all have First Aid Certificates, and it will be interesting to learn about mine rescue."

"Yes, well you will learn nothing skulking around," was Robert's tart reply. "Even if you learn nothing, the message will get back to the commies that Ottawa thought enough of the danger to send you here and is ready to prevent trouble."

Robert was far from naïve and had no illusions about either the police or the union agitators but also had no intention of having his own reputation damaged as it would be if there was any hint of secret collaboration on his part. The union situation was difficult enough at the best of times, and the war situation only increased the tension.

"Good, that's settled." The staff sergeant issued his orders, "All of you will meet with the men this week as we have discussed, and we will all be very open about our worries concerning money from Russia being used to foment unrest. What is the next step, Doctor Ross?"

"The next step is to discuss this with the miners' representatives in the mine rescue groups. We will see if you can observe the rescue class, beginning with this Sunday's practice. It is easy to set up meetings with some mine owners, and the shop stewards will be willing to talk to you. You'll certainly hear some of their complaints. Mining is not an easy job."

"During the week," the staff sergeant spoke dryly, "we'll all have our regular duties. You men can each accompany one of the corporals on his rounds and also help out with Army and Navy cadet training we run in the schools on Thursdays after the students are dismissed. We always need extra help."

He went on, "Keep your eyes and ears open on patrol. Of course, you are all capable riders. We have patrol cars, but you never know. You may have to ride. As matter of fact, horses may be necessary for you to get to some of the out-of-the way mines above the valley, where the mischief makers might be found. We'll get you all kitted out." He smiled with some satisfaction at the idea. "This will work. Thank you for your assistance, Doctor."

As the men left Robert's office, the doctor thought about the situation in the mines and hoped sincerely that if anything untoward was happening, it would come to nothing. This dratted war! The suspicion and distrust among the Allies and the Russians seemed to be getting worse and did not bode well for cooperation when the war ended.

***

The unopened letter from Victoria, British Columbia, marked "Private," lay in the middle of the green blotter on Robert's desk in the office. For a moment, he stood holding it and considering what it could mean that he, rather than Jennie, had received a communication from her cousins. "Well, if it is bad news, I'd better find out what I can do," he murmured, slitting it open.

It wasn't bad news at all but an inquiry from Horace, Nell's son, asking if it would be possible to schedule a date for Robert to perform surgery for a deteriorating ear infection.

The specialist in Victoria had told Horace that he must have surgery as his earaches had become critical, and a mastoid infection was feared. Horace had decided that he and his new wife, Blanche, would travel to Drumheller to have Robert perform the surgery.

Robert, surprised that the recently married couple were willing to make such a long trip, was nevertheless pleased at this show of confidence in his skills. Immediately after checking his schedule with the hospital, he sent a telegram informing them of an available date just two weeks hence.

He then telephoned Jennie to say they were coming, knowing that she would be both pleased to hear of their visit and alarmed that Horace's condition had deteriorated so badly. She knew that Blanche was expecting their first child and was worried that the trip would prove too stressful for her.

Nell's son had suffered from terrible earaches since childhood. The family story was that as a young boy in the 1890s, the housekeeper had accidentally shut the youngster out of his home in Sudbury in subzero weather. As a result, he had developed a massive ear infection.

Whatever the initial cause, a simple cold was always much feared by Horace and his mother as it always left him with a miserable earache. His doctor in Victoria had warned him that mastoiditis was inevitable if this latest infection was not dealt with promptly and recommended a myringotomy be performed by a specialist in Seattle. Horace much preferred to put his trust in the man who had performed his successful abdominal surgery ten years earlier and so contacted Robert and made plans accordingly.

Jennie was pleased. "Robert, this is wonderful. We shall prepare a room for them. Did you say they will be here within the week? How long will they stay, do you think?"

"I don't know, Jennie, I have no idea how severe the infection is, and it will have to be looked at before we operate, but it is a procedure I am very familiar with, so all should be well. I have been worried about his earaches for years, and I'm very glad he has chosen to deal with it at last. Also, we have recently received a small supply of penicillin, which should help with his postoperative treatment."

"Penicillin? How did you manage to acquire that? "

"Douglas's colleagues in Montreal were able to obtain a supply, and he immediately requested some for us here in Drumheller. The drug has been tested extensively on the battlefields and is said to be close to miraculous. Do you remember the journal article you gave me to read in the early thirties? What a long time it takes to get these medicines in our hands."

Jennie, somewhat impatiently, agreed. "Yes, of course, I remember Robert, but do you have any idea of how long this whole process will take? I have to prepare the house for their stay."

"Including postoperative treatment, I would guess a month. Of course, they will remain with us until he is ready to travel."

The operation was a success. Blanche, often accompanied by Jennie, spent every afternoon at the hospital until Horace returned to the Ross home to convalesce.

When Horace was feeling stronger, Jennie, who loved to entertain, hosted a special dinner party. She felt it was important for Douglas and Beth to have some time with Nell's son and his wife before they boarded the train for their return journey to the West Coast.

Douglas had already spent some time visiting with Horace while he was hospitalized, as he had assisted his father with the surgery, but Beth was pleased with this opportunity to get to know the cousins.

"We must make a trip to Vancouver Island to visit Horace and Blanche and my other Victoria cousins when the war is over, Beth." Douglas said, enthusiastically. "They have the most marvellous house near the ocean, close to a beautiful park."

Chapter 39
Churchill's Voice

Robert and Jennie along with Douglas and Beth had gathered at Robert's home on May 7, 1945, for the much anticipated radio broadcast from England. They listened as Winston Churchill's voice was heard all around the world announcing the end of the war in Europe. The enormous relief they all felt was palpable in the sitting room as they heard the longed-for words.

It was over; it was finally over. There had to be, as Churchill said, a brief time to celebrate, and the soldiers would come home from Europe. But he made it clear that there was much toil and effort still ahead.

Robert, usually an optimist, sighed. "This is my second world war, and I have a good idea of what is to come. I cannot help but worry."

Puzzled by his sadness at this joyous moment, the others looked at him as he continued, "Yes, the men and women who have survived will come home, some of them whole, some terribly injured either physically or mentally or both. The toll war takes does not end with surrender. I'm sorry to be so gloomy, but it is true."

Douglas, understanding exactly what his father was talking about, still felt it was a time for joy. "Dad, we do have reason to be happy, and we need to celebrate."

"Yes, of course, Douglas, we do. Still, I cannot help but remember 1919 and think of the dreadful waste of young lives and the rebuilding that lies ahead for us now. I wish I could be more cheerful."

Jennie, concerned about her usually positive husband's depression, spoke, "Robert, this means that Gordon will also come home. I look forward so much to his return when his work with the War Department ends."

Robert smiled at her. "Yes, it will be good to have all our family home again. We are very fortunate."

Beth, who had two younger brothers in the Canadian Navy, was thrilled at their survival and their imminent return, though her own joy was muted by thoughts of her father's illness, praying that the young men would return in time to see their father while he was still alive. She knew that he would not survive the stomach cancer that was slowly killing him. There was nothing the doctors could do, beyond helping him with the pain, but the morphine doses were becoming stronger and stronger now, and she only hoped it would not be long before he, too, found peace.

Douglas looked at her anxiously. Although he understood her deep sorrow for her father and that there was still much more war work to come, he said, "Come, Beth, we are invited to a Victory party at Brummy and Margaret's. Will you join us, Dad? Mother?"

Brummy Aiello was the anaesthesiologist at the Drumheller Hospital, and he and his wife Margaret were old friends of the Ross family.

"Not this time, Son. I think your mother and I will just have a quiet evening at home. We are very glad it is over but a bit too weary of it all to celebrate with the others."

Jennie nodded her agreement, and as Doug and Beth left, she turned to her husband and spoke quietly. "Robert, I have been praying that the war in the Pacific will also end soon, but when do you think our Canadian men will come home from the Far East? And what of those in prison camps? I can't bear to think about it."

Four months after this celebratory dinner, the war in the Pacific ended when the first atomic bomb was dropped on Hiroshima, followed three days later by the second on Nagasaki. The world was changed forever. No one yet knew what the awful power demonstrated by this weapon would mean for humanity. For many, joy at the war's ending was tempered by uneasy speculation about what might come now that mankind had unleashed the terrible power of the atomic bomb.

***

Robert and his old friends still gathered regularly for coffee and conversations midafternoon several times a week. They were fewer in number as several of the men had passed away, and others had moved to live with their children, often in the more temperate climes of the West Coast. The remaining group, retired or semi-retired, all still held vigorous opinions on matters in the valley and the world.

Today's discussion began with speculation about the horrors of the atomic bomb and the fears of where knowledge of splitting the atom could lead. No one knew what was in store, and finding the topic very unsettling they soon moved on to the rapid developments that were taking place in post-war Canada and specifically Alberta.

Nationwide, the country had changed from a largely agricultural-based rural society to a country driven by an urban industrial economy.

"I read the other day that Canada contributed over eight hundred thousand military vehicles to the war effort. Those vehicles were produced in huge factories, which employed thousands of workers. What are all those factories going to produce now? What will happen to all those jobs now that the war is over?"

"Ontario and eastern Canada are booming, but you know, there are now many factories here in Alberta. Remember, during the war years, they were mostly staffed by women. Can you believe it?"

Several of the men nodded their heads, unable to hide their disapproval of women working in factories.

"And my daughter still works and gets paid for doing a man's job in the plant near the Army base in Calgary." Bill had always been proud of his daughter but struggled with the idea of women working in a "man's job."

"I'm sure she does a fine job, too, but she still isn't paid a man's wage," came a lone voice in support of the young woman.

Willing to concede the unfairness of the situation, Bill spoke again, "Didn't seem right somehow, since she did the same job. But, no matter, that will end now that the war is over. For one thing, all those returning veterans need jobs."

"And anyway, women belong in the home," another chimed in.

"Yes, and now that the war's over, she will come home to do her proper work. She'll have a family and look after her husband and the house. She'll be glad of it," was Bill's reply, relieved to have the group's support.

"Hmmmm. Maybe." Robert mused quietly, not at all convinced that the women of Drumheller and the world would be content to return meekly to their pre-war lives.

Another man spoke up, "My youngest boy was at the University of Alberta in engineering. He spent the last few years of the war working on the Alaska Highway as part of the U.S. Defence effort. He says half the truck drivers were women, or native, or both!"

Robert smiled at this, remembering his mother. He was sure Maggie would have driven the biggest truck available. He suddenly had a vision of her tackling the ox to the sled in the winters of his boyhood in northern Ontario. The conversation circled around him as his thoughts drifted back to those times.

"Yes, once the Americans entered the war, it made a huge difference in money and manpower."

"I think," Robert rejoined the conversation, "we will continue to see plenty of change over the next few years, not all of it to our liking. War is dreadful, but from my perspective, it is also a time of accelerated medical breakthroughs. I cannot believe my eyes when I see what penicillin and streptomycin can do and surgical advances as well. Battlefield medicine is hell, but we all benefit."

"Except for those who die or lose limbs," Tom Oberlon commented bitterly. His son had lost an arm and was struggling with shell shock, one of many who were physically healing but emotionally lost.

Robert, thinking of his experiences with World War I veterans, spoke quietly. "Send him to me. Perhaps I can help a little."

For several minutes, the men were quiet, thinking of families shattered by loss and friends who would never return to the valley. The familiar figure of Reverend Moss entered the café and approached their table. He was a welcome member of their group, whatever their denomination. They were pleased he could find time to join them, especially since they knew he and his family were soon to leave for the Peace River area.

"I have some good news. I heard on the radio that the Federal government is establishing programs to build homes for returning vets and that the Alberta Legislature will be encouraging veterans to return to college or university."

Jack asked, "How are they going to do that?"

Reverend Moss replied, "By providing funding to pay for their tuition. The vets will also receive a subsistence allowance to tide them over while they study."

"That is good news. Very good news, indeed. They deserve everything we as a country can do to help. It is not easy to rebuild careers and lives interrupted by war."

"And there won't be as many farming or low-skilled jobs either. Education is going to be important."

Robert was deep in thought as he walked back to his office. He, too, needed to consider what he was going to do. Semi-retirement was fine. At seventy-six, he did tire more easily and suffered a few more aches and pains, but he needed to have something to do that fully engaged his mind.

He still found the weekly case conferences at the office interesting and enjoyed his role as a surgical consultant, though he was both encouraged and slightly worried by the vast changes in treatment during and after the war. Sometimes it was hard to grasp the enormity of them all. After nearly forty years of medical practice, a look back provided an astonishing perspective.

"Though I cannot help but be encouraged by the new discoveries," he pondered as he walked along, absentmindedly tipping his hat and nodding greetings to everyone he passed, "I'm not altogether sure that these antibiotics are the final answer to all of mankind's ills."

He and Douglas had spent hours discussing the popular fallacy that a drug can be aimed specifically at an illness. Every drug had side effects, and the more powerful the drug, the greater the possibility of adverse reactions within the body. Surely the problems with sulpha had demonstrated that. But patients were beginning to come to him now, sure that a pill was a cure.

Also, the two doctors, father and son, firmly believed in and spoke often of the body's power to heal itself and of the impossibility of separating the human body into physical, mental, and emotional components. As he trudged slowly up the stairs to his office, he thought of how important it was for doctors and patients alike to understand that. "Perhaps," he grinned to himself, "I should undertake a research study in the area of distinguishing between patients who can get well without drugs or surgery and those who need either or both. Hmmmm? There's probably a grant available."

He toyed with the idea but dismissed it when he thought of the laborious work and studies involved. But he still needed something to do.

His nurse smiled at him when, puffing slightly, he entered the office. There was no doubt those stairs were becoming a problem, especially for his back.

She informed him that he had several young people nervously waiting for their vaccinations this afternoon. Robert grinned inwardly as he imagined their faces when his slightly shaky hand holding the needle approached their arms. He knew the shaking always stopped as the needle reached its destination, but they didn't.

***

Robert recounted the vaccination story to the whole family when they gathered for Sunday dinner at Douglas and Beth's new home. After dinner, the two older grandchildren had retreated to the playroom in the basement, where Shelagh had curled up in a big chair to read the latest Nancy Drew mystery and young Robert, passionately interested in flying, had set up a table in the corner where he constructed model airplanes. The younger grandchildren were in the kitchen with Simone, who had been hired to help Beth when Helen was born in 1939. She had stayed on to help, especially through the terrible years of grief following the death of Beth's father at the war's end, and now was busy with the latest addition to Douglas's family, a little boy named James Andrew.

Robert's housewarming gift to the young couple, a Knabe grand piano, had a place of honour in the front room. Even in the midst of his fast-growing medical practice, Douglas found time to take lessons and play. For him, an hour at the piano after a strenuous and stress-filled day gave him peace, as playing the guitar still did for his father. At the older doctor's request, Douglas settled at the piano after dinner and soon the melody of a Chopin prelude filled the room.

Robert's thoughts again turned to his earlier musings about modern medicine, but as Douglas finished the piece of music, Gordon announced that he and Elsie were moving to Brockville in Ontario where Gordon had accepted a position as a financial officer with Phillips Electric.

Douglas congratulated them. "That's great news, Gordon. Have you found a house in Brockville? Is it a large city?"

Gordon nodded but said no more, and a heavy silence fell over the room. Before arriving for dinner at his younger brother's home, Gordon and Elsie had talked to Robert and Jennie about the possibility of Shelagh remaining in Drumheller. Gordon believed it would be best if they did not move the vivacious and somewhat headstrong fourteen-year-old away from her familiar surroundings and her friends.

This time, however, Robert had decided not to grant their request. "Shelagh needs more structure in her life than we as grandparents can offer. She is really too much for us, Gordon. We are very fond of her and will miss her, but she needs to be with her parents."

Douglas and Beth knew nothing of this earlier request but were certainly aware of the tension in the room. Beth, seeing the unhappiness on Jennie's face and sensitive to some discord around the topic of the move to Ontario, spoke into the awkward pause.

"How are you enjoying your semi-retirement, Dad? You were speaking of a medical research idea. Does that still intrigue you?"

Robert, glad of the change of topic, replied, "Yes, it does, Beth, but I must admit, not enough to really involve all my energies. I'm still undecided about what to do with my time."

"You are spending more time in your music room, Robert," Jennie said, also relieved at the change of topic. "And your community responsibilities still fill your evenings."

"Of course, and I enjoy both of those pursuits. I am also having a good time teaching my grandchildren how to shoot with a bow and arrows. But you understand these are all play for me. I need to have some serious work."

The family all considered his response for a few moments then Beth said, "It's time for a new career path for you, Dad. It's time for you to do what you always said you would. It's time for you to become a writer."

Douglas, who had been quietly concerned about his father's evident restlessness, was enthusiastic. "Of course, Dad, write up your Hudson's Bay adventures. Or your medical practice stories. You've told them to us for years, and they are marvellous. They are important. Get them down so everyone can enjoy them."

Gordon, deciding not to pursue the subject of Shelagh, nodded, "That's a wonderful idea, Dad. You should write them all down, or they'll be forgotten."

Robert beamed at his family, contented and pleased with their unqualified support. "You are correct. The stories will disappear if I don't get them recorded. Jennie, you will help me remember. We've had such an interesting life. But before I write those stories of our lives, I have something else that I want to do. I have long wanted to research and write about this wonderful country of Canada, because it is a great country. What I am today, my accomplishments, are all because of Canada and the Canadians who have contributed so much to the betterment and upward progress of the human family."

Douglas laughed. "Write that down, Dad, I think you have your opening sentence."

CALGARY 1950-1962

Chapter 40
Moving to Calgary

The years of peace continued to be shadowed by Cold War talk and tension while veterans returned eager to rebuild their lives; babies were born, and life went on in the small prairie town. Robert was deeply disappointed that the Canadian diplomat, Lester Pearson, was not chosen to be Secretary-General of the new organization devoted to world peace called the United Nations. Feeling more than somewhat wearied by world affairs and disillusioned about global power struggles and the bickering of politicians, he turned his mind to his dream of writing about Canada.

Robert spent less and less time at work in the medical office and more time at home and in the small local library. Mornings once taken up by surgery were now devoted to research and writing. He constantly added to his personal collection of books about Canada and Canadians and left the outside world for others to worry about. Frequent trips were made to Edmonton to the University of Alberta Library and to the library at the newly established University of Calgary. He always urged Jennie to accompany him on these trips, and she often did, enjoying the drive through the countryside and the time spent in the quiet of the campus library. When she could not accompany him, young Robert happily went along, enjoying his time with his grandfather and, under Robert's tutelage, learning to drive on the prairie roads.

The contented, busy pattern of Robert and Jennie's life continued through the late 1940s. Cartons of books ordered by mail arrived at the house in Drumheller, and once again, he and his wife spent the evenings over their tea sharing his discoveries while perusing publishers' catalogues for more volumes of Canadian history and famous Canadians.

Robert was a familiar figure at the Drumheller Library, always encouraging them to enlarge their Canadiana collection. Both he and Jennie had been library board members for years, generously donating time and money.

Reinvigorated by his passion for research and writing and delighted in 1949 when, as he put it, "This great country of Canada got bigger in so many ways when Newfoundland finally joined Confederation," he continued to write. However, this time of contentment was lessened as the decade neared its end. Jennie's health, never good, had worsened in 1947 when her beloved cousin Nell had died. Jennie mourned this loss keenly, and she became very frail. She also contracted pneumonia after a winter bout of cold and 'flu, which, given her age, was a very serious illness indeed and one from which she never fully recovered.

Their elder son and his family had returned to Drumheller in 1948 when Gordon's diabetes worsened to the point that he could no longer continue with his job in Brockville. Robert had purchased a house for them just next door, hoping that Jennie would see more of her son, but Gordon had less and less energy to do anything and spent most of his time reading and sleeping on the couch in his basement retreat. Although he came regularly to see his mother, it was obvious that the visits were tiring for both of them.

Sadly, Robert watched his wife sink into deeper and longer bouts of depression. They continued to subscribe to the medical journals, and he hoped that new advances such as the Nobel-Prize-winning discovery of a way to grow the polio virus in a test tube would interest her. Although she agreed it was a breakthrough in the fight against the ravages of poliomyelitis, it was evident that medical advances were no longer important to her. He tried to coax her into going for drives again or visiting with her friends; sometimes she was willing, but for the most part, she preferred to read quietly in her chair in the front room, only rousing for family visits or special occasions. Even then, she sat quietly at the end of the dining table, taking little part in the discussions.

Jennie spent more and more of her time in solitary prayer, no longer an active member of church groups or the board of managers. Though she always politely welcomed any of the family to the house, it was clear that she wanted to be alone with her Bible and her prayers. She showed little interest in any of her grandchildren, including Douglas and Beth's new daughter, born in 1948, and named Jean Louise after her grandmother.

Robert, who could find no way to bring Jennie out of her depression, remained full of energy and threw himself into his research and writing. He also spent hours on his other passion, music. He practised his guitars, and his playing reached the status of a highly proficient amateur. He continued to study and collect music, especially the works of the great Spanish composers.

Some afternoons each week were spent with his grandchildren, going along with young Robert to practise his driving in exchange for hauling coal into the basement. He instructed Douglas's daughter Helen on the intricacies of the guitar, even sending to Spain for a small woman's size guitar for her. The days and weeks passed swiftly, and in 1950, in his eightieth year, Robert retired completely from Associated Physicians, the medical practice he had founded thirty-one years before.

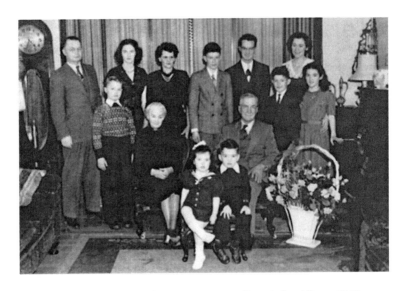

Robert and Jennie's 50th Anniversary, 1950, Drumheller, Alberta, 1950
Back Row l to r
Gordon, Shelagh, Elsie, Robert, Douglas, Beth
Middle Row, l to r
Tommy, Jennie, Robert, Colin, Helen
Front Row, l to r
Jean, James

That year was also their fiftieth wedding anniversary, and one sunny morning following their family celebration, Jennie joined Robert for an early breakfast. They lingered over their tea and talked quietly of decisions that they knew must be made.

Jennie spoke of her growing inability to manage the stairs. "I must concede that I am finding it more and more difficult to climb the stairs, Robert. I would hate to have to remain in my bedroom all day."

Robert, who already worried about Jennie's increasing isolation from family and friends, agreed that the stairs were a problem. He reluctantly admitted that he, too, was experiencing difficulties with the stairs. "You're right, my dear. We will need to look for a new home with rooms all on the same level. Where in town would you like to look? Or shall we build a new place?"

"Robert, I think at our age, it is not wise to think of building." She had obviously given the matter a lot of thought. "Also, you are spending so much time in Calgary now with your research. I think we should consider leaving Drumheller and moving there."

Robert was not really surprised. Gordon and Elsie were also talking of a move to Calgary. Gordon wanted to leave Drumheller. Shelagh was attending the University of Calgary, and Elsie wanted her to be able to live at home, and Tommy, a gregarious ten-year-old, was used to moving. Douglas and his family were planning a move to the West Coast where it had long been a dream of his younger son to establish a medical practice.

"Well, perhaps you are right. It is true that I am in Calgary a great deal of the time, and I am finding the drive somewhat tedious, especially in the winter." Still, Robert was puzzled at his own reluctance to leave Drumheller. He had always been the one to pick up and go. But he would miss the town and his good friends. Although, he admitted to himself, many of his friends were no longer in Drumheller. "It is perhaps past time to move."

"Calgary is growing so quickly, Robert; we will have no difficulty finding a new home."

It was true that the prairie city was growing rapidly. The discovery of oil in the Turner Valley, in addition to the gas wells, had made a dramatic difference to the city. Now the Leduc Oil fields had further transformed the economic base of south-central Alberta, and Calgary was at the centre of the petroleum industry.

"Jennie, you have not been well this past year or so. A move will be very disruptive. Are you sure you are strong enough?"

"Yes, I am sure. It is time, and I will manage. I always have."

The decision made, a three-bedroom house in an established neighbourhood on Calgary's North Hill was purchased. The movers came, all was packed, and almost too suddenly, in 1951 Robert and Jennie had moved again.

Jennie's bedroom was at the front of the new house, and on the increasing number of days when she felt too ill to dress after her afternoon nap, she enjoyed hearing the activities in the street as she rested. The sound of planes overhead on their way to the new Calgary Airport, named McCall Field, often roused her from her dreaming to wonder at the changes in the world. She could not help but think of the dashing young airman who had come to thrill them in Drumheller so many years ago.

On these days when she kept to her bed, Mrs. Hall would bring her afternoon tea on a tray, and her husband would sit with her.

"How is the writing progressing, Robert?"

"Very well, my dear. I am just completing my essay on how great a country Canada is, and I would be grateful if you would read it for me. I have incorporated all of your suggestions, but I need your expert eyes to review it."

"I would like to do that. And have you employed a typist for the final copy?"

"Yes, I have discovered a company in town that offers that service. When you feel it is ready, I will contact them."

"And publishing it, Robert?"

"I am exploring that as well. I need to find a publishing house that is interested in Canadiana. I also thought of the university presses. I think it should be read by young Canadians, perhaps university students."

"That is an excellent idea, Robert, and I look forward to reading it for you, but now, I am very tired. I must sleep for a time. Remember Gordon and Elsie are joining us for supper this evening."

Mrs. Hall came in to the room to remove the tea things as Robert stood up. "I'll assist Mrs. Ross, Doctor. I've planned a light supper for this evening when Gordon and Elsie are here. Will that be suitable?"

"Very suitable, thank you, Mrs. Hall," Jennie murmured as Robert left the room.

"I'm going to the university for a few hours. I'll be home well before supper. Thank you, Mrs. Hall."

Robert had not seen Gordon for a few weeks and was worried by his son's unhealthy pallor when he and Elsie arrived for dinner. "Gordon, you do not look well. Have you seen your new doctor lately?"

"Don't fuss, Dad. I saw him last week. Says I'm having a few heart palpitations, but he's adjusted my insulin dosage and given me some pills for blood pressure. Damned doctors anyway. Nobody knows what to do. Nothing seems to help."

Robert, having had this conversation with Gordon before and knowing that the new doctor was a good medical man, said nothing more about Gordon's poor colour but added, "Please don't say anything to your mother about heart problems. She worries too much as it is, and you know she is not well herself."

Jennie had dressed with Mrs. Hall's assistance and now came into the room to greet Gordon and Elsie. She, as well, was alarmed at Gordon's appearance but was too weary herself to say anything about it.

The supper table conversation was subdued; the Korean War was a blight on any discussion, though Gordon's news about the new oil pipeline taking Alberta crude to the Great Lakes for refining promised more prosperity for Calgary and Edmonton. There had been a note from Beth saying all were well on Vancouver Island and that Douglas was very busy but he hoped to visit Calgary soon. Elsie chattered happily of Shelagh's progress at university and of the new young Queen, Elizabeth II.

Robert talked a little of his research, and Jennie listened politely but said very little. Throughout the meal, everyone carefully avoided the topic of Gordon's health, and their guests did not linger, leaving shortly after supper as Gordon was very tired.

Jennie, too, retired soon after they had departed, her face drawn with anxiety and exhaustion.

Robert, recognizing the inevitability of his son's decline, and constantly worried about Jennie, picked up his favourite guitar from its stand. He had purchased the Panormo on his trip to in England twenty years ago and loved the full rich sound of this instrument. Soon the beautiful melodies of Albeniz filled the room while he played softly until the music calmed him enough to go to his own bed to sleep.

Gordon's lifelong struggle with diabetes came to an end with his death in April of 1953. In the preceding months, it seemed he had just given up, and Robert knew that if the will to live had gone, there was nothing the much vaunted new medicines could have done. Douglas flew from the West Coast to attend the simple ceremony as his older brother was buried in Burnside Cemetery in Calgary. Douglas remained in Calgary for a few days with his parents, but it was clear that he could offer little comfort to his mother.

Robert grieved deeply for Gordon, who had carried such a burden of anger at his condition all his life. Jennie, frail and white, retreated into silence and rarely left her bedroom in the year following Gordon's death.

Her husband tried to interest her in his stories and music and arranged for frequent pastoral visits from the minister of the local United Church, but it was clear that Jennie, too, had simply given up the struggle. Even the suggestion of automobile drives out to the countryside in fine weather, previously a source of pleasure, no longer roused her from her overwhelming grief and depression.

It was only ten months later when Robert phoned Douglas, telling him to come back to Calgary to see his mother, knowing that it would likely be for the last time. Shortly after this visit, and just days after Douglas's return to the West Coast, Jennie slipped into a peaceful sleep and never regained consciousness. Ten days later, Jennie Louise died. She was buried beside her beloved Gordon.

Chapter 41
Love and Loss

The predicted snowstorm had arrived, and as Robert sat at his desk looking out at the dark sky, the hard pellets of sleet rattled against the windowpane. Heavy gusts of wind tore at the black branches of the trees in the front yard and finally a curtain of white closed over the city.

A month had passed since Jennie's death in January. Family and friends had come from across Canada and the United States for the funeral, and many of them stayed on to comfort Robert. They had all now returned to their homes, and Robert knew he must deal with the slow and painful process of writing letters of thanks to those who had sent their condolences.

Mrs. Hall, who still missed Jennie dreadfully, brought the tea tray to his desk. He sipped the comforting brew before turning to the list of names and piles of envelopes, some still unopened. The tremor in his hands had worsened to the point that he could no longer hold a pen steadily enough to write, so slowly, beginning to consider his words, he slipped a clean sheet of paper into his new typewriter. But somehow, he could not seem to start.

"Not yet," he thought, "I'm not ready yet. It is just so final, writing these letters."

Casting around the room for a diversion, he saw several neat stacks of medical journals and carefully folded newspapers on the low table by his big chair. For many months, Jennie had been too ill and he had been too disinterested to look at them, but he welcomed them now. Pushing himself stiffly away from his desk, muttering "blasted arthritis," he settled himself in his comfortable reading chair where he began to go through the papers and magazines.

He was so accustomed to sharing his thoughts with Jennie that he spoke aloud as he scanned the papers. "I see that that evil man Stalin is dead, but this fool McCarthy is making everything worse with his accusations about Communism. But here is good news: The American Courts have outlawed segregated schools. How can people be so stupid as to think one race is better than another? Have we learned nothing over the centuries?"

Mrs. Hall, hearing his voice, came into the room, looking curiously at him. He smiled reassuringly at her and said, "Just thinking out loud. Thank you for the tea."

He turned to the medical journal on top of the pile. "Well, they are rediscovering Mendel, are they? I hope we're not going to have another bout of eugenics. Such harm that particular belief has done us as human beings." He read further in the article, "And now, the study of genetics seems to be focusing on something called DNA. Hmmm, I remember reading about Levene's discovery of nucleic acids in 1919 and then something else about that in the mid forties. DNA?"

Robert wondered aloud again as he read a description of its molecular structure, "What will that mean for the future if we all know exactly how we are formed? Is it all heredity now and nothing about upbringing? And what is this talk of DNA and viruses? I must read more about Wilson and Crick later on."

He marked that magazine and set it to one side, wishing sadly that he had his wife there to discuss the implications of this amazing discovery. Momentarily shaken again by grief, he made himself consider someone else he could talk to about medicine. "My good friend Doctor Williams, of course, and Douglas. Douglas will know all about DNA, and we can have some excellent talks when I see him next."

His thoughts turned to a journey to the West. "I think I must travel to the West Coast. But not just yet. Perhaps next year. Perhaps I will fly? Wouldn't that be quite something for me to do?" He had the rueful realization that he was smiling at the idea of travelling again, and then he sighed and returned to the magazines.

He continued somewhat aimlessly to leaf through the journals then stopped in astonishment when he came to an article discussing a successful kidney transplant that had been performed in Boston by two surgeons, Joseph Murray and John Harrison, with the assistance of nephrologist, John Merrill.

Robert looked with resignation at his own trembling hands, thinking of his own time as a gifted surgeon, then shrugged and returned to the article about the operation. "My word, they have finally achieved their goal. I wonder how they overcame the immune reaction problem. The medical profession has certainly been trying for long enough. What a difference that would have made to my patients. But where will the kidneys come from; who will be willing to donate a healthy kidney?"

He remembered one of his professors at Queen's long ago pointing out that people seemed to have some spare organs, and many people had managed to live on successfully with only one kidney after injury and surgery.

The thank-you letters forgotten, Robert remembered his own case studies waiting to be turned into stories. "I think it would be useful for others to know just how far we have come and how well we did without all of this knowledge." Feeling much better, he decided to use the rest of the grey afternoon to go through some of the unopened boxes stacked in his bedroom.

He had lost interest in his story of Canada when Jennie was no longer able to share it with him, but there were all those case studies and memories from his medical practice plus the Hudson's Bay stories from his youth. He was tired now but decided he would have a look and think about it after his nap.

***

He awakened from the first deep sleep he had enjoyed in many months, energized by his earlier reading. The storm had passed, and the pale late afternoon light was reflected from his desk. "It's getting colder," he thought, "This storm will turn everything to ice. Driving will be miserable."

Mrs. Hall came into the front room to bring him his tea. "You look as though you slept well, Doctor. I'm glad to see you are more rested."

"Thank you, Mrs. Hall. I did have a fine rest. I'll have my tea now and my supper here at my desk later, but would you mind helping me move the boxes from my room into here? I wish to start going through them."

"Of course, Doctor. As soon as you have had your tea, I'll be happy to help. But my goodness, there are a lot of boxes."

"I'll just start sorting, day by day, a good winter project for me. Do you know, I've really forgotten what I have here."

"Most of the boxes were packed by the movers, Doctor, I don't remember what they contain." She smiled at Robert. "You would know better than I what these labels mean."

"I hope so, but I am in no hurry; I'll figure them out. My goodness, look at that...it's a medical case study from nineteen seventeen when we were in Coleman. Now, that was before your time with us. What was the name of the young woman who looked after the boys? Emma? No, Hannah. That was it. A fine young woman. She married when we left for Drumheller. She would have grandchildren by now. Let me see what else is here."

Mrs. Hall left him to sort boxes, happy to see Robert engaged in some activity again. Over the following months, the piles of paper grew as Robert sorted and added to each carefully labelled stack. Mrs. Hall and the cleaners were forbidden to touch the boxes or the neat stacks on the table. He enjoyed the memories called forth by each case study, and the hours passed as he worked. As Robert slowly regained his verve for life, he also met with family and friends, and his medical colleagues kept in frequent touch.

By the time the busy months of winter and spring had passed, all the boxes were unpacked and sorted and the last of the thank-you notes had been written. Then it was summer, and Robert realized his old restlessness was returning. He was beginning to feel housebound.

He got the car out and began to go for long drives but found his solitary ramblings no longer gave him the pleasure they once had.

"All right," he thought, "Perhaps it's time for me to go on that promised visit to the West Coast. This back of mine means I might have difficulty with a long train trip, so it's time to try the newest method of transportation. I'll fly!"

Later that week when Mrs. Hall brought him his afternoon tea, he cheerfully told her of his plans. "Mrs. Hall, I have decided to fly to Victoria to visit with Douglas and his family."

"Fly, Doctor Ross? You are going to fly in an airplane?"

"Of course, Mrs. Hall. It is time I added flying to my travel experience. I have already spoken to a travel agent. I will go on a Canadian Pacific Airways flight to Vancouver and transfer there to a smaller airplane to Victoria. The airport is near Douglas's home."

"But you've never even been on an airplane, Doctor. How will you manage with your back problems?"

"I think it will be fine. It is a much shorter time than the train and no overnight to deal with. I can figure it out. I'm sure there will be assistance in Vancouver where I change planes. I'm just fine with a short walk, or I can get a wheelchair. The travel agent to whom I spoke said I only have to request one. I will do what is necessary to travel again."

"It's not my place to question you, Doctor, but what sort of airplane will it be? Is it big enough to go over those mountains?"

Robert laughed, "Oh, yes indeed. Douglas has flown back and forth several times. I may even be a passenger on a Super Constellation. They have been flying without incident over the North Atlantic so should have no trouble getting me to Vancouver." Robert's smile was gleeful at the prospect of flying and being able to travel again, even with his increasing physical limitations.

Mrs. Hall was pleased to see him happy and looking forward to this adventure. "Well, Doctor Ross, I will worry all the time you are away, but I am glad you are going. I will have my sister come for a visit while you are gone."

When the day of his trip to the West Coast arrived, Robert was pleased to board a Douglas DC-3, which his travel agent had assured him was the very best aircraft for the trip. Once on board, he found every aspect of the flight interesting. He had a comfortable seat at the front of the plane, which he appreciated as the aisle of the plane slanted down to the tail. He was glad that he didn't have to navigate that! He also discovered to his delight that his seat partner was the son of one of his old patients from Drumheller so the hours were passed catching up on news and sharing happy memories.

The eighty-four-year-old could barely contain his pleasure at his latest achievement when he disembarked at Patricia Bay Airport just outside of Victoria to be greeted by Douglas and his family. Douglas laughed, pleased to see his father enjoying life again. "A long way from dogsleds, Dad. We are very glad to see you. How are you?"

"I know I will be tired later, Son, but right now, I feel wonderful. I am looking forward to this visit and seeing your new home."

A happy month of visiting and telling stories followed. Robert even climbed a ladder to the roof of the new garage Douglas was building, and though his arthritis punished him every time he moved, he sat happily in the sunshine on a roof beam hammering nails as far as he could reach.

Robert's friends, Dr. and Mrs. Williams, lived in Victoria, and they were dinner guests at Douglas and Beth's on several occasions. Douglas also drove his father into Victoria for afternoon tea with his friends, especially the wife of his old friend, Sid MacMullen from Drumheller. Beth took her beloved father-in-law on frequent drives around the Saanich Peninsula.

Robert was also happy to spend time in the Associated Physicians medical practice in Sidney, where he met his son's partners and had long discussions about the current state of medicine. Everyone was cautiously delighted about Salk's discovery of a vaccine for polio, especially when Robert recounted the horror stories of earlier epidemics.

He also had an appreciative audience for his tales around the dinner table with the family. Beth, especially, was delighted to hear that he was finally writing them down. "Send them along as you finish them, Dad, they are such a valuable historical record for the family and for all Canadians."

"I shall, Beth. And Mrs. Williams has kindly offered to edit them for me. They'll get done, but I have to go home to write them. It has been a wonderful visit. Thank you all."

Later that same year, Robert made another plane trip, this time to Victoria. He had read in one of his guitar magazines, *BMG* of Manchester, England, that the guitar maestro Andre Segovia was coming to Victoria for one of his two North American appearances.

Robert immediately made plans to go to his idol's recital. "Mrs. Hall, I have just received a return phone call from the *Vancouver Sun* newspaper in response to my request to meet with Segovia. They are sponsoring the concert and have arranged for me to meet the maestro after he plays. And they will arrange for photographs to be taken! I will be featured in the Manchester magazine in next October's issue. What do you think of that?"

His devoted housekeeper was delighted. "Doctor Ross, you are becoming quite a celebrity."

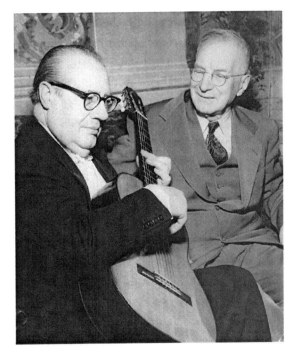

Andres Segovia and Robert, Victoria, British Columbia, 1954

Robert chuckled happily. He was quite enjoying the idea of another plane trip and was thrilled to know that he would meet Segovia. "I will enjoy another short visit with the family on Vancouver Island then return here for the winter. I must get on with my writing. I seem to be very busy with the stories and practicing my guitar and now travelling again. But I have other things I want to do outside. I've noticed our fence seems to be a bit shabby. Perhaps I'll paint it next summer when the fine weather returns."

Robert's name was in the papers again when the *Calgary Herald* published a short article about his life. The doctor had been approached by a reporter at a Queen's University Alumni reunion dinner, and the interview appeared in the newspapers of several prairie cities where he had practised medicine.

Elsie and Mrs. Hall had attended the reunion with Robert, and they all enjoyed the attention he received. He declined the request for an interview from a reporter from *The Albertan*, who wished to write the story of his life. "I told her," he wrote to the Williamses in Victoria, "that I felt I could write it myself and did not think I needed assistance. She said she would like an interview in any case, and I told her she was welcome to come along to the house any day. She has not shown up yet, and I am not worried."

Many of his old friends wrote to Robert congratulating him on the *Calgary Herald* interview. Their words gave him great pleasure and encouraged him to continue writing his life story.

He still enjoyed driving his car, and on the auspicious occasion of his first great-grandchild's christening, he and Elsie drove to Edmonton. He was pleased that Shelagh's daughter was named Janette, after her great-grandmother, Jennie. The baby was christened by Reverend Edworthy who had been a minister of the Knox United Church in Drumheller, another old friend. He wrote to Beth telling of his trip to the christening and a return letter soon arrived.

In her letter, Beth said that she had told Mrs. MacMullen about Robert painting his fence. Robert laughed when he read that the wife of his old friend President Mac, from Rotary in Drumheller days, had offered him employment painting her very long fence in Victoria. "I might get a steady job yet," he wrote to Dr. Williams, "though I would have to paint the whole thing sitting in a chair because this back of mine is playing up so badly that I can't stand for more than one or two minutes."

He looked at the pile of letters on his desk. "I must answer these before I get back to my writing. Here is one from my granddaughter Helen who is flying home from Ottawa for Christmas and will stop over here with me for a few days. Good, I will enjoy that."

He turned again to his stories, realizing that he had not yet given thought to getting his manuscripts published. "Maybe," he murmured, removing the cover from his typewriter, "I should be doing that, but I have the feeling that they could all be improved upon."

The typewriter was much used that winter, and by April of 1957, Robert had decided to send one of his Hudson's Bay stories to *The*

Beaver, the HBC house magazine, in hopes of having it published. He had also finished ten medical practice stories based on his case studies and memories. Two of those he mailed to his friends Dr. and Mrs. Williams in Victoria to read and edit for him.

Always a very social person, he once again attended the Calgary Rotary meetings and the occasional Masonic Lodge meeting, enjoying the outings and the conversation. His old friends and colleagues were happy to drive him to and from these events.

In May, accompanied by his granddaughter Helen, he flew to the West Coast to spend a month with Douglas and his family. While there, he visited again with the Williamses to discuss his medical practice stories. They were more impressed with his HBC tales, feeling the medical stories would need far more information before they were ready for a general readership.

Pleased with their honest comments, Robert agreed and said he would devote more time to the medical practice stories when he returned home. They also chatted happily of family events. The Williamses' daughter was coming to visit them, and Robert knew that would bring them great pleasure.

The old friends also spoke of what was now being called the "space race." Robert was gleeful about the launching of Sputnik. "Maybe I'll get an opportunity to travel into outer space? Who knows?"

Dr. Williams nodded, amazed at the life his old friend had lived and his eagerness to try new things. "Doctor Ross, I wouldn't be at all surprised if you did fly into space."

On his return to Calgary, Robert wrote a note to Dr. and Mrs. Williams, thanking them for their kindness and hospitality and telling them of his plans for the coming autumn.

> *I am flying to Montreal in late August to visit my brother Colin and then on to Cleveland to see my sister Sybil. I will perhaps see other family members before I return home mid-September. This will probably be my last trip East, as my arthritis is slowly crippling me to*

such an extent that locomotion is becoming extremely difficult. It is a shame, as I read that British Overseas Airlines will inaugurate trans-Atlantic flights next spring. I would enjoy flying across Canada and on to England, but I must content myself with my life here. My writing and my family and friends keep me well occupied.

By the summer of 1959, walking was extremely painful, but Robert dressed carefully every day in his suit and vest and sat at his typewriter for as long as he was able. He found that he needed to spend more and more time resting. The pain in his back and his joints was such that his physician suggested stronger pain killers. Reluctantly, Robert agreed. He knew he needed them in order to finish the stories.

Elsie moved into the house to help him for a while, but it was soon obvious that Robert would need a full-time caregiver. When he became bedridden, he insisted that a qualified nurse be hired, and Mrs. Annie Hamilton joined the household.

Lying in bed, he drifted in and out of sleep. He was aware of those who came to visit and roused himself to comment, "Another one, Shelagh?" when her latest baby Kathryn was brought for him to see him in February, but he spoke very rarely after that date.

"I have done enough and written enough and said enough," he thought drowsily. "The morphine helps with the pain. I will just rest for a while."

Epilogue
Calgary 1962

The morning sunlight was captured by tiny dust motes softly stirred by the faint breeze from the bedroom window. The sound of sprinklers swishing on the lawn and the murmur of voices in the hall roused Robert from his half sleep to drowsy thoughts. "...the nurse will be coming soon...it's time for more morphine...the pain is beginning to dig its claws into my spine again..." His mind wandered as he slipped back into sleep. "...was young James here today or was it yesterday? I remember music and a violin, but he talked to me about the guitars... where are my guitars? I wish I could speak, but I am so tired...so many stories still to tell."

The nurse arrived and gave him a sip of water and his shot of morphine. "Ahh, now the pain will go...sleep again for a while."

The golden afternoon sun was low in the sky when the old doctor next drifted back to consciousness, his trembling hands resting on the white coverlet. "...hospital bed...am I in a hospital? No, I said I wanted to die at home...yes, those are my pictures, this is my room, I'm here, but I feel so strange. I need to remember something...what? Where is Gordon? Ah, he's gone now, my poor son, he was so unhappy...I remember Banting...and travelling, always travelling...Jennie, she didn't come with me sometimes...wanted to stay home...is she gone, too? I'm very tired...mustn't sleep again until I remember...where is Douglas?...he was here just a little time ago, I know...he looked very tired and sad...it doesn't matter now. I am so very tired. I think I will sleep again." His pulse was racing, and the nurse administered more morphine to help him remain peaceful.

Darkness fell, and the nurse switched on the light beside the bed. Its golden glow threw the corners of the room into shadow as she dealt with her patient's needs without waking him. "Not long now," she whispered to Mrs. Hall who sat beside the bed, silent tears spilling from her eyes.

"I know," Robert's housekeeper and good friend of many years murmured quietly to the nurse, "the morphine keeps the pain away, but you can see that he is ready to go. It is sad, though, that he would not speak in the last months. He was the greatest storyteller I have ever known, and he had so many wonderful stories to tell."

A faint smile flickered across the old man's face. "...I remember now, Jennie, I remember it all..."

His trembling hands were still.

ACKNOWLEDGEMENTS

I owe an incalculable debt to everyone who shared his or her stories and memories with me. This book could not have been written without their generosity. While it is not possible to mention them all individually, I need to acknowledge Lisa Danesin for her constant support and peerless editing, Robert Ross QC for his endless supply of Drumheller lore and his legal expertise, and Joan Ryan who shared the treasured correspondence of her grandmother, Dr. Helen Ryan, which helped me bring Jennie Louise to life. My deepest gratitude also goes to Serge Harvey, genealogist extraordinaire, and Arthur Ross for his wonderful sense of humour and his extensive knowledge of "all things Ross." And to my husband, John, I can always count on his support. Thank you.

I also wish to thank the modern-day medical men who read and commented on the medical stories, Dr. G. Vaughan, Dr. T. Nimmon, and particularly, Dr. W. Malone for his time and timely suggestions. For their encouragement, my thanks to Dr. R. Lampard and Dr. R. Michael Giuffre of the Alberta Medical Association. Thanks also go to Marg Smith and Colin Ross, who not only enthusiastically gave of their time and expertise to proofread this large book but also provided many valuable editorial suggestions.

I thoroughly enjoyed the research involved — familial, historical, and medical. While it was a wonderful journey through many publications, archives, websites, and family histories, several volumes deserve specific mention:

A.A. Travill. *Medicine at Queen's, 1854-1920*, 1988; Carlotta Hacker, *The Indomitable Lady Doctors*, 2001; David C. Jones, *Empire of Dust*, 1987; plus a memoir, Florence R. Howey, *Pioneering on the C.P.R.,1883 to 1886*, 1938; and two social histories, *Silver Sage, Bow Island 1900 to 1920*, 1971 and *The Hills of Home, Drumheller Valley*, 1973.

—Helen Webster, Nanaimo British Columbia, October 2015

APPENDICES

i. REAL HISTORICAL CHARACTERS

The Medical Men and Women (In Order of Appearance)

Helen (Nell) Elizabeth Reynolds Ryan, MD, Queen's University, Women's Medical College, Kingston, Ont.

Thomas Robert Ross, MDCM, Queen's University, Kingston, Ont.

Emma Veale, Graduate Nurse, school of nursing unknown, Ont.

Mercilla Veale, Graduate Nurse, school of nursing unknown, Ont.

John H. Patterson, MD, McGill University, Montreal, Que.

Frank Hamilton Mewburn, MDCM, McGill Medical College, Montreal, Que.

John Westwood, MD, McGill Medical College, Montreal, Que.

Joseph Lister, MDCM, RCS, University of London, Oxford, England

John Connelly, MD, medical college unknown

John Beggs, MDCM, Queen's University, Kingston, Ont.

Sir William Osler, MDCM, FRS, FRCP, McGill University, Montreal, Que.

Alexis Carrel, MD, University of Lyon, Lyon, France

H. Winnett Orr, MD, University of Michigan, Michigan, USA

E.C. Crawford, MD, Queen's University Military Hospital, Kingston, Ont.; British Egyptian Medical College, Cairo, Egypt

S.R. McGregor, MD, Queen's University, Kingston, Ont.

D.M. Gibson, MD, medical college unknown

Sir Frederick Banting, Nobel Laureate, MDCM, University of Toronto, Toronto, Ont.; LLD, Queen's University, Kingston, Ont.; DSc, University of Toronto, Toronto, Ont.

Charles Best, MDCM, University of Toronto, Toronto, Ont.

George Munroe Ross, MD, Bellevue Medical College, New York City, New York, USA

Colin Eric Ross, MD, McGill University, Montreal, Que.

Simon Peter Ross, DO, Philadelphia College of Osteopathy, Philadelphia, Pennsylvania, USA

Sir Alexander Fleming, Nobel Laureate, MDCM, St Mary's Hospital, London, England

Douglas Robert Ross, MDCM, McGill University, Montreal, Que.

Allan Roy Dafoe, MD, OBE, University of Toronto, Toronto, Ont.

Albert Aiello, MD, University of Alberta, Edmonton, Alta.

Wilder Penfield, MDCM, University of Oxford, England; John Hopkins, Baltimore, Maryland, USA; McGill University, Montreal, Que.

Jonas Salk, MD, New York University, New York City, New York, USA; University of Pittsburgh Medical School, Pittsburgh, Pennsylvania, USA

Phoebus Levene, D. Chemistry, Rockefeller Institute, New York City, New York, USA

James Watson, D. Chemistry, Nobel Laureate, Rockefeller Institute, New York City, New York, USA

Francis Crick, D. Chemistry, Nobel Laureate, Gonville and Caius College, Cambridge, England

Herbert Wilson, MDCM, D. Physics and Biochemistry, King's College, London, England

Joseph Murray, Nobel Laureate, MDCM, Harvard Medical School, Cambridge, Massachusetts, USA

J. Hartwell Harrison, MCDM, University of Virginia, Charlottesville, Virginia, USA; Brigham and Women's Hospital, Boston, Massachusetts, USA

John Merrill, MDCM Harvard Medical School, Massachusetts, USA

Annie Hamilton, Graduate Nurse, school of nursing unknown

ii. THE ROSS FAMILY (By Generations)

Thomas Barnston Ross Family

Thomas Barnston Ross 1844-1930

Marguarite Mcleod Ross 1850-1938(T Barnston's wife - later m. Peter McKenzie)
> Simon Peter Ross 1868-1944 (T Barnston's son)
> George Munroe Ross 1870-1940 (T Barnston's son)
> Thomas Robert Ross 1871-1962 (T Barnston's son – m. Jennie Louise Ryan)

Arthur Howey Ross 1876-1969 (T Barnston's son - m. Muriel Kay)
> Rodderick Reddie Ross 1878-1894 (T Barnston's son)
> Sebbey-Mcleod (Sybil) Ross 1882-1961(T Barnston's daughter - m. Tarn Hutchinson)

Colin Eric Ross 1882-1961 (T Barnston's son - m. Ethel Currie)
> Colin James Ross 1918-1977 (Colin Eric's son)

Thomas Robert Ross Family

Dr. T. Robert Ross 1871-1962

Jennie Louise Ryan 1875-1954 (Robert's wife)

> Gordon Mcleod Ross 1904-1953 (Robert's son – m. Elsie Gabriel)
>
> Douglas Robert Ross 1908-1980 (Robert's son – m. Elizabeth Stevenson)

Gordon Mcleod Ross Family

Gordon Mcleod Ross 1904-1953

Elsie Gabriel 1904-2002 (Gordon's wife)

> Shelagh Margaret 1932-2005 (Gordon's daughter)
>
> Thomas Arthur 1940-1977 (Gordon's son)
>
> > Janette Louise (b)1956 (Gordon's granddaughter)

Douglas Robert Ross

Douglas Robert Ross 1908-1980

Elizabeth Stevenson 1913-2005 (Douglas's wife)

> Robert Douglas (b)1936 (Douglas's son)
>
> Elizabeth Ann 1938-1938 (Douglas's daughter)
>
> Helen Charlotte (b)1939 (Douglas's daughter)
>
> Colin Morris (b)1941 (Douglas's son)
>
> James Andrew (b)1946 (Douglas's son)
>
> Jean Louise (b)1948 (Douglas's daughter)

THE RYAN FAMILY

Dr. Helen (Nell) Elizabeth Reynolds Ryan 1860-1947

TJ Ryan 1858-1921 (Helen's husband)

> William Horace 1898-1987 (Helen's son m. Blanche)

iii. OTHER HISTORICAL CHARACTERS

BOW ISLAND

Emma Veale m. EC Ludtke

Ora Ludtke (Emma's daughter)

Mercilla Veale m. Howard Murray

Mrs. Whitfield, midwife

Mr and Mrs George Thomas

Chuck Chen, café proprietor

COLEMAN

Mrs. Westwood (Dr. Westwood's wife)

Miss Yuill

Sergeant Brown

Reverend Arthurs

DRUMHELLER

Captain Fred McCall, RAF

Mrs. Ewing

Mr. and Mrs. E A Toshach

Mr. and Mrs. H McVeigh

Mr. Am Rosain

Mr. Bill Crowley

Dr. Thomas Robert Ross, Australia

Morris and Charlotte Stevenson (Elizabeth's parents)

Reverend Leitch

Reverend Shortt

Reverend and Mrs. Moss

Dr. Bob Johnston, druggist

Dr. Robertson, dentist

Simone Verscheres, housekeeper

Martha Klaussen, housekeeper

Alice Hall, housekeeper

CALGARY

Mrs. Annie Hamilton, caregiver

Reverend Edworthy

VICTORIA

Andres Segovia, guitarist

iv. A Brief History of Marriage in Canada, 1900-1950

In 1900, men were considered the head of the household. A man was expected to work hard to support his wife and children, and whether factory or farm, labourer or professional, the hours were long. Clubs and organizations were an important part of men's lives, and most spent any leisure time they had with other men. To balance their responsibilities, they had many rights not available to women. Men could own property, could run for and hold political office, and they could vote. No matter what their societal status, men were considered to be superior to women, both physically and mentally. Within a marriage or business, a husband's word was law.

Women were considered to be incapable of making important decisions. At the same time, women were considered to be naturally morally superior to men, and a woman's status was linked to her moral rectitude.

The prime purpose and defining social role for women was marriage and motherhood. Abortion was illegal, and although contraception became available in the 1930s, for several decades afterwards, any form of birth control continued to be frowned upon. Divorce was an unheard of choice for a woman. While it was understood that both men and women stayed in unhappy marriages for the sake of the children, it was unlikely that a woman and her children could survive without a husband's financial support. And of course, a woman's morality would be immediately questioned if she chose to leave her marriage.

Before marriage, a woman required the consent of her father or other male relative to sign any legal document. When a woman married, all that she owned became the property of her husband, including any business that she may have owned prior to marriage. Once married, a woman required the consent of her husband to sign a legal document.

By 1925, married women in Canada had secured some of the same legal rights as men, including the right to vote in federal and provincial elections (except for Quebec). Nevertheless, women were still unable to take a full part in political life.

Women made up close to 15 percent of the workforce outside the home but still faced discrimination in employment opportunities and unequal pay. Women received 54 percent of what men earned for the same work; their unpaid work raising children, managing households, and donating time to charities was considered far less valuable than paid work.

The Second World War, 1939 to 1945, saw women running businesses and all the services necessary to keep the country going in the absence of men, including working in munitions factories and shipyards. In order to make this possible, the Government of Canada provided daycare spaces for women working for the war effort whose families were unable to care for their children. As soon as the war ended, the government closed these child-care facilities, and women were expected to return to their proper jobs as wives and mothers. The wartime jobs they had held were to be made available for the return-ing servicemen.

By 1950, although women had gained many legal rights and were becoming more vocal in their demand for social and economic equal-ity, and their competence during the war had weakened some stereo-types, popular culture still believed that "a woman's place is in the home" and the man should be the master of the household.

CPSIA information can be obtained at www.ICGtesting.com
Printed in the USA
LVOW07s1141160116

470536LV00013B/107/P